Type I Diabetes

Type I Diabetes

Molecular, Cellular, and Clinical Immunology

GEORGE S. EISENBARTH
KEVIN J. LAFFERTY

Editors

New York Oxford
OXFORD UNIVERSITY PRESS
1996

Oxford University Press

Oxford New York
Athens Auckland Bangkok Bombay
Calcutta Cape Town Dar es Salaam Delhi
Florence Hong Kong Istanbul Karachi
Kuala Lumpur Madras Madrid Melbourne
Mexico City Nairobi Paris Singapore
Taipei Tokyo Toronto

and associated companies in
Berlin Ibadan

Published by Oxford University Press, Inc.,
198 Madison Avenue, New York, New York 10016

Oxford is a registered trademark of Oxford University Press

Library of Congress Cataloging-in-Publication Data
Type I diabetes : molecular, cellular, and clinical immunology /
George S. Eisenbarth, Kevin J. Lafferty, editors.
p. cm. Includes bibliographical references and index.
ISBN 0-19-509126-4
1. Diabetes—Immunological aspects.
I. Eisenbarth, George S. II. Lafferty, Kevin.
III. Title: Type one diabetes.
[DNLM: 1. Diabetes Mellitus, Insulin-Dependent—immunology.
WK 810 T9908 1995] RC660.T97 1995
616.4'62079—dc20 DNLM/DLC for Library of Congress 94-34170

2 4 6 8 9 7 5 3 1
Printed in the United States of America
on acid-free paper

To Barbara Davis,
whose dedication for more than a decade,
has nurtured a Center devoted to the understanding and
cure of childhood diabetes.

Introduction

Type I diabetes mellitus is rapidly becoming one of the best studied autoimmune disorders. The existence of two spontaneous animal models, transgenic models where trangenes *both* create and suppress disease, coupled with the clinical importance of this illness (with millions affected and tens of thousands killed each year), has led to enormous efforts by an international group of investigators to understand, treat, and prevent type I diabetes. This book presents a synthesis of the molecular and cellular immunology of type I diabetes composed by basic immunologists and physician-investigators at the Barbara Davis Center. Thus, investigators actively engaged in basic research, clinical research, and clinical care of individuals with type I diabetes review recent progress in immunogenetics, immunopathogenesis, preventive therapy, and islet cell transplantation. As will be apparent from the individual chapters, the pathogenesis of type I diabetes is very likely a solvable puzzle, with prevention of the disorder and islet cell transplantation the prize that will derive from the puzzle's solution. In addition, the lessons learned are likely to be central to the field of autoimmunity because similar basic questions face all investigators of autoimmune diseases.

Contents

Type I Diabetes

1

Primer: Immunology/Autoimmunity

George S. Eisenbarth

Immunologists over the past decade have solved a series of fundamental genetic and biochemical questions related to immune function. Recent discoveries include elucidation of the mechanism by which antibody and T receptor diversity is generated,[1,2] the characterization of a series of lymphokines essential for lymphocyte activation,[3,4] the characterization of cell surface lymphocyte molecules (and in many cases their function),[5,6] and the definition of the crystal structure and peptide-binding properties of human leukocyte (HLA) class II[7,8] and class I molecules.[9,10] The field of immunology is now focused on defining mechanisms by which the immune system discriminates between self and nonself antigens, and therefore by necessity the determinants of autoimmunity. For some diseases and for some animal models, answers to a subset of the basic questions concerning autoimmunity posed in Table 1.1 are now available. It is clear that a single genetic or triggering mechanism to explain all autoimmune diseases affecting even a single tissue will be inadequate. For example, myasthenia gravis, which results from autoantibodies to the acetylcholine receptor, can be triggered by the drug penicillamine or the development of a thymoma, whereas for most patients no triggering factor has been defined.

Normal Immune Response

In many respects, the modern age of immunology began with the independent descriptions by Talmage and Burnet in 1957 of the clonal selection theory.[11] "The basic concept was of the immunologically competent cell . . . ; that is a

Table 1.1. Basic Questions

What genes underlie susceptibility to autoimmunity?
What triggers autoimmunity?
What are the target autoantigens?
What effector systems lead to disease?

cell which is susceptible to specific stimulation by contact with the appropriate antigenic determinant. The main possibilities of reaction are: (a) destruction, especially if physiologically immature; (b) proliferation without essential change of character—to what we would now call memory cells; and (c) proliferation and antibody production as a clone of plasma cells." In 1957 the mechanism underlying the huge diversity (which was fundamental to the clonal selection theory) of immunological reactivity of single lymphocytes was unknown. It is now understood that B cells that produce antibodies and T cells responsible for cell-mediated immunity bear on their surface unique antigen receptors created by genetic recombinatorial processes.

The receptor of B cells is immunoglobulin with the same specificity as the antibodies that will eventually be secreted by the mature plasma cell. B cells can recognize soluble antigen. Antibody genes are created by a combinatorial process in which any of a family of multiple variable-region gene segments are combined with short joining and diversity immunoglobulin gene segments and then with the constant-region gene segments of immunoglobulin. Heavy and light chains of immunoglobulin are then joined, and billions of different antibodies (differing in their amino acid sequence) are generated. Antibody genes (but not T cell receptor genes) also undergo a high degree of mutation that increases the affinity with which antigens are recognized by clones of B lymphocytes.

Although T cells have a similar genetic mechanism as B cells for the generation of T cell receptor diversity, they differ in that they react only with antigen bound to class I or class II molecules of the major histocompatibility complex (MHC) on antigen-presenting cells. In fact, for a T cell to respond to antigen, antigen must be presented on the surface of antigen-presenting cells, eg, macrophages (Fig. 1.1) in the context of MHC molecules. A crucial element of antigen-presenting cells (macrophages, dendritic cells) is the ability to present peptides of antigens in the groove of HLA molecules. These "transplantation" antigens (HLA), as they were initially termed (because differences between transplantation antigens of donor and hosts determined ability to accept grafts), function by binding short peptides for presentation to T cells. T cells expressing a T cell receptor complex that includes the co-receptor CD4 interact with class II HLA molecules (DR, DP, and DQ of man, I-A and I-E of the mouse), while the CD8 co-receptor performs a similar function for T cells that interact with class I molecules (HLA A, B, and C of man; K and D molecules of the mouse). Figure 1.1 illustrates the uptake, cleavage, and presentation of an "external" antigen to a CD4-positive T cell.

An additional name applied to the genes coding for class II HLA antigens

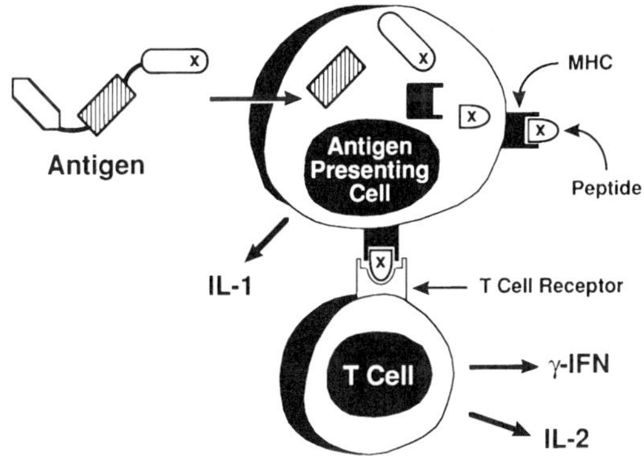

Figure 1.1. Antigen presentation by antigen-presenting cell with peptide in the groove of a major histocompatibility complex class II molecule (eg, DR, DP, or DQ).

is that of immune response genes. These molecules are highly polymorphic, differing between individuals in their amino acid sequence.[12,13] Each different sequence is given a number. Such differences are inherited in a Mendelian fashion. The sequence differences determine which peptides can be bound and presented. Thus, such inherited differences in HLA molecules between individuals can determine which antigen an individual can respond to, and importantly, which autoimmune disorder they are likely to develop. As modeled above, the developing immune system has the potential to respond to essentially every foreign antigen, but also to every self antigen.

Because the immune effector mechanisms that have evolved are capable of rapidly killing cells, the potential for response to self is a consequence of having a potent immune system (analogous to having firearms in a house to protect from burglars—weapons that may nevertheless accidentally kill family members). As stated by Burnet, "Autoimmune disease can be defined as a condition in which structural or functional damage is produced by the reaction of immunocytes or antibodies with normal components of the body . . . the central theme is the emergence of 'forbidden clones' of pathogenic immunocytes and the various ways by which these can arise and find ways of escaping the normal controls." In 1969 Burnet stated, "The most probable somagenic change responsible for the 'forbidden' quality is one which confers resistance or partial resistance to destruction when the newly differentiated immunocyte makes contact with its corresponding antigen in a thymic or equivalent environment."

Of note, such a pathogenic mechanism underlies disease of the lpr mouse.[14,15] Lpr mice have either of two independent autosomal recessive mutations of the Fas gene, which influences "programmed" lymphocyte cell death (apoptosis). Lpr mice have marked lymphoproliferation and a disorder resembling lupus erythematosus and rheumatoid arthritis. The Fas gene is the same as a human gene termed Apo-I, which is involved in the control of apoptosis. Apoptosis is the fate of more than 90% of developing thymocytes that react with self antigens in the thymus. "Central" tolerance to self antigens is determined by deletion of T cells whose T cell receptor have high affinity for self MHC antigens or self MHC antigens with bound self peptides. It is hypothesized that inhibition of the apoptotic pathway because of mutations or deletions of Fas leads to the failure to eliminate autoreactive T cells. Tolerance to self antigens is thought to result from at least three different mechanisms: deletion of autoreactive cells; clonal inactivation (anergy), where T cells reactive with self are present but cannot easily be stimulated by contact with antigen; and potential silencing of self-reactive cells by other cells. Tolerance to antigen can also be subdivided by the site of acquisition, namely central tolerance (thymus) and peripheral tolerance. The thymus is the primary site of T cell deletion, with more than 90% of T cells destroyed within the thymus. At a functional level, the breaking of "tolerance" is fundamental to concepts of autoimmunity.

In addition to the concept of "forbidden" clones arising because of mutations that bypass normal regulatory events, it has become clear that, given appropriate context of antigen presentation, "autoimmune" responses can be generated to essentially all proteins. For example, subcutaneous injection of human insulin (the current therapy for type I diabetes) almost invariably leads in man to low levels of anti-insulin autoantibodies. For most destructive autoimmune disorders, a characteristic group of autoantibodies arise. These antibodies frequently react with a series of molecules from the same subcellular localization. For lupus erythematosus, it is the ribonucleoprotein complex; for type I diabetes, insulin secretory granules and islet synaptic-like microvesicles. This suggests that once tissue destruction commences, in the context of an inflammatory lesion (insulitis), tolerance is broken to a series of autoantigens.

Genetics of Autoimmunity

The general concept that autoimmunity develops in the setting of genetic susceptibility, and in particular in association with a series of specific HLA alleles, applies to most human autoimmune disorders. It is important to note, however, that the same HLA allele may protect from one disorder (eg, HLA DR2, DQA1*0102, DQB1*0602 is rare in patients with type I diabetes but it is associated with multiple sclerosis[16,17]) and may be associated with a different disease. It appears that susceptibility encoded by alleles within the HLA region do not globally influence the development of autoimmunity but rather influence the likelihood of specific disorders.

If HLA alleles determine disease susceptibility by their function as "immune" response genes, selective targeting is likely. An alternative manner by which HLA alleles may determine susceptibility for autoimmune disease is by altering the developing T cell repertoire. This may be particularly important for diseases associated with what have been termed "superantigens," such as Kawasaki's disease. Superantigens bind to whole classes of T cells bearing specific $V\beta$ T cell receptor families. Superantigens thereby activate large numbers of T cells (many more than the usual antigen that interacts only with clones of T cells with a specific complementary binding site).

Recent experiments with transgenic mice have provided convincing evidence that the predilection of T cells for MHC is due to the way the T cell receptor repertoire is derived. Developing thymocytes express a multitude of T cell receptors, and only the infrequent thymocyte that expresses a receptor with low affinity for MHC antigens presented in the thymus matures further; the selection signal is supplied via the engaged T cell receptor complex. This selection on self MHC (termed positive selection) is potentially dangerous in that T cells with overt autoreactivity can be and most likely are selected. Those developing thymocytes with high affinity for self MHC, and which are therefore autoreactive, transduce a signal via their T cell receptor that leads to cell death rather than further differentiation.

Experiments in transgenic nonobese diabetic (NOD) mice suggest that simple skewing of the T cell repertoire is not sufficient to alter diabetes susceptibility in this animal model.[18] This observation is more consistent with the hypothesis that HLA class II alleles alter disease susceptibility because of the antigens they do or do not present to mature T cells.

In autoimmune diseases studied to date, concordance of identical twins is never 100% and is usually between 30% and 70%.[19,20] Concordance of non-identical twins is often in the range of 5% and similar to the risk of siblings. Finally, for most disorders (multiple sclerosis, type I diabetes, etc.), the concordance is higher for monozygotic twins as contrasted with HLA identical siblings. The above information strongly suggests that alleles of genes outside of the major histocompatibility complex contribute to disease susceptibility. In animal models, a number of alleles influencing disease susceptibility have been defined.[21] In humans, for example, autoimmunity is associated with complement deficiency (eg, lupus erythematosus[22]), alleles of insulin (type I diabetes[23]), and nucleoside phosphorylase deficiency (hemolytic anemia). It is likely that complement deficiencies contribute to autoimmunity by altering processing of antigen-antibody complexes. Insulin gene polymorphisms may influence the timing of insulin synthesis during embryonic development and therefore influence "tolerance" to insulin. T cells are particularly sensitive to nucleotide metabolites and it is thought that nucleoside phosphorylase deficiency may be associated with autoimmunity secondary to T cell toxicity. With refined techniques for genetic mapping, including more than 800 commercially available DNA markers to localize human genes, it is likely that in the next decade great progress will be made in the definition of alleles underlying genetic susceptibility for common autoimmune disorders.

Triggering of Autoimmunity

A large group of experimental autoimmune disorders can be induced by immunization with self proteins. To induce disease, and even to generate an

Table 1.2. "Etiologic" Classification of Autoimmunity

Classification	*Example*
Oncogenic	Ovarian carcinoma and cerebellar degeneration
Dietary	Gliadin and celiac disease
Drug	Penicillamine and myasthenia gravis
Infectious	Streptococci and rheumatic fever
Idiopathic	Type I diabetes

immune response, such molecules are usually injected in a depot form with adjuvants that activate antigen-presenting cells. A model of multiple sclerosis follows immunization with myelin basic protein[24] and there are conceptually similar models for experimental autoimmune thyroiditis (immunization with thyroglobulin), experimental myocarditis (immunization with myosin peptides), and experimental autoimmune oophoritis (immunization with the oocyte sperm cell receptor).[25] Once disease is induced in these animal models, T cell clones reacting with immunizing antigens are sufficient to transfer disease. In that disease can be induced by simple immunization with self molecules, it is clear that T cells and B cells reactive to self exist in normal animals. Thus, the context of immunization determines whether pathogenic clones are expanded. In part, the ease of inducing autoimmunity raises the question as to what mechanism prevents expansion of autoimmune clones.

In animal models, including type I diabetes, both genetic (eg, T cell immunodeficiency gene on chromosome 4 of the BB rat) and environmental manipulations of the immune system lead to autoimmunity (neonatal thymectomy, injection of anti-RT6 antibodies in nonlymphopenic BB rats, and neonatal therapy with cyclosporin A). In addition, the age at which animals are exposed to antigens, either endogenously (eg, transgenic mice expressing the T antigen in islets develop insulitis) or by neonatal oral administration, can determine enhancement of an autoimmune response.

Table 1.2 presents an "etiologic" classification of human autoimmunity based upon identified triggering factors. Infectious agents,[26] neoplasms, and drugs have all been found to induce specific autoimmune diseases. Tumors that induce autoimmunity are characterized by the expression of specific autoantigens. One of the best-characterized oncogenic autoimmune syndromes results in cerebellar degeneration. Oncogenic cerebellar degeneration is associated with specific anti-Purkinje cell antibodies and is induced by ovarian carcinomas expressing what have been termed CDR (cerebellar degeneration related) antigens.[27] Additional oncogenic autoimmune disorders include pemphigus associated with lymphoma, myasthenia gravis and pure red cell aplasia associated with thymomas, and retinopathy associated with small-cell carcinoma. It is thought that, similar to the induced autoimmune disorders of animals described above, presentation to the immune system by tumor cells of self peptides induces "remote" autoimmunity.

The drug penicillamine is associated with a large number of different

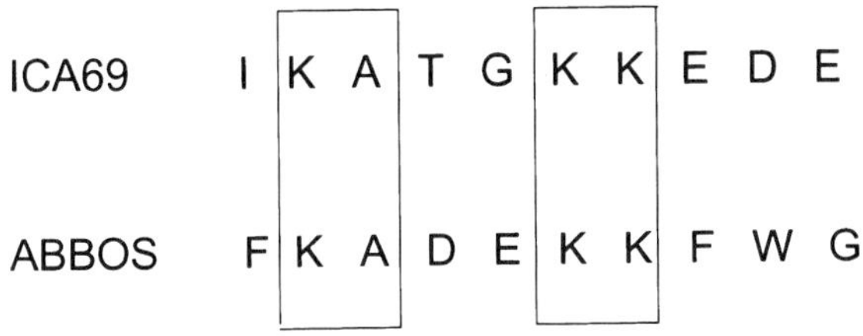

Figure 1.2. ABBOS/ICA69; homology between milk albumin peptide (ABBOS) hypothesized to be involved in diabetes induction and the islet autoantigen ICA69.

autoimmune disorders, including myasthenia gravis, bullous pemphigoid, lupus erythematosus, polymyositis, and dermatomyositis.[28] In addition to overt disease, penicillamine induces autoantibodies such as anti-insulin autoantibodies in the absence of overt pathology. It is hypothesized that penicillamine (dimethylcysteine) may induce autoimmunity by haptenation of multiple proteins.

One of the best examples of autoimmunity induced by food is celiac disease, or gluten sensitive enteropathy.[29,30] Celiac disease is characterized by marked lymphocytic infiltrates of the small bowel associated with villous atrophy. Ingestion of the wheat protein gliadin leads to the production of anti-gliadin and anti-endomysial antibodies and destruction of the villi. The disease is "cured" by elimination of wheat gluten from the diet. Like most autoimmune disorders, celiac disease occurs only in the presence of specific HLA alleles; in particular, with DQ alpha and beta sequences (DQA1*0501 and DQB1*0201) provided by HLA haplotypes DR5 (DQA1*0501) and DR7 (DQB1*0201) in *trans* or in individuals with DR3 haplotypes (DQA1*0501/DQB1*0201).

Dosch and coworkers have suggested that milk albumin introduced in a neonate's diet increases the risk of type I diabetes because of homology of bovine serum albumin to an islet molecule that we have recently cloned (ICA69).[31,32] The homology between ICA69 and milk albumin in a region thought to contain a critical T cell epitope is small (four identical amino acids) (Fig. 1.2). As few as three properly spaced amino acids in common between different peptides recognized by T cells can be enough to induce a T cell response and experimental autoimmune disorders. The minimal homology required for T cell epitopes may underlie the frequent spreading of autoimmunity (polyendocrine autoimmune syndromes) to multiple antigens and tissues.

Autoimmunity associated with mononucleosis is related to the unique ability of the virus to directly infect B cells.[33] The Epstein-Barr virus (EBV) stimulates B cell proliferation and polyclonal antibody production. These polyclonal antibodies reacting with self antigens can lead to disease. The proliferation of B cells is self-limited in the presence of an effective T cell response. The atypical lymphocytes of EBV infection are activated T cells that are essential to suppress uncontrolled B cell growth. In addition to environmental factors triggering autoimmunity, infections can suppress autoimmunity. Almost any viral infection of NOD mice prevents diabetes, as does a single injection of complete Freund's adjuvant.

Target Antigens

Studies during the past decade have led to the recognition of three major classes of antigens subdivided by the manner by which antigen presentation occurs: endogenous antigens, exogenous antigens, and superantigens. Exogenous and endogenous refer to the cell expressing the antigen. Exogenous antigens are taken into a cell by specific receptors (eg, binding of antigen to surface immunoglobulin of B cells, Fc receptor–mediated uptake of immune complexes) or non–antigen-specific mechanisms (eg, pinocytosis). Such antigens are then cleaved to peptides and coupled to class II MHC molecules for presentation on the cell surface and recognition by specific T cells (CD4-positive T cells). Endogenous antigen, synthesized by the cell (eg, viruses), is cleaved by peptidases in a proteosome complex, transported into vesicles by specific peptide transporters (TAP1, TAP2[34]), coupled to class I MHC molecules and then presented on the cell surface for recognition by T cells bearing CD8 accessory molecules. In contrast to the above usual antigen processing, superantigens are molecules that bind outside of the peptide binding "groove" of class I and class II molecules and trigger whole families of T cells by binding to common sequences of T cell receptors. Thus, for T cell responses to superantigens, it is predicted that responding cells will bear T cell receptors of limited families (eg, $V\beta8.2$), but the T cell receptor antigen-binding region ("complementarity determining region") will differ in amino acid sequence.

The antibody and T cell responses characteristic of autoimmune disorders appear to be "antigen driven." The amino acid sequences of autoantibodies are mutated relative to immunoglobulin germ-line sequences and autoantibodies are usually of high affinity. In addition, the large number of different autoantibodies to different autoantigens for even a single autoimmune disease suggests that whatever the initial lesion leading to autoimmunity, the immune response "spreads" to a series of antigenic epitopes and molecules of the involved tissue. For example, a large family of antibodies react with islet autoantigens during the beta cell destruction associated with type I diabetes. To date, these autoantibodies target molecules within two islet secretory organelles, insulin secretory granules (eg, insulin, proinsulin, carboxypeptidase H, GM2-1 ganglioside) and synaptic-like microvesicles where gamma amino butyric acid (GABA) is stored (eg, glutamic acid decarboxylase, ICA69).[35]

The detection of a family of autoantibodies for each autoimmune disease complicates the elucidation of which autoantigen (if any) is central to disease pathogenesis. In the past, the major criteria for defining such autoantigens rested primarily on the ability to immunize with the given antigen and create disease. This is probably an inadequate criterion to define pathogenic autoantigens of spontaneous autoimmune disorders of man and animal models.

It is known that for many tissues, immunization with several different autoantigens can induce disease (eg, myelin basic protein and proteolipid protein for experimental autoimmune encephalitis). With the development of molecular genetic techniques, more definitive tests of an antigen's disease relevance are now possible. For example, genes for specific autoantigens (eg, insulin) can be introduced into ectopic tissues (eg, insulin expression by pituitary cells) by creating transgenic mice with the gene coding for the autoantigen coupled to a promoter directing ectopic expression. If, for example, destruction of the ectopic tissue is induced (eg, NOD mouse model of diabetes expressing insulin in the pituitary), the single autoantigen is sufficient to target autoimmunity. In a similar manner, induction of thymic expression of an autoantigen may be sufficient to induce tolerance to the antigen. If all autoimmunity is blocked in such transgenic mice, then the given autoantigen is essential for disease pathogenesis. Finally, introduction of autoantigen synthesis by transplanted tissues (eg, adenovirus gene transfer systems) may allow a series of autoantigens to be rapidly tested to determine whether they are "sufficient" for tissue destruction.

Effector Mechanisms

In most immune disorders, both humoral and cellular arms of the immune system contribute to disease pathogenesis. Autoantibody-mediated disorders include autoimmune hemolytic anemia, immune-mediated thrombocytopenia (ITP), myasthenia gravis, Eaton-Lambert syndrome, pemphigus, and Graves' disease.[36] For each of these disorders, a transient neonatal disease follows transplacental passage of antibodies.

Autoantibodiiies can induce pathology by blocking the function of specific receptors (eg, hypothyroidism,[37] "geriatric" hypoparathyroidism[38]), stimulating receptors (Graves' disease, hypoglycemia associated with anti-insulin receptor autoantibodies), by direct cytotoxicity (hemolytic anemia), by opsonizing cells (hemolytic anemia and ITP), and by deposition of immune complexes (lupus nephritis).

Cell-mediated immunity is usually associated with tissue destruction (eg, type I diabetes, thyroiditis), either through direct cellular cytotoxicity or by indirect cytotoxic mechanisms (eg, delayed-type hypersensitivity). The classic cytotoxic pathway (that which underlies rejection of allogenic tissue) is mediated by direct recognition of antigenic peptides complexed with MHC class I molecules by CD8-positive cytotoxic T cells. Function and expansion of clones of such cytotoxic T cells are dependent upon "help" provided by CD4-positive T cells that respond to antigenic stimulation by releasing a series of lymphokines, including IL-2 (interleukin-2). Recently, CD4-positive T cells have been subdivided based on the lymphokines they produce[39,40] (and in part based on surface markers) into three groups of "helper cells": Th0, Th1, and Th2. Th0 cells constitute a small subset postulated to be related in the thymus to reactivity with autoantigens and produce IL-2 but low levels of interferon gamma (IFN-γ).[41] Th1 cells determine delayed hypersensitivity and produce IL-2 and IFN-γ, Th2 cells produce IL-4. Th2 cells predominantly lead to humoral immunity and they may even be protective relative to destructive autoimmunity (see essay by Talmage and Sanderson, Chapter 13). Killing by cytotoxic T cells involves direct cellular contact between T cells and the target cell.

An additional mechanism of cell-mediated destruction of target cells involves indirect cytotoxicity mediated by CD4-positive (Th2) lymphocytes. Such CD4-positive lymphocytes, following recognition of their target antigen presented in the context of a class II MHC molecule, secrete a group of lymphokines (eg, interferon gamma), which in turn activates cells such as macrophages to release IL-1, nitric oxide, and free radicals. Each of these molecules can directly kill selected target tissues.[42,43] This second mechanism may be primarily responsible for the autoimmune beta cell destruction of type I diabetes and for destruction of xenogeneic tissue transplants. For example, anti-islet CD4-positive clones (as will be discussed in later chapters) are sufficient to transfer diabetes.[44]

In addition to "pro-inflammatory" lymphokines, T cells also produce lymphokines that suppress cell-mediated immunity. In animal studies, such lymphokines are associated with "deviating" an immune response toward a humoral response. Both transforming growth factor–β (TGF-β) and IL-4 appear to limit immune destruction and the production of these molecules by T cells exposed to their antigen in the intestine may be important for immune regulation. In particular, the therapy of autoimmunity by ingestion of antigens of target tissues ("oral tolerance") is probably dependent on local immunosuppression by T cells secreting IL-4 and/or TGF-β.[45,46]

Therapy of Autoimmunity

A series of novel therapies for the prevention and therapy of autoimmunity are being studied. One can broadly divide therapies of autoimmunity into therapies which are antigen specific and those which are antigen nonspecific. Examples of antigen-specific therapies include prevention of diabetes in NOD mice by parenteral or oral administration of insulin,[47–49] MHC-binding peptide therapies for prevention of experimental autoimmune encephalitis,[50] and T cell or peptide vaccination strategies.[51,52] Antigen nonspecific therapies include drugs such as glucocorticoids, anti–T cell monoclonal antibodies, IL-2–diphtheria toxin conjugates,[53–55] cyclosporin A, and FK506. The disadvantage of non–antigen specific therapies is the likely suppression of important immune function with increased risk of infection and malignancy. In addition, selective drugs have unique toxicities unrelated to immunosuppression, such as osteoporosis and diabetes with glucocorticoids and the renal toxicity associated with cyclosporin A. Nevertheless it is clear that potent immunosuppressive drugs such as cyclosporin A, which appear to act by blocking lymphokine production by T cells, can prevent certain forms of autoimmunity. When it is possible to use such drugs at low doses with marked therapeutic effect (eg, cyclosporin A for psoriasis), they become important therapeutic agents. It is also hoped that certain strategies of short-term immunosuppression may lead to a state of long-term tolerance, thereby lessening the deleterious effects of immunosuppression. For example, treatment with specific monoclonals directed against the T cell coreceptor CD4 can lead to long-term engraftment of both heart transplants and islets.[56]

Antigen-specific therapies include the removal of a disease-inciting antigen (if it is identified), limiting exposure to endogenous self antigens ("isohormonal" therapy of endocrine autoimmunity), deviation of an immune response to nonpathogenic pathways (Th2 versus Th1, with oral "tolerance"[57,58] or parenteral immunization), and targeting specific autoreactive T cells or B cells through their receptors or HLA antigens.

For example, celiac disease is successfully treated by the removal of the wheat protein gluten from the diet. Studies of the effects of eliminating bovine milk products in neonates are planned for infants at high genetic risk for type I diabetes. Dosch and coworkers have advanced the hypothesis that bovine milk albumin, because of its homology to the islet ICA69 molecule, triggers diabetes.[31]

For endocrine glands it is possible to suppress cellular activity through feedback inhibitory circuits (eg, administration of thyroxine or insulin inhibits thyroid or beta cells, respectively). Therapy with insulin not only prevents development of diabetes of BB rats[59] and NOD mice,[60] but also prevents lymphocytic infiltrates into the islets and beta cell destruction. In humans, we have completed a small pilot trial of insulin therapy in high-risk relatives of patients with type I diabetes[48] (reviewed in Chapter 12 by Chase and Hayward).

Studies from Japan indicate that thyroxine therapy of patients whose Graves' disease is in remission either during pregnancy or following methimazole treatment are protected from disease recurrence.[61,62] A single report suggests that glucocorticoid therapy in patients with anti-adrenal autoantibodies leads to loss of autoantibodies and prevention of Addison's disease.[63] The mechanism by which such "isohormonal" therapy of endocrine autoimmunity is effective is unknown, but we hypothesize that in all of these disorders a component of autoantigen presentation occurs within the target gland.[69]

A single injection of Freund's adjuvant is sufficient to prevent the development of diabetes of the NOD mouse.[64,65] As reviewed in Chapter 5, such therapy may act by shifting islet-infiltrating T cells to Th2-like lymphocytes, producing IL-4 rather than interferon gamma.[65]

Pilot studies in man and experimental studies of animal models have been completed of oral antigen therapy for multiple sclerosis (myelin basic protein),[46] rheumatoid arthritis (collagen),[66] and uveitis (retinal S protein).[67] It is hypothesized that the feeding of autoantigens induces T cells, producing suppressive lymphokines TGF-β and IL-4 when such T cells encounter antigen.[68] Studies of the mechanism underlying oral tolerance are most advanced for experimental autoimmune encephalitis, where, in vivo, antibodies to TGF-β block induction of 'oral tolerance'.[45]

The trimolecular complex (MHC molecule, peptide antigen, and T cell receptor) underlyig the specificity of T cell responses is an obvious target for therapy of autoimmunity. In experimental disorders with a very limited T cell receptor response, such as experimental autoimmune encephalitis (almost exclusive use of T cells bearing Vβ8.2), targeting of a specific family of T cell receptors is efficacious in preventing disease. Another approach being actively pursued is the production of peptides that bind to MHC alleles associated with disease.[50] For example, a peptide binding to a high-risk allele for type I diabetes, DQA1*0301/DQB1*0302, might prevent diabetes by preventing the binding of "diabetogenic" peptides.

References

1. Early P, Huang H, Davis M, Calame K, Hood L. An immunoglobulin heavy chain variable region is generated from three segments of DNA: Vh, D and Jh. *Cell.* 1980; 19:091–992.
2. Davis MM, Bjorkman PJ. T cell antigen receptor genes and T cell recognition. *Nature.* 1988; 334:395–402.
3. Or R, Renz H, Terada N, Gelfand EW. IL-4 and IL-2 promote human T-cell proliferation through symmetrical but independent pathways. *Clin Immunol Immunopathol.* 1992; 64:210–217.
4. Romagnani S. Human TH1 and TH2 subsets: regulation of differentiation and role in protection and immunopathology. *Int Arch Allergy Appl Immunol.* 1992; 98:279–285.
5. Marshall LS, Aruffo A, Ledbetter JA, Noelle RJ. The molecular basis for T cell help in humoral immunity: CD40 and its ligand, gp39. *J Clin Immunol.* 1993; 13:165–174.
6. Larson RS, Springer TA. Structure and function of leukocyte integrins. *Immunol Rev.* 1990; 114:1181–217.
7. Chicz RM, Urban RG, Gorga JC, Vignali DA, Lane WS, Strominger JL. Specificity and promiscuity among naturally processed peptides bound to HLA-DR alleles. *J Exp Med.* 1993; 178:27–47X.
8. Brown JH, Jardetzky TS, Gorga JC, et al. Three-dimensional structure of the human class II histocompatibility antigen HLA-DR1. *Nature.* 1993; 364:33–39.
9. Bjorkman PJ, Saper MA, Samraoui B, Bennett WS, Strominger JL, Wiley DC. Structure of the human class I histocompatibility antigen, HLA-A2. *Nature.* 1987; 329:506–512.
10. Bjorkman PJ, Saper MA, Samraoui B, Bennett WS, Strominger JL, Wiley DC. The foreign antigen binding site and T cell recognition regions of class I histocompatibility antigens. *Nature.* 1987; 329:512–518.
11. Burnet M. *Cellular Immunology.* Melbourne: Melbourne University Press, 1969.
12. Nepom GT, Erlich H. MHC class-II molecules and autoimmunity. *Annu Rev Immunol.* 1991; 9:493–525.
13. Nepom GT. Immunogenetics and IDDM. *Diabetes Rev.* 1993; 1:93–103.
14. Watanabe-Fukunaga R, Brannan CI, Copeland NG, Jenkins NA, Nagata S.

Lymphoproliferation disorder in mice explained by defects in Fas antigen that mediate apoptosis. *Nature.* 1992; 356:314–317.

15. Lichter P, Walczak H, Weitz S, Behrmann I, Krammer P. The human APO-1 (APT) antigen maps to 10q23, a region that is syntenic with mouse chromosome 19. *Genomics.* 1992; 14:179–180.
16. Erlich HA, Griffith RL, Bugawan TL, Ziegler R, Alper C, Eisenbarth GS. Implication of specific DQB1 alleles in genetic susceptibility and resistance by identification of IDDM siblings with novel HLA-DQB1 allele and unusual DR2 and DR1 haplotypes. *Diabetes.* 1991; 40:478–481.
17. Atkinson MA, Maclaren NK. What causes diabetes? *Sci Am.* 1990; 263:62–71.
18. Lipes MA, Rosenzweig A, Tan K, et al. Progression to diabetes in NOD mice with transgenic T cell receptors. *Science.* 1993; 259:1165–1169.
19. Olmos P, A'Hearn R, Heaton DA, Risley D, Pyke DA, Leslie RDG. The significance of concordance rate of type I (insulin dependent) diabetes mellitus in identical twins. *Diabetologia.* 1988; 31:747–750.
20. Ebers GC, Bulman DE, Sadovnick AD, et al. A population based study of multiple sclerosis in twins. *N Engl J Med.* 1986; 315:1638–1642.
21. Rossini AA, Greiner DL, Friedman HP, Mordes JP. Immunopathogenesis of diabetes mellitus. *Diabetes Rev.* 1993; 1:43–75.
22. Hartung K, Baur MP, Coldewey R, et al. Major histocompatibility complex haplotypes and complement C4 alleles in systemic lupus erythematosus. *J Clin Invest.* 1992; 90:1346–1351.
23. Julier C, Hyer RN, Davies J, et al. Insulin-IGF2 region encodes a gene implicated in HLA-DR4-dependent diabetes susceptibility. *Nature.* 1991; 354:155–159.
24. Massaceso L, Joshi N, Lee-Parritz D, Rombos A, Letvin NL, Hauser SL. Experimental allergic encephalomyelitis in cynomolgus monkeys: quantitation of T cell responses in peripheral blood. *J Clin Invest.* 1992; 90:399–404.
25. Rhim SH, Millar SE, Robey F, et al. Autoimmune disease of the ovary induced by a ZP3 peptide from the mouse zona pellucida. *J Clin Invest.* 1992; 89:28–35.
26. Stollerman GH. Variation in group A streptococci and the prevalence of rheumatic fever: a half-century vigil. *Ann Intern Med.* 1993; 118:467–469.
27. Hetzel DJ, Stanhope R, O'Neill BP, Lennon VA. Gynecologic cancer in patients with subacute cerebellar degeneration predicted by anti-Purkinje cell antibodies and limited in metastatic volume. *Mayo Clin Proc.* 1990; 65:1558–1563.
28. Carroll GJ, Will RK, Peter JB, Garlepp MJ, Dawklins RL. Penicillamine induced polymyositis and dermatomyositis. *J Rheumatol.* 1987; 14:995–1001.
29. Reunala T, Salmi J, Karvonen J. Dermatitis herpetiformis and celiac disease associated with Addison's disease. *Arch Dermatol.* 1987; 123:930–932.
30. Savilahti E, Simell O, Koskimies S, Rilva A, Akerblom AK. Celiac disease in insulin dependent diabetes mellitus. *J Pediatr.* 1986; 108(1): 690–693.
31. Karjalainen J, Martin JM, Knip MM, et al. A bovine albumin peptide as a possible trigger of insulin-dependent diabetes mellitus. *N Engl J Med.* 1992; 327:302–307.
32. Kostraba JN, Cruickshanks KJ, Lawler-Heavner J, et al. Early exposure to cow's milk and solid foods in infancy, genetic predisposition and risk of IDDM. *Diabetes.* 1993; 42:288–295.
33. Ehrenstein M, Longhurst C, Isenberg DA. Production and analysis of IgG monoclonal anti-DNA antibodies from systemic lupus erythematosus (SLE) patients. *Clin Exp Immunol.* 1993; 92:39–4555.
34. Colonna M, Bresnahan M, Bahram S, Strominger JL, Spies T. Allelic variants of the

human putative peptide transporter involved in antigen processing. *Proc Natl Acad Sci USA.* 1992; 89:3932–3936.

35. Thai A-C, Eisenbarth GS. Natural history of IDDM. *Diabetes Rev.* 1993; 1:1–14.
36. Costagliola S, Swillens S, Niccoli P, Dumont JE, Vassart G, Ludgate M. Binding assay for thyrotropin receptor autoantibodies using the recombinant receptor protein. *J Clin Endocrinol Metab.* 1992; 75:1540–1544.
37. Takasu N, Yamada T, Takasu M, et al. Disappearance of thyrotropin-blocking antibodies and spontaneous recovery from hypothyroidism in autoimmune thyroiditis. *N Engl J Med.* 1992; 326:513–518.
38. Posillico JT, Wortsman J, Srikanta S, Eisenbarth GS, Malette L, Brown EM. Parathyroid cell surface autoantibodies that inhibit parathyroid hormone secretion from dispersed human parathyroid cells. *Bone Miner Res.* 1986; 5:475–485.
39. Wang R, Abrams SI, Loh DY, Hsieh CS, Murphy KM, Russell JH. Separation of CD4+ functional responses by peptide dose in Th1 and Th2 subsets expressing the same transgenic antigen receptor. *Cell Immunol.* 1993; 148:357–370.
40. Ebel F, Schmitt E, Peter-Katalinic J, Kniep B, Muhlradt PF.Gangliosides: differentiation markers for murine T helper lymphocyte subpopulations TH1 and TH2. *Biochemistry.* 1992; 31:12190–12197.
41. Romagnani S. Th1 and Th2 subsets of CD4+ T lymphocytes. *Sci Med.* 1994; 1:68–77.
42. Kolb H, Kolb-Bachofen V. Nitric oxide: a pathogenetic factor in autoimmunity. *Immunol Today.* 1992; 13:157–160.
43. Corbett JA, Wang JL, Sweetland MA, Lancaster JR, McDaniel ML. Interleukin 1B induces the formation of nitric oxide by B-cells purified from rodent islets of langerhans. *J Clin Invest.* 1992; 90:2384–2391.
44. Bradley BJ, Haskins K, La Rosa FG, Lafferty KJ. CD8 T cells are not required for islet destruction induced by a CD4+ islet-specific T-cell clone. *Diabetes.* 1992; 41:1603–1608.
45. Miller A, Lider O, Roberts AB, Sporn MB, Weiner HL. Suppressor T cells generated by oral tolerization to myelin basic protein suppress both in vitro and in vivo immune responses by the release of transforming growth factor B after antigen-specific triggering. *Proc Natl Acad Sci USA.* 1992; 421:425.
46. Weiner HL, Mackin GA, Matsui M, et al. Double-blind pilot trial of oral tolerization with myelin antigens in multiple sclerosis. *Science.* 1993; 1321–1324.
47. Gottsfredsen CF, Buschard K, Frandsen EK. Reduction of diabetes incidence of BB Wistar rats by early prophylactic insulin treatment of diabetes-prone animals. *Diabetologia.* 1985; 28:933–935.
48. Keller RJ, Eisenbarth GS, Jackson RA. Insulin prophylaxis in individuals at high risk of type I diabetes. *Lancet.* 1993; 341:927–928.
49. Zhang JZ, Davidson L, Eisenbarth GS, Weiner HL. Suppression of diabetes in nonobese diabetic mice by oral administration of porcine insulin. *Proc Natl Acad Sci USA.* 1991; 88:10252–10256.
50. Gautam AM, Pearson CI, Sinha AA, Smilek DE, Steinman L, McDevitt HO. Inhibition of experimental autoimmune encephalomyelitis by a nonimmunogenic non-self peptide that binds to I-Au. *J Immunol.* 1992; 148:3049–3054.
51. Gaur A, Wiers B, Liu A, Rothbard J, Fathman CG. Amelioration of autoimmune encephalitis by myelin basic protein synthetic peptide-induced anergy. *Science.* 1992; 258:1491–1494.
52. Haynes BF, Hemler ME, Mann DL, et al. Characterization of a monoclonal

antibody (4F2) that binds to human monocytes and to a subset of activated lymphocytes. *J Immunol.* 1981; 126:1409–1414.

53. Kelley VE, Pacha P, Pankewycz O, Nichols JC, Murphy JR, Strom TB. Interleukin 2 toxin fusion protein abolishes cell mediated immunity in vivo. *Proc Natl Acad Sci USA.* 1988; 85:3980–3984.
54. Strom TB, Kelley VR, Murphy JR, Nichols J, Woodworth TG. Interleukin-2 receptor-directed therapies: antibody- or cytokine-based targeting molecules. *Annu Rev Med.* 1993; 44:343–353.
55. Strom TB, Kelley VR, Woodworth TG, Murphy JR. Interleukin-2 receptor-directed immunosuppressive therapies: antibody- or cytokine-based targeting molecules. *Immunol Rev.* 1992; 129:131–163.
56. Shizuru JA, Taylor-Edwards C, Banks BA, Gregory AK, Fathman GC. Immunotherapy of the nonobese diabetic mouse: treatment with an antibody to T-helper lymphocytes. *Science.* 1988; 240:659–662.
57. Khoury SJ, Hancock WW, Weiner HL. Oral tolerance to myelin basic protein and natural recovery from experimental autoimmune encephalomyelitis are associated with downregulation of inflammatory cytokines and differential upregulation of transforming growth factor beta, interleukin 4, and prostaglandin E expression in the brain. *J Exp Med.* 1992; 176:1355–1364.
58. Hancock WW, Sayegh MH, Kwok CA, Weiner HL, Carpenter CB. Oral, but not intravenous, alloantigen prevents accelerated allograft rejection by selective intragraft Th2 cell activation. *Transplantation.* 1993; 55:1112–1118.
59. Gotfredsen CF, Buschard K, Frandsen EK. Reduction of diabetes incidence of BB Wistar rats by early prophylactic insulin treatment of diabetes prone animals. *Diabetologia.* 1985; 28:933–935.
60. Atkinson M, Maclaren N, Luchetta R, Burr I. Insulitis and diabetes in NOD mice reduced by prophylactic insulin therapy. *Diabetes.* 1990; 39:933–937.
61. Hashizume K, Ichikawa K, Sakurai A, et al. Administration of thyroxine in treated Graves's disease: effects on the level of antibodies to thyroid-stimulatory hormone receptors and on the risk of recurrence of hyperthyroidism. *N Engl J Med.* 1991; 324:947–953.
62. Hashizume K, Ichikawa K, Nishi Y, et al. Effect of administration of thyroxine on the risk of postpartum recurrence of hyperthyroid Graves's disease. *J Clin Endocrinol Metab.* 1992; 75:6–10.
63. De Bellis A, Bizzarro A, Rossi R, et al. Remission of subclinical adrenocortical failure in subjects with adrenal autoantibodies. *J Clin Endocrinol Metab.* 1993; 76:1002–1007.
64. Sadelain MWJ, Qin H-Y, Lauzon J, Singh B. Prevention of type I diabetes in NOD mice by adjuvant immunotherapy. *Diabetes.* 1990; 39:583–589.
65. Shahadeh NN, LaRosa F, Lafferty KJ. Altered cytokine activity in adjuvant inhibition of autoimmune diabetes. *J Autoimmun.* 1993; 6:291–300.
66. Zhang JZ, Lee CS, Lider O, Weiner HL. Suppression of adjuvant arthritis in Lewis rats by oral administration of type II collagen. *J Immunol.* 1990; 145:2489–2493.
67. Nussenblatt RB, Caspi R, Mahdi R, et all. Inhibition of S-antigen induced experimental autoimmune uveoretinitis by oral induction of tolerance with S-antigen. *J Immunol.* 1990; 144:1689–1695.
68. Miller A, Lider O, Weiner HL. Antigen-driven bystander suppression after oral administration of antigens. *J Exp Med.* 1991; 174:791–798.
69. Schloot N, Eisenbarth GS. Isohormonal therapy of endocrine autoimmunity. *Immunol Today.* 1995; 289–294.

2

The Target Organ: Embryology, Biochemistry, and Physiology

Massimo Pietropaolo,
Sunanda Babu

All vertebrates phylogenetically higher than teleosts (bony fish) have clumps of pancreatic endocrine cells scattered in the pancreatic exocrine tissue, termed islets of Langerhans after their 1869 discoverer, the medical student Paul Langerhans. The islets of Langerhans play a key role in the regulation of intermediary metabolism and in the pathogenesis of diabetes mellitus.

Pancreatic Embryology

Peptide-secreting endocrine cells, including islet cells, and neurons are closely related and it has been postulated that, during development, both have a common origin from the neural crest.[1-4] This initial hypothesis was strengthened by the fact that endocrine cells—if exposed under certain conditions in vitro—undergo neural differentiation. This phenotypic shift initially was visible upon exposure of chromaffin cells to nerve growth factor (NGF), and then spontaneously , or after experimental manipulations.[5] Direct studies of the derivation of pancreatic islet cells as well as gastrointestinal mucosa cells that secrete polypeptide hormones indicate that they do not derive from neuroectoderm, but rather from endoderm as it becomes established at the end of gastrulation.[6] It is still unclear whether islets of Langerhans grow through accumulation of cells originating from the exocrine pancreas, or by proliferation of primitive islet cells, or by both processes, although there is evidence of polyclonal origin of pancreatic islets in aggregation mouse chimeras.[7]

The pancreas is derived from two or three outpocketings of the primitive gut (digestive endoderm). The dorsal anlage appears across from the budding gut, and shortly after its appearance, one or two ventral buds form the base of the biliary floor of the gut.[3] The dorsal anlage gives rise to the splenic portion (the tail and the body) of the pancreas, and the ventral anlage (or anlagen) gives rise to the duodenal portion, or head, of the pancreas.

Islets of Langerhans appear to originate from some protodifferentiated cells at the terminal ends of the budding pancreatic tubules.[3,8] In the primordia, islet cells are scattered throughout the exocrine tissue as single cells, then as clusters within the exocrine basement membrane, and finally these clusters will be separated from the exocrine tissue to form islets. Islet mass increases significantly from the fetus to the adult. Currently two major pathways of β cell growth are implicated in the growth and regeneration of islets.[3,9] Neogenesis (ie, development of islet cells from non-islet epithelium) is responsible for most of the islet growth during fetal and perinatal stage.[8] Replication of existing islet cells occurs in the late fetus and may be related to the increasing of islet mass after birth.[10] In rodent models, increase of islet mass both by hypertrophy and replication can be readily demonstrated. In man, increase in islet mass is found in a number of physiological states associated with "insulin resistance." In humans the potential for regeneration following β cell destruction is unknown, but is likely to be limited.

During pancreas ontogeny, the four classical islet cell types derive from a common stem cell passing from a transient phase in which a coexpression of two or more hormone genes (initially glucagon and insulin) occurs.[4] This condition, called 'mixed phenotype', is followed by selective inactivation of inappropriate genes to form a mature islet cell phenotype expressing a single hormone (eg, glucagon, insulin, somatostatin, or pancreatic polypeptide).[11] This phenomenon is important in tumor biology for understanding the mechanisms of activation/inactivation of hormone genes. In an elegant study, coupling embryo microdissection with the sensitivity of the polymerase chain reaction, Gittes and Rutter[174] determined the onset of transcription of major genes of the pancreas during mouse development to within a few hours. Somatostatin mRNA was the first to appear at the 10 somite stage. Mature mRNA for insulin and glucagon appears surprisingly early at the 20 somite stage in the wall of the fore gut and is restricted to the area of the duodenum from which the pancreas will arise 10–12 hours later. In contrast, exocrine gene transcription begins 24 hours after the formation of the pancreatic diverticulum. A clonal rat islet tumor line (MSL cell line) displays the features of the stem-cell phenotype.[12] Many neuroendocrine type I diabetes autoantigens such as GAD_{65} and GAD_{67} are expressed in MSL cells. Passage of these cells results in a dramatic shift in phenotype. Such switching of phenotype is being used to study novel transcription factors that may regulate islet gene expression. Embryologically the α cells appear before the others, followed by the δ cells and then by β cells (PP cells seem to appear days before birth in the rat).[13]

Structure of the Islets

Islets of Langerhans are clusters of several endocrine cell types in a nonrandom organization.[14] Particularly in rodents (less dramatic in humans), each islet consists of a central core of insulin-producing cells (β cells) surrounded by a mantle of glucagon-producing cells (α cells), somatostatin-producing cells (δ cells) and pancreatic polypeptide-producing cells (PP cells). Reactivity for a number of other peptides (gastroinhibitory peptide or GIP, cholecystokinin or CCK, secretin, gastrin, bombesin, glicentin, endorphin, substance P, the corticotropin TRH) has been detected in islet cells, but the functional role of these peptides within islet cells is unknown.[3] Thus, mammalian islet cells have a consistent pattern of organization, with the α, δ, and PP cells surrounding a central core of β cells as a discontinuous mantle one to three cells thick. The distribution of islets is heterogeneous. α Cells are preponderant in the body and tail of the pancreas, whereas PP cells are limited to the head of the pancreas.

The islets taken together represent approximately 1%–2% of the total volume of the pancreas, weighing in an adult man approximately 1 gram and containing 1 mg of insulin. The relative volume of islet cell mass differs with age, being much greater in fetus and in young animals than in adults. Within the pancreas, small islets (up to 160 μm diameter) tend to be distributed throughout the exocrine tissue. These islets represent 75% of the islets in number but only about 15% in volume. Islets greater than 250 μm diameter are only 15% in number but 60% of the volume. These islets are localized near the larger ducts and blood vessels and are not surrounded by acinar tissue.[15] A human pancreas may contain over 1 million islets, and each islet consists of several thousand cells.[3,15]

It has been postulated that islets may have a trophic and a regulatory effect on acinar tissue,[16] and that acinar-islet interactions may be of importance for the normal function of both tissues. Although acinar-islet interactions have not yet been clearly demonstrated, intracellular communication between islet cells occurs. Injection of lucifer yellow dye into a single β cell within an islet results in a visualization of the dye to adjacent β cells and α cells.[17] This type of communication occurs by cell connections termed gap junctions. Electrical activity between neighboring islet cells has been demonstrated electrophysiologically using two electrodes simultaneously recording changes in membrane potential from separate cells within a single islet.[18]

Another interesting observation is that when islets are disrupted and dispersed as single cells in culture, these single cells tend to form islet-like clusters with the same nonrandom characteristics of native islets, providing additional evidence of the importance of islet cell–cell interactions.[19] Both β cells and non-β cells have high levels of Ca^{2+}-dependent cell adhesion molecules (cadherins), but non-β cells contain also Ca^{2+}-independent cell adhesion molecules. It is thought that this different expression of cell adhesion molecules may be responsible for the segregation of β cells and non-β cells.[19]

Heterogeneity within the Islets

Besides the difference in the size of islets mentioned before, there is a regional distribution of islet cellular composition: in addition to the heterogeneity of the anatomical distribution of islets of Langerhans, it is likely that islets are heterogeneous in function. The tail, body, and the superior part of the head is glucagon poor and pancreatic polypeptide rich, whereas most of the pancreatic head (unacinated process) is glucagon rich and pancreatic polypeptide poor. There is evidence that splenic islets release more insulin in response to glucose than duodenal islets.

Islets are also functionally heterogeneous.[20] Experiments with single β cells indicated that intracellular differences in glucose responsiveness occur.[21] At glucose levels as low as 1 mM, 5% of the β cells are in active biosynthesis, whereas the remaining 95% are inactive. A rise in glucose increases the number of biosynthetically active β cells. At greater than 10 mM glucose, 70% of β cells are able to release insulin, but 30% remain inactive.[22] These experiments suggest that in vitro β cell populations are functionally heterogeneous because of differences in glucose sensitivity (Fig. 2.1). The causes of this metabolic variability have not been completely clarified, but potential key regulatory candidates include glucose transporters, glucokinase (GK), and other glucose-induced signals.[11,22] Using specific antibodies to glucokinase, significant differences in GK immunoreactivity among pancreatic β cells of euglycemic rats are found. This observation was confirmed in transgenic mice expressing fusion genes driven by the upstream GK promoter, suggesting that β-cell heterogeneity in GK expression is regulated at the transcriptional level.[11] Although the role of GK in β cells is still unclear, this heterogeneity in GK expression suggests that individual β cells may secrete insulin in an "all or none" fashion, similar to the generation of action potential in neurons, and that the ability to secrete insulin may depend on levels of glucose and particularly may reflect a recruitment of individual β cells into an active secretory state. If Newgard's hypothesis is correct, namely that GK levels in AtT20 cells are critical to determine glucose sensitivity of insulin secretion,[23] one can speculate that low GK-expressing β cells may respond at lower glucose levels, whereas high GK-expressing β cells may respond at higher glucose concentrations. Such β cell heterogeneity may relate to differential infiltration and destruction of islet cells over time.

Heterogeneity of β cells may explain why in type I diabetes mellitus, β cells do not simultaneously undergo the same pathological process. It is known that the clinical features of the disease occur when less than 10% of the β cell mass remains. It is unclear what makes different islets and their β cells more or less vulnerable to the immune-mediated pathological process. Experiments

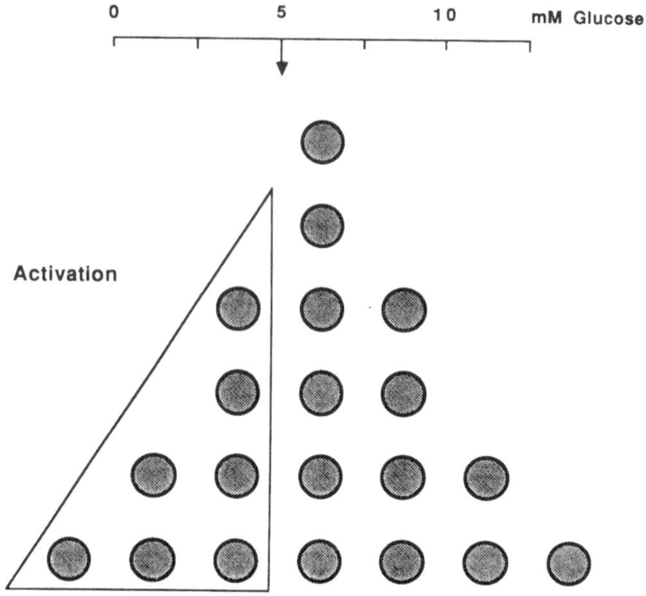

Figure 2.1. Hetogeneity of glucose sensitivity. Model of β cell population composed of subpopulations with different sensitivities to glucose. The percentage of activated cells varies with glucose concentration. The figure shows a subpopulation of β cells already active in the absence of glucose, plus those recruited between 0 and 5 mM glucose. (From Pipeleers D. *Diabetes*, 41:778, 1992.)

with rat cells have indicated that intracellular differences in oxidative state can explain differences in the sensitivity of β cells to cytotoxic agents and in their defense reactions.[24]

Relationship with Pancreatic Exocrine Tissue

A putative functional effect of islets of Langerhans on pancreatic exocrine tissue has been postulated since 1899 when Jarotzky noted that acinar cells close to the islets of Langerhans had more zymogen granules than those at a distance from islets. More recent morphological findings indicate that peri-insular acinar cells are twice as big as teleinsular cells.[3] Nevertheless, in type I diabetes the functional loss of β cells does not lead to a clinical reduction of exocrine function. There is evidence that in the perfused pancreas model, low insulin levels are associated with a significant reduction in stimulated acinar cell enzyme secretion. A high number of insulin receptors is found on pancreatic acini.[25] Somatostatin and pancreatic polypeptide, but not glucagon,[26] also affect pancreatic acinar function.[27] Both somatostatin and pancreatic polypeptide inhibit pancreatic acinar function in vitro [28] and in vivo.[29] To date the main evidence for a functional relationship between islets and acinar tissue derives from studies on endocrine hormones on exocrine function, but acinar-islet relationships can also be affected by neural reflexes that cause a redistribution of blood supply between exocrine and endocrine tissue.[30]

Blood Supply and Innervation of Islets

The islets of Langerhans are richly vascularized, receiving 5 to 10 times the blood supply of a comparable portion of exocrine pancreatic tissue.[31] The blood flow to islets has been estimated as 10%–15% of the total pancreatic blood flow. Islets have fenestrated capillaries, unlike capillaries surrounding the exocrine tissue. Afferent arterioles enter the islets through discontinuities of the mantle of non-β cells and branch into capillaries that form a glomerular-like structure.[3] The direction of the blood is from the β cell core capillaries to the α and δ cells. In large islets (>260 μm in diameter) efferent capillaries coalesce at the edge of the islet and run along the mantle as collecting venules. In islets smaller than 160 μm in diameter, efferent capillaries pass through the exocrine tissue before coalescing into collecting venules.

The islets are innervated by sympathetic fibers from the celiac ganglion and by parasympathetic fibers from the vagus nerve. Cholinergic stimulation increase insulin, glucagon, and pancreatic polypeptide release. Beta-adrenergic stimulation increases insulin, glucagon, pancreatic polypeptide, and somatostatin secretion. Alpha-adrenergic stimulation appears to inhibit insulin release.

Ultrastructure of the Islets

β Cells, Insulin Secretory Granules, Synaptic-Like Microvesicles

β cells are polyhedral and are arranged in tubes of 8 to 10 cells surrounding capillaries. In well-granulated β cells the rough endoplasmic reticulum (RER) is scanty and scattered among numerous secretory granules.[32] Two major forms of granule are currently described: a mature granule that has an electron-dense core, and an immature granule that has moderately electron-dense contents. The insulin secretory granule of the pancreatic β cell is a complex intracellular organelle composed of many proteins with different enzymatic and physiological functions, and measures 200–300 nm in diameter.

With the aid of tumor models of β cells and the development of molecular cloning techniques, significant progress has been made over the past decade to elucidate the structure and function of granule proteins. The proteolytic conversion of proinsulin is an event that occurs in the secretory granules (see below). The β cell secretory granule is far more than a static structure of hormone storage. It is the site of proteolytic cleavage of proinsulin. Approximately 10% of the granule population turns over every hour during active secretion.[32] Granule membrane proteins represent approximately a tenth of the granule mass. These membranes are recovered by endocytosis and then delivered either to the lysomal compartment for degradation or returned to the site of granule assembly. Lysosomal degradation of entire secretory granules by crinophagy is a pathway of granule disposal that may be regulated. At least twelve proteins whose molecular mass ranges from 5 to 60 kilodaltons (kd) have been observed to be released along with insulin. One of the more abundant of these peptides is a 21-kd protein termed betagranin.[33] Betagranin is also present in the secretory granules of pituitary and adrenal, and also in isolated cells in the gut. By pulse-chase labelling experiments it has been reported that betagranin is synthesized as a larger precursor that is then converted to a 21-kd fragment. This conversion apparently requires carboxypeptidase H activity, as well as a type II–like endopeptidase activity.[34] Other secretory granule proteins include pancreastatin, which has been found in δ cells, insulin-associated polypeptide (IAPP), substrates (P10, P29, and P100), enzymes (C-kinase) involved in granule membrane protein phosphorylation, enzymes of phosphatidylinositol metabolism, cathepsin B–related proteins, Ca^{2+}-binding proteins, and membrane antigens (SGM 80 and SGM 110).[32] In insulin-dependent diabetes mellitus (IDDM) the β cell secretory granule is considered a prominent target organelle involved in the induction of an islet-specific autoimmune response. The autoimmune response to different autoantigens such as insulin, carboxypeptidase H, or ICA69[35] may well be driven by aggregates of granule molecules recognized as non-self. Moreover, disturbances of secretory granule regulation may lead to increased concentrations of proinsulin and processing intermediates in type II diabetic patients.[36]

Many biochemical similarities between neurons and endocrine cells have become clear. The identification of synaptic-like microvesicles (SLMVs) in endocrine cells and in particular in pancreatic β cells represents a new and important element of general similarity between endocrine cells and neurons.[37] SLMVs are very similar to neuronal synaptic vesicles in morphology, membrane compostion, and life cycle. The function of SLMVs appears to be related to the storage and secretion of nonpeptide signaling molecules (eg, GABA in islets), and possibly to the uptake, storage, and secretion of neurotransmitters or neurotransmitter-like molecules.[38] SLMVs contain several synaptic vesicle proteins including synaptophysin, synaptobrevin (neuronal isoforms),[38] and the proteins p29, SV2, and rab3A.[39] It is still unclear whether β cell SLMV membranes contain synaptotagmin.[37]

α Cells

α Cells are smaller than β cells and their shape is columnar. α cells are well granulated, with granules 200 to 250 nm in diameter. The granules are electron dense with a little halo of less dense material. α cells in humans, but not in the rat or mouse, express glutamic acid decarboxylase. The reason why human α cells (expressing GAD) are not destroyed in the autoimmune process leading to type I diabetes is unclear.

δ Cells

δ Cells are usually smaller than α or β cells, well granulated, and their shape is dendritic. The granules, whose diameter is 200–250 nm, contain moderately electron-dense material.

PP Cells

PP cells in humans contain very electron-dense granules whose diameter is 120–160 nm. The granules' shape is elongated. The function of pancreatic polypeptide within islets is unknown.

Biochemistry/Physiology

Insulin Gene Structure

The product of the insulin gene, insulin, was the first peptide hormone molecularly cloned. DNA recombinant technology has led to large scale production of human insulin in bacteria, and its use is primarily for the treatment of insulin-dependent diabetes mellitus. Moreover, cloning of the insulin gene has provided new insights on its structure, regulation, biosynthesis of insulin, and its involvement in the pathophysiology of diabetes.

The human insulin gene is localized on chromosome 11 between the tyrosine hydroxylase and IGFII genes (Fig 2.2). The structure of the insulin gene is remarkably conserved among species, and most animals have a single copy of the insulin gene.[40] Three exons with a total of 446 base pairs (bp) form the mature preproinsulin mRNA. The two introns between the exons are removed from the primary transcript during the process of RNA splicing and polyadenylation. This process takes place in the nucleus. The first intron, termed IVS1, is located between exon 1 and exon 2 and starts 42 bp downstream from the transcription start site. The second intron, IVS2, located between exon 2 and exon 3, splits the coding sequence for the C peptide. When completely processed, the preproinsulin mRNA codes for preproinsulin. In the mRNA coding for the preproinsulin peptide, there are 59 bp on the 5′ end, 73 bp on the 3′ end, and a long polyadenosine 3′ tail that are not translated into protein. Sequence comparisons among mammalian insulin genes revealed significant conservation in the 5′ flanking regions, especially up to about 350 bp from the transcription start site,[41,42] indicating that cell-specific transcription patterns are directed by DNA sequences in this region. In addition, further upstream of the human insulin gene is a region of variable nucleotide tandem repeats, which varies in size between individuals. Of note, the size of these repeats has been associated with diabetes susceptibility, suggesting that such upstream repeats may influence insulin gene expression.[43–45,177]

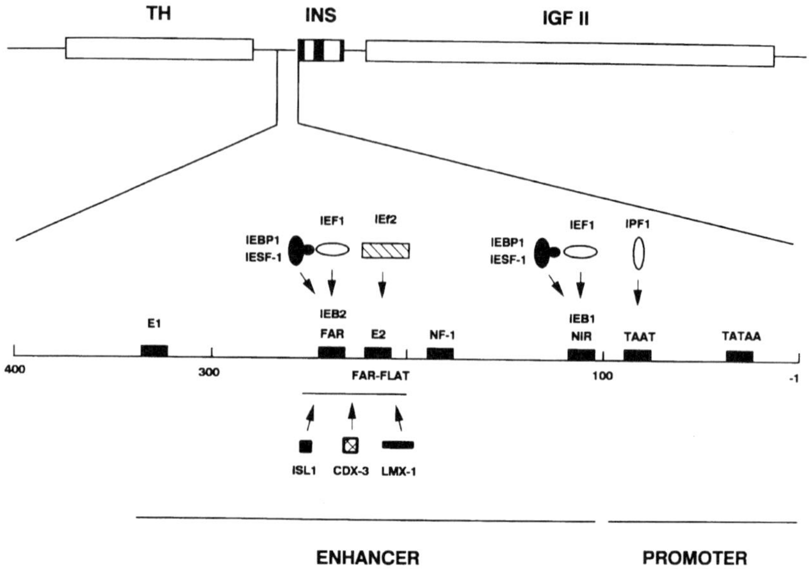

Figure 2.2. Rat insulin gene. Between the TH and IGF II genes. Enlarged promoter/enhancer region, indicating some of the DNA binding sites and the factors that bind to them.

Regulation of Insulin Gene Expression

5′ Flanking Regulatory Sequences. At least three distinguishable elements determining cell specifity are contained within the 5′ flanking region—a gene specific promoter, a cell-specifying enhancer region, and a negative regulatory element that prevents transcription of insulin in non-insulin-producing cells.

A proximal fragment promotes cell-specific transcription when coupled with a nonspecific viral enhancer.[46] This element is located within sequences from +1 to −113 and appears to be an integral part of the insulin promoter. In the rat insulin II gene, Hwung and coworkers[47] reported that the chicken ovalbumin upstream promoter transcription factor bound to the region −53 to −46 of the promoter, although the binding sequences showed limited similarities.

Several *cis*-acting sequences involved in conferring tissue-specific expression of the rat and human insulin genes are located within a region up to 350 bases from the transcription start site.[48] Deletion mutants in the 5′ flanking region of the human insulin gene linked to a reporter gene revealed the presence of positive and negative regulation.[49]

Karlsson and coworkers identified two structurally related elements that were important for transcriptional activation, by a series of block mutation replacements in the rat insulin I promoter expressed in HIT cells (an insulin-producing hamster insulinoma cell line). These elements are located at −104 to −112 (now called the Nir box or IEB1 insulin enhancer box) and −233 to −240 (called the Far box or IEB2) (Fig 2.2). When mutated individually, they significantly reduced activity; the double mutant virtually abolished it.[50]

These two regions were protected in DNAase 1 footprinting assays, indicating that regulatory proteins were bound to them.[51] They contain an 8-bp homology GCCATCTG and act as enhancers, directing β-cell–specific transcription on heterologous promoters.[52] In addition, these sequences share similarities with enhancers of the immunoglobulin heavy chain μE1,μE2 and μE3.[53] A DNA-binding nuclear protein found in insulin-producing cell lines but absent in nonendocrine cells, termed IEF1, binds to both of these segments (Fig. 2.2).[54] Another 25-kd protein (IESF-1) has been shown to bind to these elements.[55] In the human insulin gene enhancer, there is a motif (GCII) with 75% similarity and a comparable location to the IEF-1 binding site.[49]

The IEB sequences are part of a family of transcriptional control elements with a consensus sequence CANNTG, identified in genes expressed in lymphoid cells, muscle cells, and exocrine pancreas.[56] Factors containing the basic helix-loop-helix dimerization domain bind to the sequences. Such proteins have been cloned from mouse β-cell line, the A1 protein,[57] HIT cells,[58,59] the Pan-1 and Pan-2 proteins[60] and from a RIN cell (rat insulinoma cell line) library, IEBP1.[61] They are all similar to the previously reported human immunoglobin enhancer E47/E12 proteins.[62]

Another enhancer-binding protein, Isl-1, has been cloned from RIN cell and shares similarities with a metal-binding protein isolated from *C. elegans*, including a homeo domain and a Cys-His domain.[63] This protein binds to sequences −199 to −252 of the enhancer. Proteins with the homeo domain are important for the establishment of developmental lineages and bind to motifs containing TAAT sequences. Two other proteins containing homeo domains have been cloned that bind to the TAAT element, cdx-3 and lmx-1.[64] In addition, lmx-1 also contains two Cys/His domains like the Isl-1 protein.

A promoter proximal TAAT box is located at −86 [65] and binds a pancreatic β cell factor IPF-1 not present in α cell lines. Three more TAAT elements are found in the distal region of the rat insulin 1 gene enhancer termed FLAT element.[53] Proteins cdx-3 and lmx-1 can activate transcription of a Far/FLAT–linked gene when expressed in a non–insulin producing fibroblast cell line.[64] The addition of a Far-binding helix-loop-helix protein causes a synergistic activation in fibroblasts expressing transfected lmx-1. In combination with the Far element, but not separately, the FLAT element functions as a β-cell–specific mini-enhancer. Sequences similar to the mini-enhancer are also present in the 5′ flanking DNA of the human, islet amyloid polypeptide (IAP) and the rat β cell–specific glucokinase genes, two proteins that are synthesized in the β cells of the islet but also in other cells. Similar mini-enhancer constructs from the insulin and AP genes function as cell-specific transcriptional activators and compete for binding of the same nuclear factors.[66]

Sharing of transcriptional regulators is seen in the hepatocyte nuclear factor

1 α, which is expressed in a hamster insulinoma cell line and transactivates the rat insulin I gene.[67] Pan-1 and Pan-2 bind chymotrypsin and the viral AP-4 enhancer motifs in addition to insulin.[60]

Transient expression of the rat insulin gene II has revealed that there are differences in the regulatory elements used by the two genes.[47] Whelan and coworkers[68] identified both positive and negative elements in the rat insulin II gene with one element between −100 and −91 regulated by positive and negative factors; this element alone can impart β-cell specific expression. The distal element essential for rat insulin gene I is dispensable for rat insulin gene II expression.[69] In the rat insulin II gene, the region between −126 and −86, termed the rat insulin promoter element (RIPE3), binds three factors that interact for maximum enhancer activity.[59]

In the human insulin gene, sequences from −339 upstream of the start site are sufficient to activate transcription in reporter systems.[49] This region contained a CRE-like motif (cAMP response element) and three CT binding sites at −82 (CT1 box), −215 (CT2 box), and −319 (CT3 box); GC-binding sites (similar to the IEB sequences of the rat I gene); and a negative regulatory element. Boam and Docherty[70] identified a factor, IUF-1 (insulin upstream factor), that binds to the CT2 site, in the human insulin gene enhancer. IUF-1 was present only in mouse pancreas β cells but not in α cells. This may be important in β cell–specific expression.[71]

While studying the binding of nuclear proteins from insulinoma cells to the −258/+241 region of the human insulin gene, Reibel and coworkers[72] discovered a protein-binding site in the intron 1 region +160 to +175 with a core sequence GGGCCC. Binding activity was present only in insulin-producing cell lines, including RIN and HIT lines, and to a related sequence in the rat and mouse insulin genes contiguous with the Far element.

Kennedy and Rutter[73] isolated Pur-1, a zinc finger protein binding to another kind of element, a GAGA box, in the rat insulin genes I and II and the human islet amyloid polypeptide gene. It is a potent transactivator and activates an intact insulin promoter in HeLa cells, where it is normally inactive. At least four different proteins bind to these elements located about −57 to −40 of the rat insulin I gene promoter.

Negative Regulatory Elements. In the human insulin gene enhancer, the GAGA motif (−278 to −268) was associated with a powerful negative element found in β cells that could downregulate a heterologous promoter.[49] Nir and coworkers[74] reported negative trans-acting factors that repress the insulin enhancer activity in cells not expressing insulin.

Cell-specific repressor activity is also associated with the E-boxes IEB1 and IEB2 (Fig. 2.2). Plasmids bearing four or six copies of the IEB motif showed sharply reduced activity as compared with those with two copies. Moreover, multiple copies of the IEB sequence were able to inhibit activity of a heterologous promoter upon transfection into β cells but not other cell types.[75]

A potent negative regulatory element (NRE)[11] is also present upstream of the insulin gene. The NRE function on β cells seems to be as a silencer (ie, functions independently of position and orientation). NRE is not simply responsible for repression of insulin gene expression because it is expressed in other neuroendocrine cells. An adjacent positive element modulates the activity of NRE.

Studies in Transgenic Mice. The first transgenic experiments with the insulin gene were performed by Hanahan, who injected the rat insulin II gene promoter region linked to the SV40 large T antigen.[76] He found expression of large T antigen was restricted to the β cells of the islets. Transgeneic strains with delayed expression of the T antigen developed insulitis.

In transgenic mouse cell lines carrying the human insulin gene with various lengths of the 5′ flanking sequences, deletions upstream from positions −353, −258, and −168 allowed correct initiation of transcripts and specificity of expression but diminished quantitative expression.[77] With any of the deletions used, expression of the transgene was not observed in cell types other than β cells.

In transgenic mice the −345 to −103 fragment of the rat insulin I promoter linked to a reporter gene was sufficient for expression of the transgene in the pancreas and brain.[78] However, the DNA sequences IEB1 and IEB2 were not enough for specific expression in transgenic mice although they confer about 40% of the activity in HIT cells.

It is likely that in the near future a number of additional transcription factors will be identified, and this will shed light on the mechanisms of islet development as well as understanding the specific phenotype of islet cells. German and coworkers[79] have recently simplified the nomenclature of the insulin gene promoter, but the interactions remain complex.

Insulin Gene Polymorphism and Insulin-Dependent Diabetes Mellitus. Polymorphism in the human insulin gene exists. Variations in sequence are reported in the variable-sized insert (HVR) at −360 bp in the promoter. Three HVR inserts of the promoter region have been described[40]: the class 1 allele, whose HVR size is less than 600 bp; the class 2 allele, whose size is between 600 and 1600 bp; and the class 3 allele, whose size is greater than 1600 bp. Among whites HVR inserts are class 1 and class 3. Class 2 allele is rare except in African and African-American populations.

The size of the HVR can be used as a genetic marker to study the linkage of this region of chromosome 11 with clinical evidence of insulin-dependent diabetes. It has been reported that HVR class 1 alleles are significantly associated with insulin-dependent diabetes.[43,170,176] This initial observation has been recently confirmed by Julier and coworkers[80] in a study of French, American, and North African patients that analyzes families with heterozygous parents. This linkage was strongest when the class 1 allele was inherited from the father and when the affected family member was HLA-DR4 positive. Other studies from England,[81] Norway,[81] and Belgium[82] have not reported any significant association between insulin locus polymorphism and HLA-DR haplotype in insulin-dependent diabetes.

Although there is conclusive evidence of linkage between the HVR/insulin locus and insulin-dependent diabetes mellitus, the molecular mechanism that might underlie the disease process is unknown. One possibility is that the insulin polymorphic locus might be in linkage disequilibrium with another gene (eg, IGF2 gene[83]), or a group of unknown genes, which may be involved in the pathogenesis of the disease because of mutations that result in abnormal gene products. Moreover, polymorphism in the insulin gene may affect the expression of insulin.[176] It has been shown by Jolicoeur and coworkers that transient thymic expression of insulin occurs in mice.[175] If we assume that insulin is one of the major autoantigens associated with insulin-dependent diabetes, a mutation in the promoter region of the insulin gene could play a role in the pathogenesis of type I diabetes. This mutation may result in a defective expression of insulin in the thymus during the first stage of development. If this hypothesis is correct, autoimmunity to insulin may be explained by failure of the mechanisms that normally generate self-tolerance to insulin; such failure may result from abnormalities in the gene regulation of insulin in the early stage of development.

Biosynthesis of Insulin

A normal adult human pancreas is able to secret approximately 40/50 units of insulin per day. The basal concentration of insulin in the bloodstream in the fasting state is approximately 10 μU/mL. In a normal control subject after a standard meal, insulin rises about 10-fold (100 μU/mL). Insulin secretion varies in basal conditions and after stimuli.

Basal Insulin Secretion. In the fasting state, with plasma glucose levels below 80–100 mg/dL, significant pulses of insulin release occur every 10–15 minutes. Both insulin secretion and β cell electrical activity display cyclic oscillations.[84,85] These normal regular pulses are not observed in some cases of non–insulin-dependent diabetes mellitus (NIDDM)[86,87] and in relatives of patients with type II diabetes.This oscillatory insulin secretion does not appear to be neurally controlled because it is preserved either in vitro in the perfused pancreas model, or in vivo after pancreas transplantation. What controls the pancreas pulsatility and its significance in the regulation of carbohydrate metabolism is not clear.

Stimulated Insulin Secretion. Glucose is the most potent stimulant of insulin release. When the glucose concentration is increased rapidly, the kinetics of the insulin response to glucose is biphasic. An initial short-lived burst of insulin release occurs (the early phase) within 1 minute upon glycemic stimulus, reaches a peak within 2 minutes and declines over the ensuing 3 to 5 minutes. A second phase (the late phase) is characterized by a more gradual increase in insulin levels that begins 5 to 10 minutes after the initiation of insulin infusion and continues over the next hour. These observations led to the concept that within the β cell, insulin is segregated in a two-pool system.[88] Immediately releasable presynthesized insulin is rapidly discharged in the early phase. A continuing release pool, which is mostly newly synthesized insulin, including small amounts of proinsulin, is discharged during the late phase. Other factors involved in the regulation of insulin secretion are summarized in Table 2.1. These factors can be summarized in three categories: direct insulin secretagogues (which are known to stimulate insulin release directly); amplifiers of glucose-induced secretion, which seem to amplify the insulin secretion in response to glucose; and inhibitors of insulin secretion, such as somatostatin and some drugs.

The gene that encodes insulin is localized on chromosome 11p. The product of the insulin gene, insulin, is abundantly expressed only in pancreatic β cells.[89,90] Transient thymic expression of insulin detected with PCR gene amplification has been seen to occur in mice.[175] Insulin production is initiated by transcription of the gene in the nucleus of the beta cell. The translation product of proinsulin mRNA is a peptide of 11,500 daltons termed preproinsulin, which is converted to proinsulin (molecular weight [MW] about 9,000) by microsomal proteases. Preproinsulin has a very short half-life. Proinsulin is then transported by an energy-dependent process from the rough endoplasmic reticulum (RER) to the Golgi complex, thereafter accumulating along with zinc in the mature secretory granule (Fig. 2.3).[91–93] All or most of the enzymatic processing of proinsulin to insulin occurs in a subpopulation of secretory granules (Fig. 2.3) that are coated with clathrin (a complex aggregate of protein subunits that appear to facilitate intracellular shuttling.[94] The result of post-transcriptional processing leads to an equimolar production of insulin

Table 2.1. Regulation of Insulin Release

STIMULANTS OF INSULIN SECRETION
Glucose, mannose
Leucine
Vagal stimulation
Sulfonylureas
AMPLIFIERS OF GLUCOSE-INDUCED INSULIN SECRETION
1. Enteric hormones:
Gastrin inhibitory polypeptide
Cholecystokinin
Gastrin
Secretin
2. Neural: Beta-adrenergic stimulation
3. Amino acids: Arginine
INHIBITORS OF INSULIN SECRETION
Neural: Alpha-adrenergic effect of catecholamines
Humoral: Somatostatin
Drugs: Diazoxide, colchicine, phenytoin, vinblastine

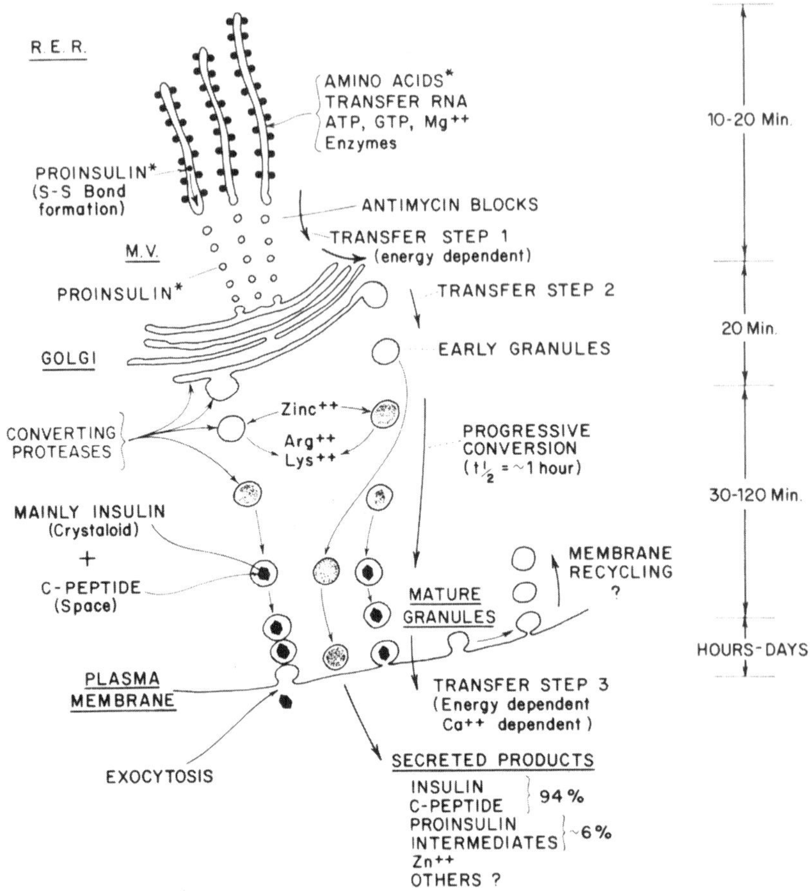

Figure 2.3. Conversion of pre-proinsulin to insulin in pancreatic β cells. Pre-proinsulin after its synthesis in the rough endoplasmic reticulum (RER) and rapid cleavage to proinsulin (within one or two minutes), is then released into the cisternal spaces of the RER. In RER, proinsulin folds to form the native disulfide bonds of insulin and is then transported to the Golgi apparatus. Processing mainly occurs in the granules.[89,94] The release of newly synthesized proinsulin and insulin begins approximately one hour after synthesis in the RER. The granules undergo a maturation process that leads to their exocytosis. Exocytosis of granules, which results in the release of insulin and C-peptide in equimolar proportions, is the outcome of proinsulin biosynthesis, which can be stimulated at both transcriptional and translational levels.[94,95,112,114] (From Steiner DF. In: *Endocrinology*, De Groot, 1269, 1989)

with its alpha and beta chains linked by disulfide bonds and a connecting peptide termed C peptide.[94-96,114]

Secretory granule converting enzymes, such as carboxypeptidase H, carboxypeptidase B–like and trypsin-like proteases, cleave off two pairs of amino acids (Arg31, Arg32, Lys64, Arg65) from the proinsulin molecule (Fig. 2.4A).[97] The result is a 51–amino acid molecule, which represents insulin, and the 31–amino acid C peptide. The proinsulin processing of an endo-

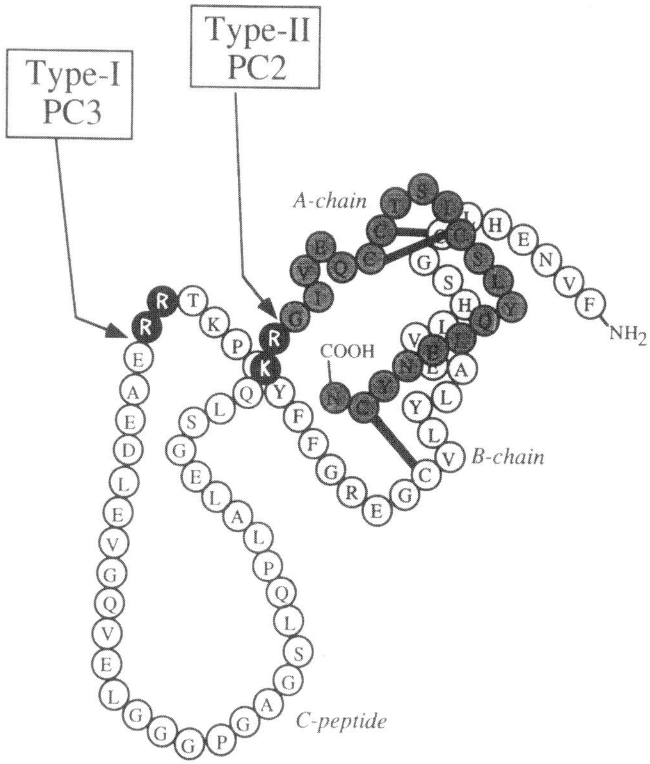

Figure 2.4A. Cleavage sites of the two distinct proinsulin-processing endopeptidases on human proinsulin. (From Rhodes CJ et al., *Diabetes*, 43:511–517, 1994.)

peptidase activity was first observed as a Ca^{2+}-dependent B-granule–specific proteinase activity with an acidic pH optimum.[98] Two distinct endopeptidases are involved in the processing of proinsulin (Fig. 2.4A).[99] One, termed type I, cleaves exclusively at Arg31, Arg32 site, whereas the other, termed type II, cleaves preferentially at Lys64, Arg65 (Fig. 2.4B).[97] Over the past few years, a number of proprotein-processing endopeptidases have been identified.[100-102] Among these novel neuroendocrine enzymes, two appear to be involved in the processing of proinsulin. The first is a specific proteinase named PC2,[103,104] and the second is named PC3[105] (PC3 has also been named PC1).[106] Recently it has been demonstrated that PC2 and the type-II proinsulin-processing activity are equivalent,[107] and that the PC3 is immunologically[107] and bio-chemically[108,109] identical to the type-I proinsulin-processing activity. Proinsulin biosynthesis can be stimulated by glucose at both transcriptional and translational levels.[110-112] It is likely that PC3 initiates the majority of sequential processing leading to proinsulin conversion in human β cells (Fig. 2.4B).[113] As a matter of fact, the biosynthesis of PC3, unlike PC2 and carboxypeptidase-H biosynthesis (which is not glucose-related)[114] is stimulated by a short-term glucose stimulation (<2 h) in parallel of proinsulin at a translational level.[113] Therefore, PC3 appears to be the key peptidase that regulates proinsulin processing in β cells.

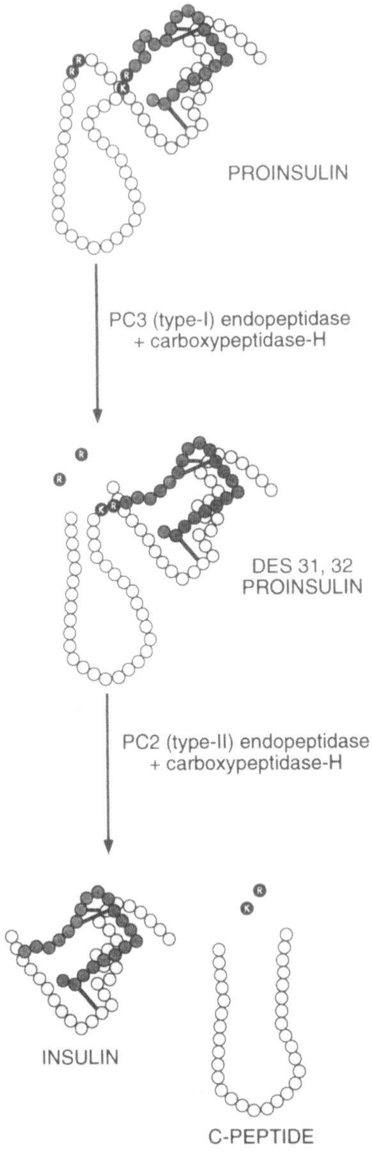

Figure 2.4B. Sequential processing of proinsulin. (From Rhodes CJ et al., *Diabetes.*, 43:511–517, 1994.)

The secretory granules store large amounts of insulin, which is extremely concentrated (10^{-2} M) within secretory granules. Secretory granules also have a zinc concentration 50-fold higher than in plasma, which appears to be involved in the cellular storage of the hormone. Insulin release is achieved in β cells by exocytosis of granule contents. The granule membrane fuses with the plasma membrane of β cells, and its contents are released from the cells (Fig.

2.3). Endogenous insulin (MW 5,808) has a circulatory half-life of 3–5 minutes. It is catabolized mainly by a number of enzymes such as the insulin-degrading enzyme (IDE) mainly in liver, kidney, and placenta.[115] The region of insulin responsible for its high-affinity interaction with IDE has been recently identified.[116,117] Approximately 50% of insulin is removed in a single pass through the liver.

There is no convincing evidence of a biological role for C peptide (MW 3,000), although it is released into the bloodstream in the same quantity as insulin. Its half-life is 3 to 4 times that of insulin, probably because proinsulin is not metabolized by the liver. In the basal state, after an overnight fast, the average concentration of C peptide is approximately 1000 pmol/L.

Proinsulin can be released from β cells, reflecting incomplete conversion of insulin in the secretory granules, and is approximately 3%–5% of immunoreactive insulin extracted from human pancreas. Human proinsulin has about 7%–8% of the biological activity of insulin. Kidney is the principal site of proinsulin catabolism.

Signal Transduction

Glucose Sensing. Both glucose uptake and metabolism are required for insulin secretion. Glucose-stimulated insulin release is critical for the maintenance of glucose homeostasis. The current hypothesis is that glucose transporter of β cells known as GLUT-2 and the enzyme glucokinase (GK) are key components of the "glucose sensing apparatus."[118,119] GLUT-2 is expressed in β cells, as well as intestine, kidney, and liver, but it is not expressed by other pancreatic endocrine cells. Both GLUT-2 and GK have lower affinities and higher capacities for glucose transport and glucose phosphorylation, respectively.[120–122] The presence of a high K_m (~18 mM), high capacity and low affinity for glucose[120] of GLUT-2, a high K_m for GK (~9 mM) lead to glucose uptake and phosphorylation proportional to a wide variety of extracellular glucose concentrations. Therefore, β cell insulin secretion responds to the wide physiological glycemic changes that occur in the postprandial state. In view of these kinetic properties, it has been suggested that both GLUT-2 and GK play a role in the β cell glucose sensing. Under certain physiological conditions, GK rather than GLUT-2 appears to be rate limiting for glucose utilization in β cells.[123]

Chronic exposure to high glucose in HIT pancreatic cells down-regulates GLUT-2 mRNA levels, glucose transport, and glucose-induced insulin secretion.[124] In addition, reduction of the number of GLUT-2 transporters in islets has been observed in a spontaneous animal model of NIDDM.[125] The extent of reduction of GLUT-2 expression correlates with the severity of diabetes as determined by the glycemic levels. To date there is no evidence that GK levels fall in tandem with GLUT-2 in rodent NIDDM.

Ca^{2+}, K^+, Na^+ Channels, ATP:ADP Ratio, cAMP, DAG, IP_3, GLP-1. Intracellular calcium concentrations are believed to influence insulin release.

Increased Ca^{2+} uptake appears to be regulated by glucose metabolism and apparently is dependent on a decrease in K^+ membrane permeability, resulting in depolarization of the β cells. The resulting rise in cytosolic Ca^{2+} induces insulin release.[126,127]

The membrane potential of the pancreatic β cells is controlled by an ATP potassium channel (K-ATP channels) (Fig. 2.5). In the absence of glucose the membrane potential is at -70 to -80 mV. When extracellular glucose rises (eg, 10 mM) the ATP content of β cell increases. This rise in ATP content (or the change in ATP/ADP ratio) seems to inhibit K^+ efflux through specific channels in the plasma membrane.[126,128–130] Mitochondrial metabolism likely plays an important role in insulin secretion. It is known that agents that block islet cell respiration and agents that block mitochondrial electron transport or oxidative phosphorylation also block glucose-stimulated insulin secretion.[118,131,132] Thus, it is hypothesized that glucose induces depolarization of the membrane through closure of specific K channels, leading to a decrease of K^+ permeability.[126] The membrane potential ranges from approximately -55 mV in basal levels of glucose and depolarizes to about -30 mV in the presence of higher concentrations of glucose (above 7 mM). As a consequence of this membrane depolarization, dihydropyridine-sensitive Ca^{2+} channels open (Fig. 2.5).[127] The resulting influx of Ca^{2+} leads to an increase in the submembrane Ca^{2+} concentration, $[Ca^{2+}]_{sm}$.[133,134] This rise in $[Ca^{2+}]_{sm}$ causes

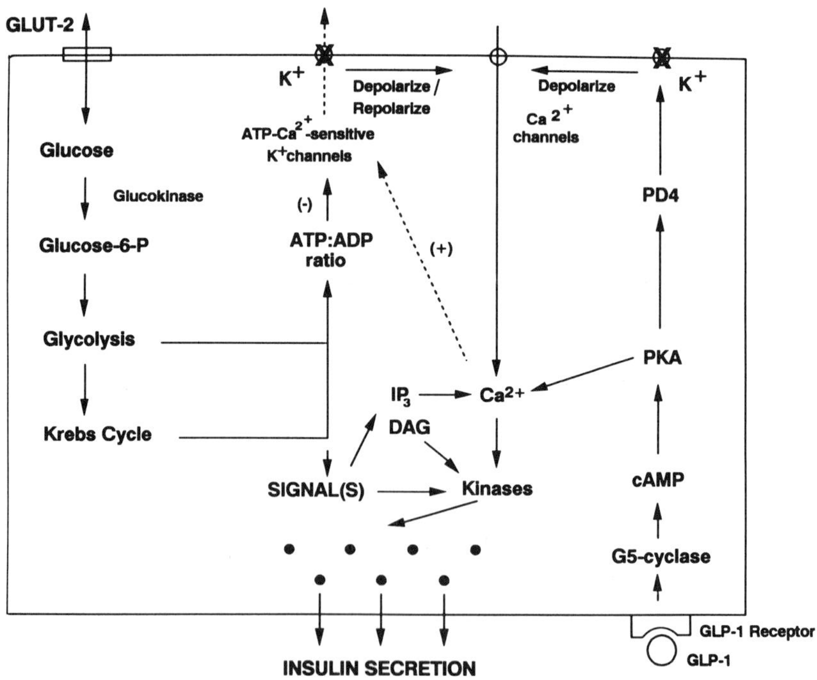

Figure 2.5. Schematic representation of biochemical events involved in glucose-stimulated insulin secretion in the β cell.

the opening of Ca^{2+} -sensitive K^+ channels in the membrane,[135,136] resulting in an increase K^+ efflux, therefore leading to a repolarization of the plasma membrane thereby closing the voltage-dependent Ca^{2+} channels. In addition, a rise in $[Ca^{2+}]_{sm}$ leads to the calmodulin-dependent activation of the plasma membrane pump.[137] Thus, by repolarizing the membrane and enhancing Ca^{2+} pump activity, the rise in $[Ca^{2+}]_{sm}$ is a self-limiting process. As the $[Ca^{2+}]_{sm}$ falls back to its original values, another cycle of Ca^{2+} influx and efflux follows. Thus, extracellular glucose levels induce firing of Ca^{2+} action potentials, which can be recorded as repetitive bursts of electrical activity. Whereas stimulated insulin secretion is strictly dependent on Ca^{2+} entry into β cells, basal insulin release is not dependent on Ca^{2+} entry.

It is noteworthy that glucose, under certain conditions, leads to intracellular sequestration and extrusion of Ca^{2+}.[138–140] Therefore, high glucose levels may, paradoxically, cause an inhibition of insulin secretion, which may explain an impaired β cell function in some forms of type II diabetes.

The possible role of Na^+ channels in the physiology of insulin release has been postulated in view of the fact that tetrodoxin (TTX), a specific inhibitor of voltage-sensitive Na^+ channels, has been shown to partially inhibit insulin secretion in the rat, whereas veratidine, which induces opening of Na^+ channels, stimulated insulin secretion.[141] Misler and coworkers[142,143] reported that in human and rat β cells, trains of Na^+-dependent action potentials are seen, and that in the majority of rat β cells Na^+ channels are inactivated.

Voltage-dependent Na^+ channel membrane proteins have been identified by cloning using cDNA libraries from mammalian brain, heart, and skeletal muscle.[144–146] Recently Philipson and coworkers[147] have identified a Na^+ channel α_1-subunit mRNA expressed in human, rat, and canine islets by RT-PCR mRNA amplification. The cDNA sequence of this molecule is closely related to the brain III α_1-subunit isoform, primarily expressed in fetal rat brain. Pressel and Misler[142] have hypothesized that the "early train" of Na^+-dependent action potentials may induce an early phase of insulin secretion by transiently activating Ca^{2+} channels leading to pulsatile Ca^{2+} entry. Na^{2+} and Ca^{2+} make significant contributions to first-phase insulin secretion and second-phase or sustained insulin release, respectively. The addition of TTX, which blocks Na^+ channels, reduced in vitro initial peak glucose-induced insulin secretion by nearly twofold as compared with the control. No effect of TTX was seen in one experiment where a control lacked initial peak secretion. Addition of the Ca^{2+} channel agonist BAY K 8644 during the plateau produces a dramatic increase in insulin release, both in the presence and absence of TXX.[127]

Cyclic AMP is thought to participate in the insulin secretory process. It is considered a positive synergistic modulator of a glucose-sensitive secretory step in view of the fact that theophylline (a potent inhibitor of phosphodiesterase that increases cAMP concentration) has a weak stimulatory effect on insulin secretion that is enhanced in presence of glucose.[118,146,148] It is commonly thought that cAMP has an important effect on Ca^{2+} at glucose concentrations at or above 6.5 mM.[135]

Phospholipids, in particular the *myo*-inositol 1,4,5 triphosphate (IP_3), appear to play a significant role on stimulus-secretion coupling in β cells,[149] although the mechanism is not yet completely understood. IP_3 likely mobilizes Ca^{2+} directly from the endoplasmic reticulum (ER), and a second product of the action of phospholipase C on phosphatidylinositol biphosphate, diacylglycerol (DAG), is involved in stimulus-secretion coupling by stimulating protein kinase C (PKC) (Fig. 2.5). (In pituitary PKC phosphorylated peptides are involved in the excoytosis of secretory granules of hormones such as TSH.)

There is evidence that glucagon-like peptide-1 (GLP-1) (proglucagon 78 to 107) is a potent stimulator of insulin secretion.[150] This seems to be due to induction of depolarization of the β cell membrane through a closure of specific K^+ channels, and the effect of protein kinase A (PKA) on the Ca^{2+} mobilization from the ER (Fig. 2.5).

Artificial β Cells. One alternative to islet transplantation for diabetes therapy is to genetically engineer insulin-secreting artificial β cells. Newgard and coworkers have attempted to create an artificial β cell from the anterior pituitary cell line AtT20.[120,121,151,153] A stable transfectant of AtT20 cells with the GLUT-2 cDNA confers on these cells the ability to secrete insulin in response to glucose. A major current drawback of this system is that maximal insulin secretion occurred at subphysiological glucose concentrations. One potential explanation is that although AtT20 cells express the glucose phosphorylating enzyme GK, the hexokinase:GK ratio is greater in these cells than in islets. Further studies are under way to genetically manipulate the hexokinase:GK ratio in AtT20 cells in order to elevate the K_m for glucose-stimulated insulin secretion closer to the physiological range. The general strategy to address this issue, shown in Fig. 2.6, uses recombinant adenovirus[23,152,153] to transfer genes necessary to enhance the glucokinase activity. Over the past few years significant progress has been made in the area of cellular engineering and gene therapy strategies in an attempt to create glucose-stimulated insulin secretion in cell lines that might serve as artificial islets for insulin replacement in IDDM. It is of importance that RIN1046-38 cells overexpress human insulin and can secrete approximately half as much as freshly isolated rat islets (S. Ferber, S. Clark, H. Constandy, C.B. Newgard, unpublished observations). If the adverse immunological responses of grafting engineered cell lines are overcome, gene therapy could be a potential candidate for the treatment of syndromes of β cell dysfunction.

The GABA System in Pancreatic β Cells

Pancreatic islets contain high concentrations of γ aminobutyric acid (GABA), glutamic acid decarboxylase (GAD), and GABA transaminase. The latter two enzymes are responsible for GABA synthesis and metabolism (Fig. 2.7). It is noteworthy that the enzyme GAD is an autoantigen related to insulin-dependent diabetes mellitus. Within islets GABA, GAD and GABA transaminase are found in β, and possibly in α-cells (from human but not

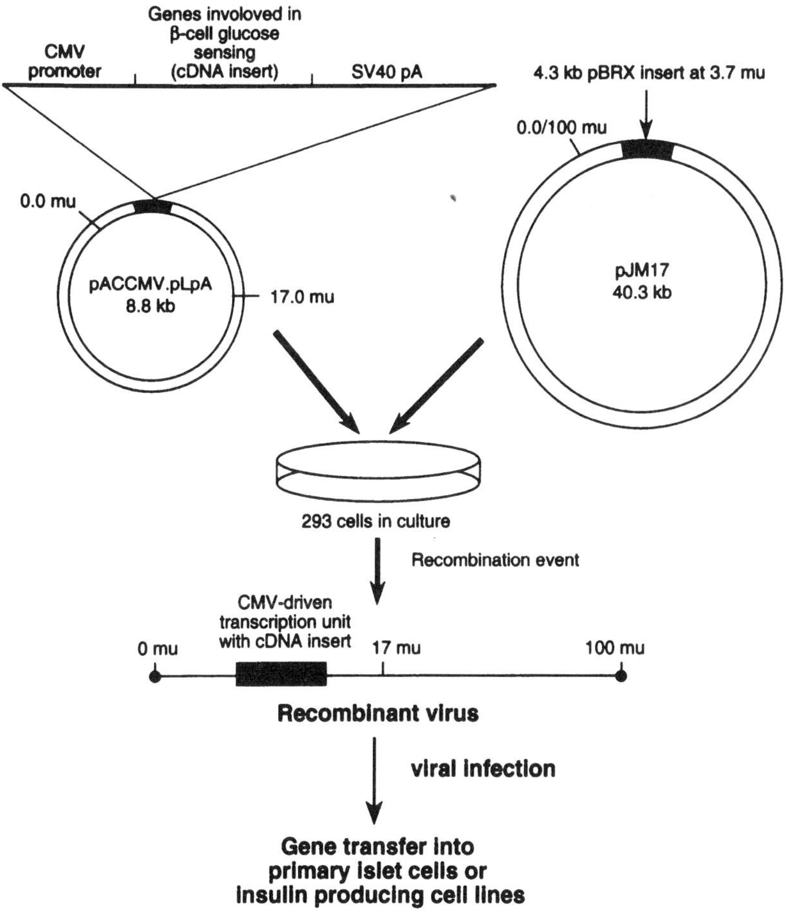

Figure 2.6. Preparation of recombinant adenoviruses. Genes involved in glucose-stimulated insulin release, such as glucokinase or GLUT-2, are cloned into the pACCMV.pLpA vector adjacent to the CMV promoter. The pAC plasmid is then cotransfected with plasmid pJM17 into 293 cells. pJM17 consists of the adenovirus genome interrupted by a fragment of pBR that prevents production of wild-type virus because the size of the plasmid exceeds the packaging limit. Recombination of the plasmids produces virions that are infectious but replication-defective, because of deletion of the adenovirus E1A gene from the pACCMV.pLpA plasmid. The recombinant adenovirus is then amplified and maintained, and provides a highly efficient vehicle for gene transfer into islet cells or insulin-secreting cell lines. (From Newgard CB, *Diabetes*, 43:341–350, 1994.)

rat islets). Immunocytochemical findings have indicated that GAD is contained in β-cell synaptic-like microvesicles (SLMVs).[38,154] Two distinct genes encode for GAD_{65} and GAD_{67}[155], both of which are expressed in nervous system and in β-cells. Only GAD_{65} appears to interact with membranes both in neurons and pancreatic β-cells. This interaction is thought

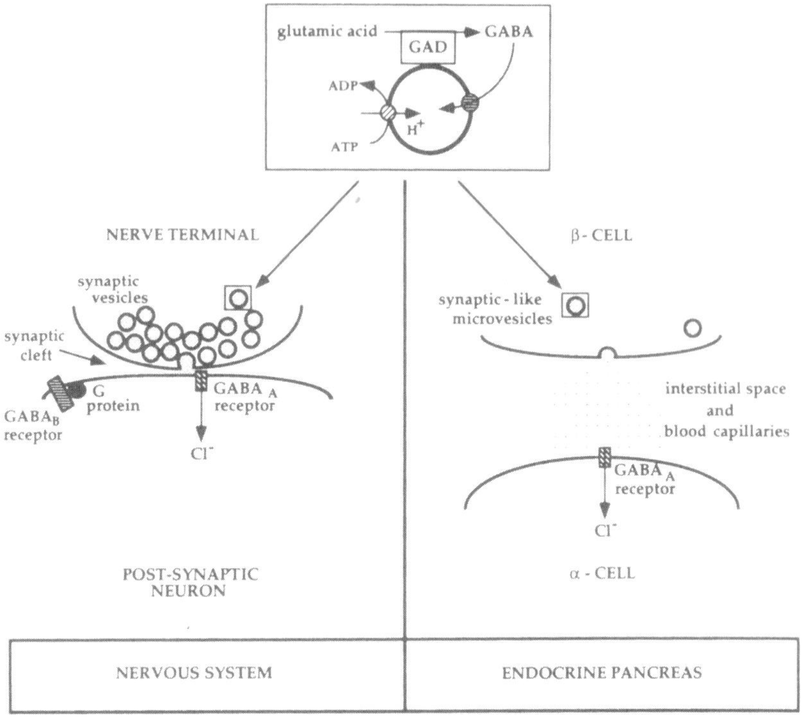

Figure 2.7. Schematic representation of the components of the GABA system in neurons and pancreatic α and β cells. (From De Camilli et al., *FASEB J*, 8:209–216, 1994.)

to be mediated by the NH_2-terminal domain, which is the only region where GAD65 and GAD67 are not identical.

GABA serves as a paracrine signal molecule in either neurons or pancreatic β-cells[37] (Fig. 2.7). In neurons GABA is secreted into the synaptic cleft and then binds to either $GABA_B$ or $GABA_A$ receptors located on postsynaptic neurons. $GABA_B$ are G protein–linked receptors. $GABA_A$ receptors are GABA-gated chloride channels.[156,157] The interaction of GABA with $GABA_A$ receptors leads to opening of the chloride channels, allowing an influx of chloride ions, and therefore leading to hyperpolarization and inhibition of the target neuron[39] (Fig. 2.7). Immunocytochemical studies carried out in islet cells and islets showed the presence of the β-subunit of the $GABA_A$ receptors in a subpopulation of α and δ cells. The current hypothesis based on electrophysiological studies in α cells[156] is that $GABA_A$ receptors may be involved in the inhibition of glucagon secretion mediated by β-cells. In addition, a modulatory action of GABA on α and δ cells was reported.[39,158]

Therefore, these studies suggest that GABA is secreted from β-cells and regulates the function of the mantle cells of islet of Langerhans by binding to $GABA_A$ receptors on their surface, a hypothesis that partially explains the functional interrelationship between pancreatic islet cells.

Pathology

Insulitis in Humans

Insulitis is an inflammatory infiltrate affecting the islets of Langerhans that is considered to be a characteristic lesion of type I diabetes. However, its exact incidence in humans is somewhat controversial because of the small number of cases reported in the literature due to problems of autolysis of the pancreatic tissue during the interval between death and autopsy.[159]

The relative frequency of lymphocytes, macrophages, and interferon gamma-positive cells has been studied in formalin-fixed pancreata of 12 patients who died of recent-onset type I diabetes and one prediabetic patient who had died of cardiomyopathy.[160] In the 87 islets that were examined, the ratio of lymphocytes to macrophages was 9.7:1, and approximately 40% of lymphocytes were interferon gamma-positives.

One study, in which frozen pancreas from an autopsy was available, circumvented the problem of formalin fixation.[161] The majority of cells in the insulitis lesions were T lymphocytes with a predominance of CD8 over CD4 cells.[159,160] However, the number of macrophages was not conspicuous in this single human case.[161]

Recently, the nucleotide sequence of the T cell infiltrate of islets of two children who died of ketoacidosis revealed identity with $V_{\beta}7$ T cell receptor skewing.[162] This observation led to the speculation that a superantigen may play a role in the pathogenesis of IDDM.

Other histopathological findings in type I diabetes include the aberrant expression of class II, and class I major histocompatibility complex (MHC) by β cells and expression of interferon alpha.[160] Aberrant expression of class II MHC was demonstrated immunohistochemically in insulin-secreting cells in 21 out of 23 patients with recent-onset disease, whereas no such expression was seen on glucagon- or somatostatin-staining cells.[163] A marked degree of hyperexpression of class I MHC on insulin-containing islets from newly diagnosed diabetic patients was observed. Furthermore, it appears that when glucagon- and somatostatin-secreting cells are adjacent to insulin-containing cells they hyperexpress class I MHC, but when they are functionally disrupted from β cells during the late time course of the disease, they cease to hyperexpress class I MHC.[163]

The current hypothesis is that interferon gamma or interferon alpha could possibly cause expression of class I and rarely class II MHC of beta cells in IDDM. (There is some controversy as to the expression of class II molecules; in the BB rat model, such cells are apparently macrophages having engulfed insulin-containing granules.) This hypothesis is consistent with the observation in vitro that a high dose of interferon gamma, alone or in combination with tumor necrosis factor, can induce class II MHC overexpression on normal cultured human β cells.[164] However, aberrant expression of class II MHC was also seen on α cells in vitro, something which is never seen in vivo in diabetes.[165] Recently Stewart and coworkers have reported that transgenic mice induced to produce interferon alpha in beta cells develop type I diabetes.[166] With the finding by Foulis and coworkers of interferon alpha–containing beta cells in islets of new-onset patients,[167] it appears that interferon alpha produced by beta cells may contribute to the disease immunomediated process.

The embryology and molecular biology of beta cells are likely to have an impact on the pathogenesis of type I diabetes in terms of the regulation of expression of key autoantigens. Hanahan and coworkers have demonstrated—utilizing a transgenic mouse model with the SV40 T antigen driven by the insulin promoter—that insulitis develops in transgenic strains of mice with a delayed expression of beta cell T antigen.[76] Thus the timing of expression of islet molecules may influence the development of autoimmunity. It is noteworthy that polymorphisms mapped to the 5′ untranslated region of the insulin gene are associated with type I diabetes risk.[44,176] These polymorphisms associated with variable lengths of tandem repeats apparently are able to influence expression of the insulin gene. In addition, studies from populations of France[80] and the United States[168] (but not an English population studied by Todd and coworkers),[81] indicate that such insulin gene polymorphisms appear to influence diabetes risk only when a "protective" haplotype is inherited from a father and not from a mother. Such sexual dimorphism in transmission of disease risk suggests imprinting of gene function. Insulin gene expression within beta cells is apparently not imprinted, as mutant insulin alleles resulting in hyperproinsulinemia are expressed in a codominant manner. We hypothesize that the insulin gene is expressed during development in extra-islet tissue such as the thymus,[178] and that such expression may induce tolerance to insulin, influence diabetes risk, and be imprinted.

Another manner by which regulation of islet function may determine diabetes risk relates to the ability of exogenous insulin therapy to prevent type I diabetes in animal models and, potentially, in humans. Insulin therapy of an animal, through feedback inhibition of beta cell activity, decreases not only the expression of insulin by beta cells, but a series of other molecules including autoantigens such as GAD.[169,170] Morphologically, the volume of beta cells is markedly reduced in animals with chronically insulin-induced hypoglycemia. For the BB rat model of type I diabetes, induction of hypoglycemia is apparently important for the prevention of insulitis and diabetes.[171] The amounts of insulin utilized in pilot trials of insulin therapy for prevention of type I diabetes do not induce apparent hypoglycemia,[172] and thus are unlikely to suppress beta cell metabolism to the degree associated with the above animal studies. If part of the potential ability of insulin to prevent type I diabetes of man is due to suppression of beta cell function, it probably relates to the differential sensitivity of different beta cells to stimulation by glucose (Fig. 2.1). Thus, one can hypothesize that if initiation of insulitis in a single islet is dependent upon a rare event such as seeding by an anti-islet T cell coming in contact with an actively secreting beta cell, a small change in beta cell activity may have a profound effect on a process that in some individuals requires decades to produce overt diabetes.[173]

References

1. Pearse W. 5-hydroxytryptophan uptake by dog thyroid "C" cells, and its possible significance in polypeptide hormone production. *Nature.* 1966; 211(49):598–600.
2. Henderson JR. Why are the islet of Langerhans? *Lancet.* 1969; 2(618):469–470.
3. Bonner-Weir S, Smith FE. Islet of Langerhans: morphology and its implications. In: *Joslin's Diabetes Mellitus.* Philadelphia: Lea & Febiger; 1994: 15–28.
4. Alpert S, Hanahan D, Teitelman G. Hybrid insulin genes reveal a developmental lineage for pancreatic endocrine cells and imply a relationship with neurons. *Cell.* 1988; 53:295–308.
5. Sundler F, Bottcher G. Islet innervation, with special reference to neuropeptides. In: Samols E, ed, *The Endocrine Pancreas.* New York: Raven Press; 1991:29-52
6. Le Douarin NM. On the origin of pancreatic endocrine cells. *Cell.* 1988;53:169–171.
7. Deltour L, Leduque P, Paldi A, Ripoche MA, DuBois P, Jami J. Polyclonal origin of pancreatic islets in aggregation mouse chimaeras. *Development.* 1991: 112:1115–1121.
8. Pictet R, Rutter WJ. Development of the embryonic pancreas. In: Geiger SR, Greep RO, Astwood EB, eds. *Handbook of Physiology: A Critical Comprehensive Presentation of Physiologic Knowledge and Concepts.* Baltimore: Williams & Wilkins; 1972:25–66.
9. Bonner-Weir S, Baxter LA, Schuppin GT, Smith FE. Two pathways for beta cell regeneration after 90% pancreatectomy. *Diabetes.* 1991; 40:163A.
10. Hellerstrom C, Swenne I, Andersson A. Islet cell replication and diabetes. In: Lefebvre PJ, Pipeleers DJ, eds. *The Pathology of the Endocrine Pancreas in Diabetes.* Heidelberg, FRG:Springer-Verlag; 1988:141–170.
11. Steiner DF, James E. Cellular and molecular biology of the beta cell. *Diabetologia.* 1992; 35 (Suppl 2):S41–S48.
12. Madsen OD, Neilsen JH, Michelsen B, Westermark P, Betscholtze C, Nishi M, Steiner DF. Islet amyloid polypeptide and insulin expression are controlled differently in primary and transformed islet cells. *Mol Endocrinol.* 1991; 5:143–148.
13. Fujii S. Development of pancreatic endocrine cells in the rat fetus. *Arch Histol Jpn.* 1979; 42:467–479.
14. Orci L, Baetens D, Ravazzola M, Stefan Y, Malaisse-Lagae F. Pancreatic polypeptide and glucagon:non-random distribution in pancreatic islets. *Life Sci.* 1976; 19:1811–1816.
15. Williams JA, Goldfine ID. The insulin-pancreatic acinar axis. *Diabetes.* 1985; 34:980–986.
16. Weir GC, Bonner-Weir S. Islets of Langerhans; the puzzle of intraislet intersections and their relevance to diabetes. *J Clin Invest.* 1990; 85:983–987.
17. Meda P, Santos RM, Atwater I. Direct identification of electrophysiologically monitored cells within intact mouse islet of Langerhans. *Diabetes.* 1986; 35:232–236.
18. Eddlestone GT, Goncalves A, Bangham JA, Rojas E. Electrical coupling between cells in islets of Langerhans from mouse. *J Membr Biol.* 1984; 77:1–14.
19. Halban PA, Powers SL, George KL, Bonner-Weir S. Spontaneous reassociation of dispersed adult rat pancreatic islet cells into aggregates with three-dimensional architecture typical of native islets. *Diabetes.* 1987; 36:783–790.
20. Van Schravedijk CFH, Kiekens R, Pipeleers DG. Pancreatic B cell heterogeneity in glucose-induced insulin secretion. *J Biol Chem.* 1992; 267:21344–21348.
21. Schuit F, In't Veld P, Pipeleers D. Glucose stimulates proinsulin biosynthesis by a

dose-dependent recruitment of pancreatic beta cells. *Proc Natl Acad Sci U S A.* 1988; 85:3865–3869.
22. Pipeleers DG. Heterogeneity in pancreatic beta-cell population. *Diabetes.* 1992; 41:777–781.
23. Newgard CB. Cellular engineering and gene therapy strategies for insulin replacement in diabetes. *Diabetes.* 1994; 43:341–350.
24. Pipeleers D, Van De Winkel M. Pancreatic beta-cell possesses defense mechanisms against cell-specific toxicity. *Proc Natl Acad Sci USA.* 1986; 83:5267–5271.
25. Korc M, Sankaran H, Wong KY, William JA, Goldfine ID. Insulin receptors in isolated mouse pancreatic acini. *Biochem Biophys Res Commun.* 1978; 84:293–299.
26. Pandol SJ, Sutliff VE, Jones SW, Charlton CG, O'Donohoe TL, Gardner JD, Jensen RT. Action of natural glucagon on pancreatic acinii: due to contamination by previously undescribed secretagogues. *Am J Physiol.* 1983; 245:G703–G710.
27. Jung G, Louie DS, Owyang C. Pancreatic polypeptide inhibits pancreatic enzyme secretion via cholinergic pathway. *Am J Physiol.* 1987; 253:G706–G710.
28. Taparel D, Susini C, Esteve JP, Diaz J, Cazaubon C, Vaysse N, Ribet A. Somatostatin analogs: correlation of receptor affinity with inhibition of cyclic AMP formation in pancreatic acinar cells. *Peptides.* 1985; 6:109–114.
29. Boden G, Sivitz MC, Owen OE, Essa-Koumar N, Landor JH. Somatostatin suppresses secretin and pancreatic exocrine secretion. *Science.* 1975; 190:163–165.
30. Trimble ER. Pancreatic islet. Acinar relationships. In: Ricordi C, ed. *Pancreatic Islet Cell Transplantation.* Austin, TX: R.G. Landes Co.; 1992:19–25.
31. Bonner-Weir S, Orci L. New perspectives on the microvasculature of the islet of Langerhans in the rat. *Diabetes.* 1982; 31:883—889.
32. Hutton JC. The insulin secretory granule. *Diabetologia.* 1989; 32:271–281.
33. Hutton JC, Hansen F, Peshavaria M. Betagranins: 21 kDa co-secreted peptides of the insulin granule closely related to adrenal medullary chromogranin A. *FEBS Lett.* 1985; 188:336–340.
34. Hutton JC, Davidson HW, Peshavaria M. Proteolytic processing of Chromogranin A in purified insulin granules. Formation of a 20000 dalton fragment (betagranin) by the concerted action of Ca^{2+}-dependent endopeptidase and carboxypeptidase H. *Biochem J.* 1987; 244:457–464.
35. Pietropaolo M, Castano L, Babu S, Buelow R, Kuo YL, Martin S, Martin A, Powers AC, Prochazka M, Naggert J, Leiter EH, Eisenbarth GS. Islet cell autoantigen 69 kDa (ICA 69): molecular cloning and characterization of a novel diabetes associated autoantigen. *J Clin Invest.* 1993; 92:359–371.
36. Ward WK, LaCava EC, Paquette TL, Beard JC, Wallum BJ, Porte D. Disproportionate elevation of immunoreactive proinsulin in type 2 (non-insulin dependent) diabetes mellitus and in experimental insulin resistance. *Diabetologia.* 1987; 30:698–702.
37. Thomas-Reetz Ac, De Camilli P. A role for synaptic vesicles in non-neuronal cells: clues from pancreatic B cells and from chromaffin cells. *FASEB.* 1994; 8:209–216.
38. Reetz A, Solimena M, Matteoli M, Folli F, Takei K, De Camilli P. GABA and pancreatic beta-cells: colocalization of glutamic acid decarboxylase (GAD) and GABA with synaptic-like microvesicles suggests their role in GABA storage and secretion. *EMBO J.* 1991; 10:1275–1284.
39. Thomas-Reetz A, Hell JW, During MJ, Walch-Solimena C, Jahn R, De Camilli P. A gamma-aminobutyric acid transporter driven by a proton pump is present in synaptic-like microvesicles of pancreatic beta cells. *Proc Natl Acad Sci U S A.* 1993; 90:5317–5321.

40. German, MS. Insulin gene structure and regulation. In: Draznin B and LeRoith D, eds. *Molecular Biology of Diabetes.* Totowa, NJ. Humana Press Inc. 1994; 91–117.
41. Steiner DF, Chan SJ, Welsh JM, Kwok SCM. Structure and evolution of the insulin gene. *Annu Rev Genet.* 1985; 19:463–484.
42. Hanahan D. Heritable formation of pancreatic beta-cell tumors, in transgenic mice expressing recombinant insulin/simian virus 40 oncogenes. *Nature.* 1985; 315:115–122.
43. Bell GI, Horita S, Karam JH. A polymorphic locus near the human insulin gene is associated with insulin dependent diabetes mellitus. *Diabetes.* 1983; 33:176–183.
44. Lucassen A, Julier C, Beressi J-P, Boitard C, Froguel P, Lathrop M, Bell JJ. Susceptibility to insulin dependent diabetes mellitus maps to a 4.1 kb segment of DNA spanning the insulin gene and associated VNTR. *Nature Genetics.* 1993; 4:305–310.
45. Owerbach D, Gabbay KH. Localization of a type 1 diabetes susceptibility locus to the variable tandem repeat region flanking the insulin gene. *Diabetes.* 1993; 42:1708–1714.
46. Edlund T, Walker MD, Barr PJ, Rutter WJ. Cell specific expression of the rat insulin gene: evidence for the role of two distinct 5′ flanking elements. *Science.* 1985; 230:912–916.
47. Hwung Y-P, Crowe DT, Wang L-H, Tsai M-J. The COUP transcription factor binds to an upstream promoter element of the rat insulin II gene. *Mol Cell Biol.* 1988; 8:2070–2077.
48. Walker MD, Edlund T, Boulet AM, Rutter WJ. Cell specific expression controlled by the 5′ flanking region of insulin and chymotrypsin genes. *Nature.* 1983; 306:557–561.
49. Boam DSW, Clark AR, Docherty K. Positive and negative regulation of the human insulin gene by multiple trans-acting factors. *J Biol Chem.* 1990; 265:8285–8296.
50. Karlsson O, Edlund T, Moss JB, Rutter WJ, Walker MD. A mutational analysis of the insulin gene transcriptional control region: expression in beta cells is dependent on two related sequences within the enhancer. *Proc Natl Acad Sci USA.* 1987; 84:8819–8823.
51. Ohlsson H, Edlund T. Sequence specific interactions of nuclear factors with the insulin gene enhancer. *Cell.* 1986; 45:35–44.
52. Karlsson O, Walker MD, Rutter WJ, Edlund T. Individual protein-binding domains of the insulin gene enhancer positively activate beta-cell-specific transcription. *Mol Cell Biol.* 1989; 9:823–827.
53. Moss LG, Moss JB, Rutter WJ. Systemic binding analysis of the insulin gene transcription control region: insulin and immunoglobulin enhancers utilize similar transactivators. *Mol Cell Biol.* 1988; 8:2620–2627.
54. Ohlsson H, Karlsson O, Edlund T. A beta cell specific protein binds to two major regulatory sequences of the insulin gene enhancer. *Proc Natl Acad Sci USA.* 1988; 84:8819–8823.
55. Park CW, Walker MD. Subunit structure of cell-specific E Box-binding proteins analyzed by quantitation of electrophoretic mobility shift. *J Biol Chem.* 1992; 267:15642–15649.
56. Clark AR, Docherty K. Cell-specific gene expression in the islets of Langerhans: E boxes and TAAT boxes. *Biochem Soc Trans.* 1993; 21:154–159.
57. Walker MD, Park CW, Rosen A, Aronheim A. A cDNA from a mouse pancreatic beta cell encoding a putative transcription factor of the insulin gene. *Nucleic Acids Res.* 1990; 18:1159–1166.

58. German MS, Blanar MA, Nelson C, Moss LG, Rutter WJ. Two related helix-loop-helix proteins participate in separate cell-specific complexes that bind the insulin enhancer. *Mol Endocrinol.* 1991; 5:292–299.
59. Shieh S-Y, Tsai M-J. Cell-specific and ubiquitous factors are responsible for the enhancer activity of the rat insulin II gene. *J Biol Chem.* 1991; 266:16708–16714.
60. Nelson C, Shen L-P, Meister A, Fodor E, Rutter WJ. Pan: a transcriptional regulator that binds chymotrypsin, insulin, and AP-4 enhancer motifs. *Genes Dev.* 1990; 4:1035–1043.
61. Shibasaki Y, Sakura H, Takaky F, Kasuga M. Insulin enhancer binding proteins has helix-loop-helix structure. *Biochem Biophys Res Commun.* 1990; 170:314–321.
62. Murre C, McCaw PS, Baltimore D. A new DNA binding and dimerization motif in immunoglobin, enhancer binding, daughterless, Myo and myc proteins. *Cell.* 1989; 56:777–783.
63. Karlsson O, Thor S, Norberg T, Ohlsson H, Edlund T. Insulin gene enhancer binding protein Isl-1 is a member of a novel class of proteins containing both a homeo- and a Cys-His domain. *Nature.* 1990; 344:879-882.
64. German MS, Wang J, Chadwick RB, Rutter WJ. Synergistic activation of the insulin gene by a LIM-homeo domain protein and a basic helix-loop-helix protein: building a functional insulin minienhancer complex. *Genes Dev.* 1992; 6:2165–2176.
65. Ohlsson H, Thor S, Edlund T. Novel insulin promoter- and enhancer binding proteins that discriminate between pancreatic alpha and beta cells. *Mol Endocrinol.* 1991; 5:897–904.
66. German MS, Moss LG, Wang J, Rutter WJ. The insulin and islet amyloid polypeptide genes contain similar cell specific promoter elements that bind identical beta-cell nuclear complexes. *Mol Cell Biol.* 1992; 12:1777–1788.
67. Emens LA, Landers DW, Moss LG. Hepatic nuclear factor 1 alpha is expressed in hamster insulinoma line and transactivates the insulin I gene. *Proc Natl Acad Sci USA.* 1992; 89:7300–7304.
68. Whelan J, Poon D, Weil A, Stein R. Pancreatic beta-cell-specific expression of the rat insulin II gene is controlled by a positive and negative cellular transcriptional elements. *Mol Cell Biol.* 1989; 9:3253–3259.
69. Crowe DT, Tsai M-J. Mutagenesis of the rat II 5′ flanking region defines sequences important for expression in HIT cells. *Mol Cell Biol.* 1989; 9:1784–1789.
70. Boam DSW, Docherty K. A tissue specific nuclear factor binds to multiple sites in the insulin-gene enhancer. *Biochem J.* 1989; 264:233–239.
71. Clark AR, Peterson HV, Read ML, Scott V, Michelsen BK, Docherty K. Human insulin gene enhancer binding protein in pancreatic alpha and beta cell lines. *FEBS Lett.* 1993; 329:139–143.
72. Reibel L, Bernard C, Lares L, Jami J, Gabon G. An insulinoma nuclear factor binding tp GGGCCC motifs in human insulin gene. *Nucleic Acids Res.* 1993; 21:1595–1600.
73. Kennedy GC, Rutter WJ. Pur-1, a zinc finger protein that binds to purine-rich sequences, transactivates an insulin promoter in heterologous cells. *Proc Natl Acad Sci USA.* 1992; 89:11498–11502.
74. Nir U, Walker MD, Rutter WJ. Regulation of rat insulin 1 gene expression: evidence for negative regulation in nonpancreatic cells. *Proc Natl Acad Sci USA.* 1986; 83:3180–3184
75. Leshkowitz D, Aronheim A, Walker MD. Insulin producing cells contain a cell

specific repressor activity that functions through multiple E-box sequences. *DNA Cell Biol.* 1992; 11:549–558.

76. Hanahan D. Transgenic mice as probes into complex systems. *Science.* 1990; 246:1265–1275.
77. Fromont-Racine M, Bucchini D, Madsen O, Desbois P, Linde S, Nielsen JH, Saulnier C, Ripoche M, Jami J, Pictet R. Effect of 5′ flanking sequence deletions on expression of the human insulin gene in transgenic mice. *Mol Endocrinol* 1990; 4:669–677.
78. Dandoy-Dron F, Monthioux E, Jami J, Bucchini D. Regulatory regions of rat insulin I gene necessary for expression in transgenic mice. *Nucleic Acids Res.* 1991; 19:4925–4930.
79. German M, Ashcroft K, Docherty K, Edlund H, Edlund T, Goodison S, Imura H, Kennedy G, Madsen o, Melloul D, Moss L, Olson K, Permutt MA, Philippe I, Robertson RP, Rutter WJ, Serup P, Stein R, Steiner D, Tsai MJ, Walker MD. The insulin gene promoter: a simplified nomenclature. *Diabetes.* 1995; 44:1002–1004.
80. Julier C, Hyer RN, Davies J, Merlin F, Soulare P, Briant L, Cathelineau G, Deschamps I, Rotter JI, Froguel P, Boitard C, Bell JI, Lathrop GM. Insulin-IGF2 region on chromosome 11p encodes a gene implicated in HLA-DR4-dependent diabetes susceptibility. *Nature.* 1991; 354:155–159.
81. Bain SC, Prins JB, Hearne CM, Rodrigues NR, Rowe BR, Pritchard LE, Ritchie RJ, Hall JRS, Undlien DE, Ronningen KS, Dunger DB, Barnett AH, Todd JA. Insulin gene region-encoded susceptibility to type I diabetes is not restricted to HLA-DR4-positive individuals. *Nature Genetics.* 1992; 2:212–215.
82. van der Auwera BJ, Heimberg H, Schrevens AF, Van Waeyenberge C, Flament J, Schuit FC. 5′ insulin gene polymorphism confers risk for IDDM independently of HLA class II susceptibility. *Diabetes.* 1993; 42:851–854.
83. DeChiara TM, Robertson EJ, Efstratiadis A. Parental imprinting of the mouse insulin-like growth factor II gene. *Cell.* 1991; 64:849–859.
84. Lang DA, Matthews DR, Peto J, Turner RC. Cyclic oscillations of basal plasma glucose and insulin concentration in human beings. *N Engl J Med.* 1979; 301:1023–1027.
85. Rosario LM, Atwater I, Scott AM. Pulsatile insulin release and electrical activity from single ob/ob mouse islet of Langerhans. *Adv Exp Med Biol.* 1986; 211:413–425.
86. Polonsky KS, Given BD, Hirsch LJ, Tillil H, Shapiro ET, Beebe C, Frank BH, Galloway JA, van Canter E. Abnormal patterns of insulin secretion in non-insulin dependent diabetes mellitus. *N Engl J Med.* 1988; 318:1231–1239.
87. O'Rahilly S, Turner RC, Matthews DR. Impaired pulsatile secretion of insulin in relatives of patients with non insulin-dependent diabetes. *N Engl J Med.* 1988: 318:1225–1230.
88. Porte D Jr, Pupo AA. Insulin response to glucose: evidence for a two-pool system in man. *J Clin Invest.* 1969; 48:2309–2319.
89. Steiner DF, Kemmler W, Tager HS, Rubenstein AH, Lernmark A, Zuhlke H. Proteolytic mechanisms in the biosysnthesis of polypeptide hormones. In: Reich E, et al, eds. *Proteases and Biological Control.* Cold Spr Har Lab 1975; 531–549.
90. Steiner DF, Docherty K, Carroll R. Golgi/granule processing of peptide hormone and neuropeptide precursors (a minireview). *J Cell Biochem.* 1984; 24:121–130.
91. Grodsky GM. A new phase of insulin secretion. How will it contribute to our understanding of B-cell function? *Diabetes.* 1989; 38:673–678.

92. Weigle DS. Pulsatile secretion of fuel-regulatory hormones. *Diabetes.* 1987; 36:764–775.
93. Draznin B, Melmed S, LeRoith D, eds. *Molecular and Cellular Biology of Diabetes Mellitus.* New York: Alan R. Liss, Inc., 1989.
94. Orci L, Ravazzola M, Amherdt M, Madsen O, Vassalli JD, Perrelet A. Direct identification of prohormone conversion site in insulin-secreting cells. *Cell.* 1985; 42:671–681.
95. Permutt MA, Kipnis DM. Insulin biosynthesis: studies of islet polyribosomes. *Proc Natl Acad Sci USA.* 1972: 69:505–509.
96. Orci L. The insulin factory: a tour of the plant surroundings and a visit to the assembly line. *Diabetologia.* 1985; 28:528–546.
97. Rhodes CJ, Alarcon C. What beta-cell defect could lead to hyperproinsulinemia in NIDDM? *Diabetes.* 1994; 43:511–517.
98. Davidson HW, Peshavaria M, Hutton JC. Proteolytic conversion of proinsulin into insulin: identification of a Ca^{2+}-dependent acidic endopeptidase in isolated insulin secretory granules. *Biochem J.* 1987; 246:279–286.
99. Davidson HW, Rhodes CJ, Hutton JC. Intraorganellar Ca^{2+} and pH control proinsulin cleavage in the pancreatic B-cell via two site-specific endopeptidases. *Nature.* 1988; 333:93–96.
100. Steiner DF, Smeekens SP, Ohagi S, Chan SJ. The new enzymology of precursor processing endopeptidases. *J Biol Chem.* 1992; 267:23435–23438.
101. Hutton JC. Subtilisin-like proteinases involved in the activation of proproteins of the secretory pathway of eukaryotic cells. *Curr Opin Cell Biol.* 1991; 2:1131–1142.
102. Lindberg I. The new eukaryotic precursor processing proteinases. *Mol Endocrinol.* 1991; 5:1361–1365.
103. Smeekens SP, Steiner DF. Identification of a human insulinoma cDNA encoding a novel mammalian protein structurally related to the yeast dibasic processing KEX2. *J Biol Chem.* 1990; 265:2997–3000.
104. Seidah NG, Gaspar L, Mion P, Marcinkiewiez M, Mbikay M, Chretien M. cDNA sequence of two distinct pituitary proteins homologous to Kex2 and furin gene products: tissue specific mRNAs encoding candidates for pro-hormone processing proteinases. *DNA Cell Biol.* 1990; 9:415–424.
105. Smeekens SP, Avruch AS, LaMendola J, Chan SJ, Steiner DF. Identification of a cDNA encoding a second putative prohormone convertase related to PC2 in AtT20 cells and islets of Langerhans. *Proc Natl Acad Sci USA.* 1991; 88:340–344.
106. Seidah NG, Marcinkiewiez M, Benjannet S, Gaspar L, Beaubien G, Mattei MG, Lazure C, Mbikay M, Chretien M. Cloning and primary sequence of a mouse candidate convertase PC1 homologous to PC2, furin, and Kex2: distinct chromosomal localisation and messenger RNA distribution in brain and pituitary compared to PC2. *Mol Endocrinol.* 1991; 5:111–122.
107. Bennett DL, Bailyes EM, Neilson E, Guest PC, Rutherford NG, Arden SD, Hutton JC. Identification of the type-II proinsulin processing endopeptidase as PC2, a member of the eukaryotic subtilisin family. *J Biol Chem.* 1992; 267:15229–15236.
108. Bailyes EM, Shennan KIJ, Seal AJ, Smeekens SP, Steiner DF, Hutton JC, Docherty K. A member of the eukaryotic subtilisin family (PC3) has the enzymic properties of the type-I proinsulin-converting endopeptidase. *Biochem J.* 1992; 285:391–394.
109. Smeekens SP, Montag AG, Thomas G, et al. Proinsulin processing by the subtilisin-related proprotein covertases furin, PC2 and PC3. *Proc Natl Acad Sci USA.* 1992; 89:8822–8826.

110. Nielsen DA, Welsh M, Casadaban MJ, Steiner DF. Control of insulin gene expression in pancreatic beta-cells and in an insulin-producing cell line, RIN-5F cells. Effects of glucose and cAMP on the transcription of insulin mRNA. *J Biol Chem.* 1985; 260:13586–13589.
111. Welsh M, Nielsen DA, MacKrell AJ, Steiner DF. Control of insulin gene expression in pancreatic beta-cells and in an insulin-producing cell line, RIN-5F cells. Regulation of insulin mRNA stability. *J Biol Chem.* 1985; 260:13590–13594.
112. Welsh M, Schernberg N, Gilmore R, Steiner DF. Translational control of insulin biosynthesis: evidence for regulation of elongation, initiation and signal-recognition particle-mediated translational arrest by glucose. *Biochem J.* 1986; 235:459–467.
113. Alarcon C, Lincoln B, Rhodes CJ. The biosynthesis of the subtilisin related proprotein covertase PC3, but not that of the PC2 convertase, is regulated by glucose in parallel to proinsulin biosynthesis in rat pancreatic islets. *J Biol Chem.* 1993; 268:4276–4280.
114. Guest PG, Rhodes CJ, Hutton JC. Regulation of the biosynthesis of insulin secretory granule proteins: coordinate translational control is exerted on some but not all granule matrix constituents. *Biochem J.* 1989; 257:431–437.
115. Affholter JA, Fried VA, Roth RA. Human insulin-degrading enzyme shares structural and functional homologies with E. coli protease III. *Science.* 1988; 242:1415–1418.
116. Affholter JA, Casceri MA, Bayne ML, Brange J, Casaretto M, Roth RA. Identification of residues in the insulin molecule important for binding to insulin-degrading enzyme. *Biochemistry.* 1990; 29:7727–7733.
117. Ding L, Becker AB, Suzuki A, Roth RA. Comparison of the enzymatic and biochemical properties of human insulin-degrading enzyme and Escherichia coli protease III. *J Biol Chem.* 1992; 267:2414–2420.
118. Meglasson MD, Matschinsky FM. Pancreatic islet gucose metabolism and regulation of insulin secretion. *Diabetes Metab Rev.* 1986; 2:163–214.
119. Matschinsky FM. Glucokinase as glucose sensor and metabolic signal in pancreatic beta-cells and hepatocytes. *Diabetes.* 1990; 39:647–652.
120. Johnson JH, Newgard CB, Milkburn JL, Lodish HF, Thorens B. The high Km glucose transporter of islets of Langerhans is functionally similar to the low affinity transporter of liver and has identical primary sequence. *J Biol Chem.* 1990; 265:6548–6551.
121. Hughes SD, Quaade C, Milburn JL, Cassidy L, Newgard CB. Expression of normal and novel glucokinase mRNA in anterior pituitary and islet cells. *J Biol Chem.* 1991; 266:4521–4530.
122. Johnson JH, Ogawa A, Chen L, Orci L, Newgard CB. Underexpression of beta-cell high Km glucose transporters in noninsulin-dependent diabetes. *Science.* 1990; 250:546–549.
123. Thorens B, Charron MJ, Lodish HF. Molecular physiology of glucose transporters. *Diabetes Care.* 1990; 13:209–218.
124. Purrello F, Buscema M, Rabuazzo AM, et al. Potential role of glucose transport in the mechanism of glucose-induced insulin release. *Diab Nutr Metab.* 1992; 5(Suppl. 1):9–14.
125. Unger RH. Diabetic hyperglycemia: link to impaired glucose transport in pancreatic beta cells. *Science.* 1991; 251:1200–1205.
126. Ashcroft FM, Harrison DE, Ashcroft SJH. Glucose induces closure of single potassium channels in isolated rat pancreatic beta-cells. *Nature.* 1984; 312:446–448.

127. Pressel DM, Misler S. Role of voltage-dependant ionic currents in coupling glucose stimulation to insulin secretion in canine pancreatic islet B-cells. *J Membr Biol.* 1991; 124:239–253.
128. Rajan AS, Aguillar-Bryan L, Nelson DA, Yaney GC, Hsu WH, Kunze DL, Boyd AE III. Ion channels and insulin secretion. *Diabetes Care.* 1990; 13:340–363.
129. Cook DL, Hales CN. Intracellular ATP directly blocks K^+ channels in pancreatic beta cells. *Nature.* 1984; 311:271–273.
130. Ghosh A, Ronner P, Cheong E, Khalid P, Matschinksky FM. The role of ATP and free ADP in metabolic coupling during fuel-stimulated insulin release from islet beta cells in the isolated perfused pancreas. *J Biol Chem.* 1991; 266:22887–22892.
131. Hellestrom C. Effects on carbohydrates on the oxygen consumption of isolated pancreatic islets in mice. *Endocrinology.* 1967; 81:105–112.
132. Zawalich WS, Dye ES, Rognstad R, Matschinsky FM. On the biochemical nature of triose- and hexose-stimulated insulin secretion. *Endocrinology.* 1978; 103:2027–2034.
133. Arkhammar P, Nilsson T, Rorsman P, Berggren PO. Inhibition of ATP-regulated K^+ channels precedes depolorization-induced increase in cytoplasmic free Ca^{2+} concentration in pancreatic beta cells. *J Biol Chem.* 1987; 262:5448–5454.
134. Arkhammar P, Nilsson T, Berggren PO. Glucose- induced changes in cytoplasmic free Ca^{2+} concentration and the significance for the regulation of insulin release. *Cell Calcium.* 1989; 10:17–27.
135. Koranyi L, Bourney R, Turk J, Mueckler M, Permutt MA. Differential expression of rat pancreatic islet B-cell glucose transporter (GLUT 2), proinsulin and islet amyloid polypeptide genes after prolonged fasting, insulin-induced hypoglycaemia and dexamethasone treatment. *Diabetologia.* 1992; 35:1125–1132.
136. Findlay I, Dunne MJ, Peterson OK. High-conductance K^+ channel in pancreatic islet cells can be activated and inactivated by internal calcium. *J Membr Biol.* 1985; 83:169–175.
137. Hellman B. Calcium transport in pancreatic beta-cells: implications for glucose regulation of insulin release. *Diabetes Metab Rev.* 1986; 2:215–241.
138. Nakhooda AF, Like AA, Chappel CI, Wei CN, Marliss EB. The spontaneously diabetic Wistar rat (the "BB" rat). *Diabetologia.* 1978; 14:199–207.
139. Colle E, Guttmann RD, Seemayer TA, Mechel F. Spontaneous diabetes mellitus syndrome in the rat. *Metabolism.* 1983; 32(suppl 1):54–61.
140. Zawalich WS, Rasmussen H. Control of insulin secretion: a model involving Ca^{2+}, cAMP and diecylglycerol. *Mol Cell Endocrinol* 1990; 70:119–137.
141. Donatsch P, Lowe DA, Richardson BP, Taylor P. The functional significance of sodium channels in rat pancreatic beta cell membranes. *J Physiol.* 1977; 267:357–376.
142. Pressel DM, Misler S. Role of voltage-dependent ionic currents in coupling glucose stimulation to insulin secretion in canine pancreatic beta cells. *J Membr Biol.* 1990; 124:239–253.
143. Misler S, Barnett DW, Gillis KD, Pressel DM. Electrophysiology of stimulus-secretion coupling in human beta cells. *Diabetes.* 1992; 41:1221–1228.
144. Kayano T, Noda M, Flockerzi V, Takahashi H, Numa S. Primary structure of rat brain sodium channel III deduced from the cDNA sequence. *FEBS Lett.* 1988; 228:187–194.
145. Noda M, Ikeda T, Kayano T, Suzuki H, Takeshima H, Kurasaki M, Takahashi H, Numa S. Existence of distinct sodium channel messenger RNAs in rat brain. *Nature.* 1986; 320:188–192.

146. MacDonald MJ. Exclusive proximal signals of beta cells for insulin secretion. *Diabetes.* 1990; 39:1461–1466.
147. Philipson LH, Kusnetsov A, Larson T, Zeng Y, Westernmark G. Human, rodent and canine pancreatic B-cells express a sodium channel alpha1-subunit related to a fetal brain isoform. *Diabetes.* 1993; 42:1372–1377.
148. Charles MA, Laweck J, Pictet R, Grodsky GM. Insulin secretion. Interrelationships of glucose, cylic adenosine 3'5'-monophosphate and calcium. *J Biol Chem.* 1976; 250:6134–6140.
149. Metz SA. Role of phospholipase activation in signal transduction in the pancreatic beta cell. In: Drazin B, Melmed S, LeRoith D, eds. *Molecular and Cellular Biology of Diabetes Mellitus.* New York: Alan R. Liss Inc., 1989:81–92.
150. Schmidt WE, Siegel EG, Creutzfeldt W. Glucagon-like peptide-1 but not glucagon-like peptide-2 stimulates insulin release from isolated rat pancreas islets. *Diabetologia.* 1985; 28:704–707.
151. Moore H-P, Walker MD, Lee F, Kelly RB. Expressing a human proinsulin cDNA in a mouse ACTH-secreting cell. Intracellular storage, proteolytic processing, and secretion on stimulation. *Cell.* 1983; 35:531–538.
152. Becker TC, Noel RJ, Coats WS, Gomez-Foix AM, Alam T, Gerard RD, Newgard CB. Use of recombinant adenovirus for metabolic engineering of mammalian cells. *Meth Cell Biol.* 1994; 43:161–189.
153. Gomez-Foix AM, Coats WS, Baque S, Alam T, Gerard RD, Newgard CB. Adenovirus-mediated transfer of the muscle glycogen phosphorylase gene into hepatocytes confers altered regulation of glycogen metabolism. *J Biol Chem.* 1992; 267:25129–25134.
154. Christgau S, Aanstoot HJ, Schierbeck H, Begley K, Tullin S, Hejnaes K, Baekkeskov S. Membrane anchoring of the autoantigen GAD65 to microvesicles in pancreatic beta-cells by palmitoylation in the NH2-terminal domain. *J Cell Biol.* 1992; 118(2):309–320.
155. Edelhoff S, Grubin CE, Karlsen AE, Alder DA, Foster D, Disteche CM, Lernmark A. Mapping of glutamic acid decarboxylase (GAD) genes. *Genomics.* 1993; 17:93–97.
156. Rorsman P, Berggre P-O, Bokvist K, et al. Glucose-inhibtion of glucagon secretion involves activation of $GABA_A$-receptor choride channels. *Nature.* 1989; 341:41–44.
157. Olsen RW, Tobin A. Molecular biology of $GABA_A$ receptors. *FASEB J.* 1990; 4:1469–1480.
158. Sorenson RL, Garry DG, Brelje TC. Structural and functional considerations of GABA in islet of Langerhans beta-cells and nerves. *Diabetes.* 1991; 40:1365–1374.
159. Foulis AK, McGill M, Farquharson MA. Insulitits in type 1 (insulin-dependent) diabetes mellitus in man. Macrophages, lymphocytes, and interferon-gamma containing cells. *J Pathol.* 1991; 165:97–103, 161.
160. Bottazzo GF, Dean BM, McNally JM, Mackay EH, Swift PGF, Gamble DR. In situ characterization of autoimmune phenomena and expression of HLA molecules in the pancreas in diabetic insulitis. *N Engl J Med.* 1985; 313:353–360.
161. Itoh N, Hanafusa T, Miyazaki A, et al. Mononuclear cell infiltration and its relation to the expression of major histocompatibility complex antigens and adhesion molecules in pancreas biopsy specimens from newly diagnosed insulin-dependent diabetes mellitus patients. *J Clin Invest.* 1993; 92:2313–2322.
162. Conrad B, Weidmann E, Trucco G, Rudert WA, Behboo R, Ricordi C, Rodriguez-

Rilo H, Finegold D, Trucco M. Evidence for superantigen involvement in insulin-dependent diabetes mellitus etiology. *Nature.* 1994; 371:351–355.

163. Foulis AK, Farquharson MA, Hardman R. Aberrant expression of Class II major histocompatibility complex molecules by B cells and hyperexpression of class I major histocompatibility complex molecules by insulin containing islets in type I (insulin-dependent) diabetes mellitus. *Diabetologia.* 1987; 30:333–343.

164. Pujol-Borrell R, Todd I, Doshi M, Bottazzo GH, Sutton R, Gray D, Adolph GR, Feldman M. HLA class II induction in human islet cells by interferon gamma plus tumor necrosis factor of lymphotoxin. *Nature.* 1987; 326:304–306.

165. Bottazzo GF, Pujol-Borrell R, Hanafusa T, Feldman M. Role of aberrant HLA-DR expression and antigen presentation in induction of endocrine autoimmunity. *Lancet.* 1983; 2:1115–1118.

166. Stewart TA, Hultgren B, Huang X, Pitts-Meek S, Hully J, Maclachan NJ. Induction of type I diabetes by interferon-alpha in transgenic mice. *Science.* 1993; 260:1942–1946.

167. Foulis AK, Liddle CN, Farquharson MA, Richmond JA, Weir RS. The histopathology of the pancreas in type I diabetes (insulin-dependent) mellitus: a 25-year review of deaths in patients under 20 years of age in the United Kingdom. *Diabetologia.* 1986; 29:267–274.

168. Pugliese A, Awdeh ZL, Alper CA, Jackson RA, Eisenbarth GS. The paternally inherited insulin gene B allele (1,428 Fok1site) confers protection from insulin-dependent diabetes in families. *J Autoimmunity.* 1994; 7:687–694.

169. Appel MC, Dotta F, O'Neill J, Eisenbarth GS. Beta cell activity regulates the expression of islet antigen determinant. *Diabetologia.* 1989; 32:461A.

170. Aaen K, Rygaard J, Josefsen K, Petersen H, Brogren CH, Horn T, Buschard K. Dependence of antigen expression on functional state of B-cells. *Diabetes.* 1990; 39:697–701.

171. Gottlieb PA, Handler ES, Appel MC, Greiner DL, Mordes JP, Rossinig AA. Insulin treatment prevents diabetes mellitus but not thyroiditis in RT-6-depleted diabetes resistant BB/Wor rats. *Diabetologia.* 1991; 34:296–300.

172. Keller RJ, Eisenbarth GS, Jackson RA. Insulin prophylaxis in individuals at high risk of type I diabetes. *Lancet.* 1993; 341:927–928.

173. Srikanta S, Ganda OP, Soeldner JS, Eisenbarth GS. First degree relatives of patients with type I diabetes mellitus: islet cell antibodies and abnormal insulin secretion. *N Engl J Med.* 1985; 313:461–464.

174. Gittes GK, Rutter WJ. Onset of cell specific gene expression in the developing mouse pancreas. *Proc Natl Acad Sci USA.* 1992; 89:1128–1132.

175. Jolicoer C, Hanahan D, Smith KM. T-cell tolerance toward a transgenic β-cell antigen and transcription of endogenous pancreatic genes in thymus. *Proc Natl Acad Sci USA.* 1994; 91:6707–6711.

176. Bennett ST, Lucassen AM, Gough SCL, Powell EE, Undlien DE, Pritchard LE, Merriman ME, Kawaguchi Y, Dronsfield MJ, Pociot F, Nerup J, Bouzekri N, Cambon-Thomsen A, Ronnigen KS, Barnett AH, Bain SC, Todd JA. Susceptibility to human type I diabetes at *IDDM2* is determined by tandem repeat variation at the insulin gene minisatellite locus. *Nature Genetics.* 1995; 9:284–291.

3

NOD Mouse and BB Rat: Genetics and Immunological Function

Donald Bellgrau
Alberto Pugliese

The ancient Egyptians described diabetes several millennia ago, but the first major breakthrough in the understanding of the physiopathology of the disease came in 1922 with the discovery of insulin by Banting, Macleod, and Best. Because of the problems of performing pathological studies in the human pancreas, the development in the past decade of the two inbred animal models described in this chapter has provided an invaluable tool to investigate the pathogenic mechanisms of diabetes.

The Nonobese Diabetic (NOD) Mouse

The nonobese diabetic mouse is an animal model of diabetes remarkably similar to insulin-dependent diabetes mellitus (IDDM) in man. NOD mice spontaneously develop pancreatic autoimmunity[1–3]; like IDDM patients,[4] they show T cell infiltration of the endocrine pancreas (insulitis), and autoantibodies against β-cell antigens can be demonstrated in their sera preceding diabetes onset.[5–14] As in man, genetic susceptibility appears to be polygenic, with a strong predisposing effect deriving from genes within the major histocompatibility complex (MHC).[15,16] The NOD model differs from human diabetes in that sex influences IDDM incidence, with NOD females developing the disease with a higher frequency (70%) than males (40%).[17]

IDDM incidence is also affected by environmental conditions (being higher in sterile-maintained colonies and conversely reduced by infectious agents).[18,19] The disease can be prevented in several ways, including immunological or genetic manipulations of NOD mice. This allows researchers to investigate the immunogenetic mechanisms underlying the disease in the mouse and to test several experimental preventive approaches before starting clinical trials in humans. In this chapter we will summarize the current available knowledge on the NOD mouse, concentrating on its immunological and genetic features.

Immunology of IDDM in the NOD Mouse

One of the most prominent features of the autoimmune process leading to insulin-dependent diabetes in humans is the inflammatory infiltrate invading the islets of Langerhans. This phenomenon is called insulitis and it can be observed also in the NOD mouse.[1–3] In fact, a periductal and perivascular T cell infiltrate can be histologically demonstrated at 4–6 weeks of age. This particular stage of the process is called perinsulitis and it is followed at 6–8 weeks of age by invasion of the islets and selective β-cell destruction (insulitis). Following insulitis, overt diabetes develops beginning at 3 months of age and within 7 months at least 70% of female NOD mice will be diabetic.[17] Faustman and coworkers[20] reported that NOD mice have a defective antigen presentation associated with a reduced expression of MHC class I molecules on the lymphocyte surface and suggested that these abnormalities may impair the development of self-tolerance. Similarly, Serreze and co-investigators[21] have recently described that NOD mice are characterized by a quantitative defect in generating mature bone marrow myeloid cells and by a deficient expression of MHC class I molecules by macrophages. This should lead to the generation of antigen-presenting cells (APCs) unable to interact with CD8 positive (+) T cells and to activate tolerogenic mechanisms. Since pancreatic β-cells express high constitutive levels of MHC class I antigens and these levels can be increased by interferon gamma (IFN-γ),[21–24] autoreactive CD8+ T cells that were not clonally deleted by class I-deficient APCs will recognize and target MHC class I positive pancreatic cells.[25] Indeed, macrophages appear to be essential in initiating the diabetogenic process because neither diabetes nor insulitis was observed in silica-treated NOD mice (silica is selectively toxic to macrophages).[26] Although the hyperexpression of MHC class I antigens on the pancreatic endocrine (and exocrine) tissue suggests that β-cells are destroyed by CD8+ T cells,[27] disease-transfer experiments have shown that both CD4+ and CD8+ T cells are involved in the autoimmune process.[28–30] It is still controversial whether CD8+ T cells facilitate intra-islet migration of CD4+ T cells and macrophages[27] or instead CD4+ T cells represent the main immunological effector promoting migration of CD8+ T cells into the islets and their subsequent differentiation into killer cells. Recent studies on islet isograft destruction in NOD mice by Wang and coworkers[31] suggest that the autoimmune process is CD4+ and not CD8+ T cell dependent. Moreover, there is evidence that CD4+ T cell clones can induce islet tissue damage in the absence of CD8+ T cells.[32] These findings are in agreement with the hypothesis that the role of CD4+ T cells is recruitment of other cell types that are the final effectors of β-cell destruction.[27,31] According to this model, CD4+ T cells are responsible for islet cell damage by initiating the inflammatory process. Toxic agents such as oxygen-free radicals and cytokines would be the final mediators of the destructive lesion whose specificity derives from the sensitivity of β-cells to radical damage.[31]

Although all NOD mice show insulitis, this is not always followed by diabetes; the disease penetrance is 0.4 for male and 0.7 for female NOD mice.[17] This sex difference may be explained by a suppressive or regulatory effect on the immune system exerted by male androgens.[33] Of interest, pancreatic tissue from mice treated with complete Freund's adjuvant (CFA) who did not become diabetic show a nondestructive insulitic lesion that is qualitatively different from classic destructive insulitis. In nondestructive insulitis, infiltrating T cells seem to preferentially release interleukin-4 (IL-4) and not IFN-γ. This may induce the deviation of the autoimmune response with the preferential recruitment of the Th2 T helper cells rather than Th1. Th2 cells produce more IL-4, IL-5, and IL-10 and may inhibit IFN-γ–producing Th1 cells.[34] This immune deviation could hypothetically downregulate class I expression on the surface of pancreatic islet cells, making β-cells less visible to the immune effectors.[25] A reduced class I expression on islet cells can also be achieved by administration of anti–IFN-γ antibodies.[23]

As in IDDM in humans, antibodies against several islet antigens are associated with diabetes in the NOD mouse. Autoantibodies have been described against insulin[5–8] and their levels correlate with progression to overt diabetes.[6] Of note, insulin autoantibodies cross-react with the retroviral antigen p73.[9] other target molecules include a 65-kd heat shock protein,[13] and 52-kd and 58-kd RINm5F cell-specific membrane proteins.[10–12,35] The 58-kd molecule has been recently identified as peripherin, a filament protein present in neurons and in neuroblastomas. This molecule cross-reacts with MHC class II antigens and it may contribute to defective self-tolerance in the NOD mouse.[12] In general, these antibodies appear to be specific for the NOD mouse and to correlate with the onset of diabetes although fewer studies than in humans are available on their relation with insulitis and β-cell function and predictive power.[14] However, two independent reports have recently suggested a central role for the enzyme glutamic acid decarboxylase (GAD), which is a target autoantigen also in human IDDM.[36] In these studies, autoantibodies and T cell responses against GAD were detected in 4-week-old NOD mice and seem to precede the broadening of the immune response to other target molecules.[37,38]

Genetics of Diabetogenesis in the NOD Mouse

Genetic susceptibility to IDDM appears to be controlled by several genes both in humans and in the NOD mouse. Although a significant portion of

Table 3.1. Diabetogenic Loci in the NOD Mouse

	Locus	*Candidate Genes*	*Mouse Chromosome*	*Human Chromosome*
Idd-1	D17	I-A, I-E, /	17	6
Idd-2	D9Nds6	Thy-1	9	11
Idd-3	D3Nds6	IL-2	3	1 or 4
	D3Nds1	?		
	D3Nds12	GLUT-2?		
Idd-4	D11Nds1	?	11	17
Idd-5	D1Nds6	IL-1r1	1	2
		Lsh/Ity/Bcg		
Idd-6	D6Mit14	Ins-1?	6	11
Idd-7	D7Nds6	?	7	
Idd-8	D14Nds1	?	14	
Idd-9	D4Nds16	?	4	
Idd-10	D3Nds7	?	3	1 or 4
	D3Nds11	?		
	D3Nds8	?		

susceptibility may be linked to the MHC with striking similarity between humans and mice,[15,16] the relatively small contribution of many other genes may be difficult to assess and thus their identification is not an easy task, especially in man. The major current approach to delineating determinants of genetic susceptibility consists of screening the genome with genetic markers such as restriction fragment length polymorphisms (RFLPs) and more abundant locus-specific microsatellites, with the possibility, in the mouse, of improving the analytical power of this method by creating experimental crosses and congenic mouse strains. By following this procedure, it has been suggested that the MHC (Idd-1) and at least nine additional non-MHC loci (Idd-2 through Idd-10, Table 3.1) may contribute to create diabetes susceptibility in the NOD mouse with a polygenic mode of inheritance. None of these loci has a fully recessive inheritance and they all encode partially dominant effects. However, the complex of non-MHC susceptibility genes acts in a fully recessive manner and it is essential for diabetes development.[39–41]

Idd-1 has been located within the mouse MHC on chromosome 17.[15,17] The I-A^{g7} (formerly I-A^{nod}) molecule influences diabetes development, as suggested by studies in transgenic mice,[22,42–44] and the genetic sequence of its first external domain is different from other mouse strains.[45] The NOD I-A corresponds to the DQ-β locus in the human MHC, which is also associated with IDDM in man. Of note, both human DQ and mouse I-A diabetes-associated sequences (DQB1*0302 and I-A^{g7}) carry serine at position 57 of their β-chain instead of the aspartic acid residue conserved on other mouse strains and on other DQB1 alleles conferring low diabetes risk in humans.[16,45] These findings have suggested that this particular residue may influence diabetes susceptibility, but it is likely that other amino acids of DQ or I-A and other MHC loci both in humans and mice may be important. In fact, population studies[46] and experiments in transgenic mice[22,44] have failed to show position 57 alone as a susceptibility factor and supported a significant role for alleles at the DRB1 locus in humans and for the corresponding I-E molecule in mice. The NOD mouse lacks surface expression of the I-E molecule and its expression as a transgene prevents diabetes.[22,42,44] Therefore, Idd-1 may act as a gene complex with at least two susceptibility loci, I-A and I-E.[44] It must be noted that even the combination of the two loci may not be sufficient, because CTS mice share the same class II genes with NOD mice but do not develop diabetes.[47,48] However, CTS MHC is diabetogenic in the presence of an NOD background.[49,50] A recent report suggests that diabetes susceptibility also maps to a region flanked by class I and class III Bat5 loci.[51] This region contains genes (tap1 and tap2) encoding for peptide transporters. These molecules play a major role in the delivery of endogenous peptides into the endoplasmic reticulum, and thus they allow the correct MHC class I assembly and expression on the cell surface.[52] NOD tap genes contain several mutations, and although their relation to diabetes is still controversial, it has been suggested that these mutations may be associated with the deficient class I expression reported for lymphocytes and macrophages.[20,21,53] The same region also harbors the tumor necrosis factor (TNF) gene,[51] and there is a report that administration of human TNF-α suppresses insulitis and diabetes in the NOD mouse, which is normally a low TNF-α producer.[54] In any case, the NOD MHC complex (probably including all the above loci) is essential[17] even if both MHC and non-MHC genes are required for diabetes development as shown by studies with experimental crosses.[55] Although the NOD MHC seems to act in a recessive fashion,[15,17] diabetes has also been reported in crosses heterozygous for the NOD MHC, suggesting that it may actually be dominant with incomplete penetrance.[17,56,57]

Idd-2 (D9Nds6) has been assigned to mouse chromosome 9 and linked to the T lymphocyte marker Thy-1[58,59] although a significant association with diabetes has not been found in other studies.[40]

Originally, Idd-3 was linked to both diabetes and insulitis severity and frequency and mapped to a 48-centimorgan interval on chromosome 3 between the IL-2 and Adh-1 genes (D3Nds6, D3Nds9).[40] Diabetes was observed in approximately 10% of heterozygous mice, suggesting that Idd-3 was not a simple recessive trait. Further studies have shown that susceptibility on chromosome 3 is encoded by at least two distinct loci: one locus (Idd-3) maps to the proximal portion (D3Nds12–D3Nds1 region) and the other one (Idd-10) maps to a distal portion (D3Nds7–D3Nds9 region).[39] Moreover, even within the proximal portion, susceptibility may be associated with more than one locus. One of the candidate genes in this region is the IL-2 gene (D3Nds6), for which the evidence of linkage is dependent on the age of diabetes onset. Of note, studies in transgenic mice (discussed in the next section of this chapter) have shown an important role for IL-2 in the induction of autoimmune diabetes,[60] and there is now evidence that the IL-2 gene of the NOD mouse has a different sequence from that of the B10 control strain.[39] Another potential candidate in this region is the GLUT-2 gene (D3Nds12) coding for a glucose transporter.

Idd-4 (D11Nds1) maps on chromosome 11 and may influence the frequency and severity of insulitis and progression to diabetes.[17,40] In particular, Idd-4 homozygosity determines the age of onset of diabetes and Idd-4, Idd-3, and Idd-2 may accelerate progression to overt diabetes.[39] Similar to what is described for Idd-1 and Idd-3, the penetrance of the Idd-4 NOD allele may be influenced by other genetic and environmental factors.[40]

Idd-5 (D1Nds6) has been localized on chromosome 1 and it is linked to genes encoding the interleukin-1 receptor (IL-1r1) and Lsh/Ity/Bcg.[61] Il-1r1 is a candidate susceptibility gene because IL-1 is involved in T cell activation and its administration in vivo can prevent diabetes.[62] The Lsh/Ity/Bcg gene represents another possible candidate because it influences macrophage activation and the immune response to several organisms, including mycobacteria[63–65] expressing a 65-kd heat shock protein that has been reported to be a target antigen in the NOD mouse.[13] There has been a suggestion that Idd-5 may be represented by a 65-kd heat shock protein gene because in man such a gene maps on chromosome 2 within the region homologous to the mouse one linked to diabetes on chromosome 1.[66] Idd-5 appears to influence the development of insulitis, in particular its early stages (peri-insulitis).[67] Also, Idd-5 seems not to be recessive and it has been suggested that Idd-5, Idd-3, and Idd-4 may act in an additive way with an epistatic component.[61]

Idd-6 (D6Mit14) has not been precisely mapped on chromosome 6 and it is possible that Idd-6 is the one of the two mouse insulin genes (Ins-1).[39] Of note, the insulin gene has been associated with diabetes susceptibility in man.[68–72] Idd-6 may interact with Idd-5 and Idd-8 and influence insulitis.[39]

Little information is available on Idd-7 (D7Nds6), Idd-8 (D7Nds1), and Idd-9 (D7Nds16). Surprisingly, Idd-7 and Idd-8 seem to be protective in homozygosity, suggesting that even for the NOD mouse the diabetes trait is genetically heterogeneous.[39]

Finally, Idd-10 maps to a distal portion (D7Nds7–D3Nds9 region) of chromosome 3.[39] A fully penetrant immunological defect maps to this region being encoded by the high-affinity receptor for immunoglobulin G (IgG), Fc-gammaRI. The Fc-gammaRI NOD allele has 24 single-base differences from control mice with 17 changes in the amino acid sequence of the receptor, which result in a deletion of the cytoplasmic tail and a profound reduction in the turnover of receptor-antibody complexes on the cell surface. This defect may alter some macrophage functions (such as phagocytosis) but the phenotype may not be dominant, because one dose of the wild-type allele in heterozygous mice is sufficient for a normal receptor function and provides protection from diabetes.[41]

Table 3.1 shows the above loci, candidate genes, and the corresponding chromosomal localization in mouse and human.

Transgenic Mouse Models of Type I Diabetes

The development of techniques for the insertion of functional genes into mouse germ lines has become a powerful tool to study the immune system.[73] This technology has been widely applied in diabetes research to investigate the role of several different molecules and immune effectors in the autoimmune process and several colonies of mice expressing different transgenes are now established.[74]

The initial studies were focused on the role of MHC class I and class II antigens in the pathogenesis of diabetes, especially after a report suggesting that aberrant expression of class II molecules could enable pancreatic β-cells to function as antigen-presenting cells and trigger autoimmunity.[75] To test this hypothesis, mice were made transgenic for the class I H-2K^{b} [76] antigen and for the class II molecules I-E$^{\beta}$ [77] and I-A^{d}.[78] Expression of these molecules was targeted to β-cells using the rat insulin promoter. All these experiments resulted in expression of high levels of these molecules in the β-cells and development of severe diabetes. However, there was no evidence of autoimmunity in the pancreas, and the occurrence of diabetes was explained as the result of the disruption of the normal protein synthetic and secretory pathways caused by the hyperproduction of class I or class II molecules in β-cells.[79] This explanation was also supported by the finding that a different colony of transgenic mice designed to express lower levels of class II molecules did not show any sign of autoimmunity or develop diabetes.[80] Moreover, it was shown that I-E transgenic islets require the presence of conventional antigen-presenting cells providing lymphokines and costimulatory signals in order to be destroyed after being transplanted into naive I-E negative recipients.[81] Therefore, studies with transgenic mice have shown that aberrant expression of class I or class II molecules is likely not responsible for initiating the autoimmune process leading to diabetes.

As detailed in the previous paragraph, MHC alleles strongly influence diabetes susceptibility, both in mouse and human, and transgenic mice have provided important evidence that the I-A molecule is essential for diabetes development.[22,42–44] In particular, NOD mice are homozygous for the I-A^{g7} molecule. The NOD I-A β-chain sequence is unique and differs from that of the I-A^{k} molecule found in other mouse strains. Like the corresponding IDDM susceptibility allele DQB1*0302 in man, the I-A of NOD mice carries serine at position 57 of the β-chain instead of the more conserved aspartic acid residue and it has a histidine residue instead of proline at position 56.[16,45] The essential role of I-A^{g7} was confirmed by the finding that diabetes could be prevented in transgenic mice by expressing the I-A^{k} molecule.[42,44] However, studies with mice transgenic for a modified I-A^{k} molecule where position 57 had been mutated to serine by site-directed mutagenesis showed no diabetes, suggesting that position 57 alone may not entirely explain the MHC genetic contribution.[44] The same conclusion was suggested by another study where mice were made transgenic for a modified I-A^{g7}, in which the histidine residue at position 56 was mutated to proline and this transgene prevented diabetes.[22]

Transgenic mice have also demonstrated that other MHC molecules are involved in diabetogenesis. In fact, the NOD mouse lacks surface expression of the I-E molecule. Interestingly, when C57B1/6 mice transgenic for the I-E α-chain were backcrossed to NOD mice, diabetes was not observed in those NOD mice expressing a complete I-E molecule.[22] The mechanisms by which I-E protects from diabetes are not completely understood, but no evidence was found for thymic deletion of autoreactive T cells.[82] The same hypothesis is supported by studies showing that the skewing of the T cell receptor repertoire in transgenic mice does not influence diabetes development.[83] More recent studies have shown that the expression of class I L^d molecules also can reduce diabetes incidence in NOD mice.[44] Moreover, a transgenic NOD mouse expressing a class II I-A^d molecule (together with the endogenous I-A^{g7}) showed reduced incidence of IDDM, and the proposed mechanisms of protection include thymic selection and/or proliferation in the periphery of regulatory T cells.[84]

Transgenic mice have also been used to investigate the role of different immune cell subtypes and effectors in the autoimmune process. Two independent studies have shown that viral infection may trigger pancreatic autoimmunity and lead to β-cell destruction in viral antigen transgenic mice by an anti-viral cytotoxic (CD8+) T cell response.[85,86] Therefore, CD8+ T cells may be involved in β-cell destruction also in spontaneously developing diabetes. In another study, diabetes could be induced also in class II deficient transgenic C57B1/6 mice.[87] Class II deficient mice were obtained by targeted disruption of class II loci and such mice were crossed with transgenic mice carrying the lymphocytic choriomeningitis virus (LCMV) glycoprotein under the control of the rat insulin promoter. The pancreatic expression of the LCMV glycoprotein antigen drove a cytotoxic immune response against β-cells resulting in overt diabetes. These findings suggest that diabetes may develop also in the absence of CD4+ T cells and that CD8+ T cells may not always need T helper cells to mount an autoimmune response.[88]

Besides T cells, it is thought that lymphokines also may be important in the autoimmune process and they may even be the final mediators of β-cell destruction.[31] Studies in transgenic mice with sustained IFN-γ expression (targeted to β-cells via the human insulin promoter) showed that IFN-γ overexpression (either directly or indirectly by recruiting and activating immune effector cells) was sufficient to mediate pancreatic destruction.[78] The role of interleukin-2 (IL-2) has also been studied in triple transgenics expressing IL-2, the class I Rip-K^b antigen, and a K^b specific T cell receptor (TCR) in the pancreatic β-cells.[60] Interestingly, the presence of IL-2 was associated with the induction of autoimmune diabetes. The infiltrating T cells were predominantly CD8+, expressing also the K^b TCR and the IL-2 receptor (IL-2R). This study suggested that induction of autoimmunity by CD8+ T cells may be dependent on IL-2 and this lymphokine could be supplied by CD4+ T cells or even produced by CD8+ T cells if affinity for the target antigen is high.[88]

Prevention of Diabetes in the NOD Mouse

The NOD mouse is a good model for testing the feasibility of experimental therapies in the attempt to prevent the disease. Diabetes onset can be prevented in the NOD mouse in several ways by immunological or genetic manipulation.

Among aspecific immunological therapies, the treatment with complete Freund's adjuvant,[89] nicotinamide,[90] corticosteroids and antioxidants,[91] or monoclonal antibodies against different T cell subsets[92,93] have proven to be effective in preventing diabetes or at least have modified the natural course of the disease. However, several of these therapies are not very effective in man and their important side effects pose serious concerns on their safety.

More specific immunological approaches of potential application in man include T cell or peptide vaccination. For T cell vaccination, T cells are primed with a specific antigen epitope, attenuated by gamma-irradiation, and inoculated into mice. A T cell vaccine specific for a 65-kd heat shock protein (HSP65) was reported to be effective in preventing diabetes in the NOD mouse by Elias and coworkers.[94] The same HSP65 peptide used to prime T cells prevented diabetes when administered in incomplete Freund's adjuvant.[94]

Among other antigen-specific therapies, insulin administration was recently shown to prevent diabetes both when administered orally[95] or subcutaneously.[96] Also, the administration of bacillus Calmette-Guérin (BCG) vaccine prevents diabetes in the NOD mouse.[97] These encouraging results have led to the planning of preventive trials with oral insulin or BCG vaccination soon to begin in man. Meanwhile, a randomized insulin trial with subcutaneous insulin has already shown positive effects.[98]

Recent studies in the Bio Breeding (BB) rat have shown that diabetes can also be prevented by inducing tolerance to pancreatic islets by their intrathymic transplantation.[99] Similar experiments in newborn NOD mice have also shown a dramatic reduction in diabetes incidence,[100] and recently intrathymic injection of GAD has been shown to prevent diabetes in NOD mice and was associated with reduced T cell responses to GAD.[37,38]

The recent development of more refined gene manipulation techniques has not only made it possible to evaluate the contribution of individual genes to the disease,[22,42] but it has also provided tools for experimental gene therapy. In particular, transgenic NOD mice can be used to study the potential or protective genes and their mechanism of action. For instance, interesting experiments by Nishimura and coworkers[101] have shown that the human diabetes-protective HLA-DQw6 antigen can be introduced as a transgene into the mouse and function properly as a class II molecule. Although this approach has failed to prevent diabetes in the NOD mouse,[102] several aspects need to be worked out before the inefficacy of such protective gene transfers can be demonstrated. In this particular model, human class II molecules may not find in the NOD immune system other accessory molecules or factors essential to their proper and complete function. If these obstacles can be overcome, the

NOD mouse will also allow find testing of potential gene therapy in human type I diabetes.

The Bio Breeding (BB) Rat

The first inbred animal model for spontaneous, insulin-dependent diabetes mellitus (IDDM) evolved from the discovery of diabetic animals in an outbred colony of Wistar rats maintained at the Bio Breeding Research Laboratories in Ottawa, Canada. Selective breeding led to the first paper on the Bio Breeding (BB) rat[103] wherein the clinical description of insulin-dependent diabetes was documented. Prevention of diabetes with antiserum to rat lymphocytes[104] suggested an autoimmune pathogenesis for disease. Further support for this hypothesis was provided by studies describing the linkage of the disease with the major histocompatibility complex (MHC).[105] The disease is now known to have a polygenic basis for susceptibility[106] and abnormalities in T cell function have been described.[107,108] In this section we will focus on the genetics and immune status of the BB rat, with a special emphasis on the relationship between T cell function and disease susceptibility.

Derivation of BB Rats

All BB rat colonies worldwide were derived from a progenitor stock in Ottawa. As there was considerable genetic heterogeneity in the original Ottawa stock, inbreeding at other locations has predictably led to genetically distinct but related, inbred BB rat lines. In a recent study of 11 different BB rat colonies describing over 20 different BB sublines,[109] inbred lines could be classified as belonging to one of four groups, distinguished by eight protein markers from at least three linkage groups. Selected for sensitivity or resistance to diabetes, BB rats can be further subdivided into diabetes prone (BB-DP) or diabetes resistant (BB-DR).[110] As described later, the BB-DR subline progeny are designated by their ability to develop diabetes following experimental manipulations that do not induce diabetes in other animals.

Genetic Susceptibility Loci

Three genetic loci have been implicated in the pathogenesis of diabetes in the BB rat: the MHC, as mentioned; a gene responsible for the development of a severe T cell lymphopenia, assigned to chromosome 4[62] (Fig. 3.1); and at least one other yet to be identified locus.

Linkage to the MHC was first defined by Colle and coworkers[105] in an analysis of diabetes incidence among F2 animals from a cross of BB-DP with Lewis strain animals. Lewis animals are not prone to diabetes and are incompatible with the BB-DP at the MHC. All diabetic F2 animals were shown to be homozygous for the BB-DP MHC.

One of the most pronounced T cell abnormalities in the BB-DP is a severe

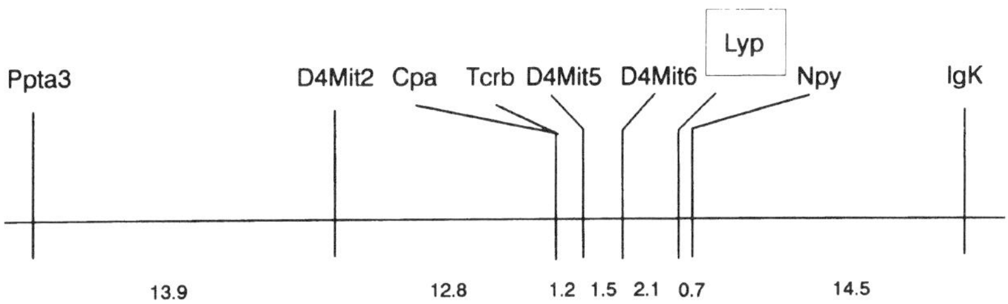

Figure 3.1. Schematic representation of the lymphopenia gene (Lyp) on chromosome 4 in the BB rat. (Modified from Jacob et al., *Nature Genetics*, 2:56–60, 1992.)

lymphocytopenia, first described by Jackson and coworkers,[111] measured in absolute terms by as much as an 80% reduction in T cell numbers. While earlier reports suggested that nonlymphopenic BB animals could develop spontaneous disease,[112] more recent studies indicate an absolute requirement for the lymphopenia gene, when other environmental factors are considered.[113] In an analysis of BB-DP×BB-DRF2 animals, it was concluded that the only diabetes susceptibility gene that was not shared by BB-DP and BB-DR was lymphopenia, as approximately one in four F2 animals developed diabetes and all the diabetic animals were also lymphopenic.

Homozygosity at the BB-DP MHC and lymphopenia loci was not sufficient for spontaneous disease development when the BB-DP was crossed with the diabetes-resistant strain Fischer rat. Although it was concluded that lymphopenia was required for disease, a third locus was proposed.[62] Its location and function are not known. A subline of lymphopenic BB DP has also been reported to be disease free. Whether this is due to heterozygosity at this third locus or is due to some other genetic factor has not been determined.[114]

Immune Dysfunction and Its Relationship to the Major Histocompatibility Complex

Type I diabetes is a T cell–dependent disease.[115] Antibody depletion studies indicate that T cells are both necessary[116] and sufficient for disease[117] but the way in which T cells contribute to disease is not yet understood. T cells have a predilection for antigens coded for by the MHC. They are MHC restricted[118]; ie, they do not respond to antigen unless it is presented in association with MHC antigens presented by antigen-presenting cells. T cells also respond in unusually high frequency to allogeneic MHC antigens from genetically distinct members of the same species.[119] The most likely explanation for MHC restriction and high frequency alloreactivity is that the T cell receptor repertoire is selected on the basis of reactivity to the MHC antigens presented in the host thymus where the maturing thymocytes develop.[120,121] Thus the dual specificity of T cells for antigen and MHC can be in part explained on this basis. The T cell repertoire is selected for reactivity to self MHC (MHC restriction) and these receptors bear significant cross-reactive potential for closely related MHC antigens of the species (high-frequency alloreactivity).

Both the class I[122] and class II[123] MHC antigens are dimeric molecules with antigen-binding clefts. Short peptides from 9 to 14 amino acids in length are bound in these clefts. In the absence of an external source of antigen, the MHC molecules are most probably occupied with self peptides. The dominant presenters of external antigen presented to the immune system are class II MHC molecules. Therefore, one obvious explanation for the mapping of a diabetes susceptibility trait to the class II MHC locus is that certain class II molecules are more effective in presenting self peptides that can induce the activation of T cells with self-reactive potential. The recent crystallographic analysis of the structure of MHC class II molecules[123] indicates a dimerization of MHC class II heterodimers with an orientation that could allow simultaneous interactions with two T cell receptor complexes. It is conceivable that the MHC class II association with disease could involve the facility with which dimer pairs are formed either spontaneously or following TCR engagement, possibly by influencing in a quantitative fashion the nature of the T cell signaling.[124]

Because the major targets for autoimmune diabetes are islet β-cells that express little or no class II MHC antigens, it may be that class II MHC restricted autoreactive T cells do not destroy class II negative β-cells directly but perform their effector role either through the production of cytotoxic cytokines or through the activation of macrophages or natural killers that go on to destroy the β-cells (Lafferty, Chapter 13). An alternative explanation is that the genetic mapping to the class II locus does not necessarily indicate the involvement of the class II genes. Genes controlling processing and presentation of class I–associated antigens map to the class II region of the MHC. Suggestive evidence for their potential involvement in diabetes has been described for the NOD mouse[20] and is discussed in the section devoted to the NOD mouse.

Immune Dysfunction and Its Relationship to Lymphopenia

Lymphopenia was first defined in 1981 by Jackson and colleagues.[111] An early important characteristic distinguishing lymphopenic from nonlymphopenic animals was the absence of the RT6+ subset of peripheral T cells.[125,126] The underrepresentation of the CD45R+ T cell subset isoform was also documented.[127] The absence of RT6+CD45R+ T cells correlated well with the overall reduction in the numbers of peripheral t cells found in the BB-DP. Since thymocytes are both RT6−[125] and 98% CD45R−[128] a plausible role of the lymphopenia gene is to retard T cell maturation to a stage prior to the expression of these peripheral T cell antigens. Combined with the conclusion that the autoreactive potential may exist in all animals, regardless of sensitivity to autoimmune disease,[129] one way in which retarded T cell maturation might influence autoreactivity is through a failure in the maturation of regulatory T cells. However, it seems unlikely that the association of RT6 with lymphopenia indicates that a defect in RT6 gene transcription is the cause of the lymphopenia, as the BB-DP RT6 allele is expressed in F1's between BB-DP and other diabetes-resistant strains expressing the other RT6 allele.[130] This demonstrates that the gene is intact. Further, more recent analyses indicate significant RT6 expression on BB-DP intraepithelial lymphocytes[131] as well as low-level RT6 expression by BB-DP T cells.[132] Taken together these results indicate that the RT6 phenotype leading to a paucity in RT6 positive T cells is due to the impact of the lymphopenia on the capacity of BB-DP T cells to mature to the point where RT6 would normally be significantly expressed. This would also provide an explanation for the relative absence of CD45R+ peripheral T cells.

Another T cell phenotype unique to the BB-DP that appears to segregate with the lymphopenia gene is short T cell lifespan. Within 2 weeks of adult thymectomy, BB-DP peripheral T cell numbers are dramatically reduced.[129] Similar reductions do not occur following thymectomy of diabetes-resistant animals. Perhaps the short lifespan is another indicator of immaturity brought on by the lymphopenia gene's influence on T cell maturation. Adult thymectomy protects against disease,[133] indicating that the effector population involved in β-cell destruction may also be short lived.

Additional Susceptibility Loci

Although lymphopenia is a requirement for spontaneous disease in the BB-DP rat, nonlymphopenic BB-DR animals can be induced to develop disease. this was first shown by depleting BB-DR animals of RT6+ T cells,[134] thus implicating RT6 expression in disease pathogenesis. More recent analyses designed to understand the basis of spontaneous disease observed in some BB-DR animals indicated that Kilham rat virus (KRV) was the inducing agent in the nonlymphopenic BB-DR line[135] and that depletion of RT6 positive T cells could only enhance this inductive effect.[133] The way in which KRV induces diabetes in the BB-DR is unknown but it is not due to direct tropism for islet β-cells and most probably involves activation of T lymphocytes. Poly IC, a polyclonal activator of T cells, also induces diabetes in the BB-DR.[136] Ironically, KRV infection of BB-DR animals protects against the development of spontaneous disease.[135] The inductive effects of KRV or poly IC appear to be effective only when BB-DR animals are 25–35 days of age. Thus an age-related effect may be involved in disease pathogenesis.

One of the more paradoxical observations in the pathogenesis of diabetes in the BB-DP rat is the association between weak T cell–mediated responses and diabetes propensity. BB-DP T cells respond poorly to cell-bound antigen assessed by weak proliferative[107] and cytotoxic[137] responses to alloantigen. Improved proliferative responses correlate both directly and indirectly with disease protection.[138,139] BB-DR T cells proliferate normally to alloantigen[140] and their adoptive transfer to BB-DP animals protects the recipient from disease.[141] Other experimental procedures associated with improved T cell responsiveness are also protective, including bone marrow[142] and thymus transplantation.[140,143]

While the poor cytotoxicity can be attributed to a near absolute absence of CD8+ T cells, with the remaining CD8+ T cells expressing abnormally low levels of CD8,[144,145] CD4+ T cells appear phenotypically normal. The majority of the proliferative response to alloantigen in the rat has been attributed to the CD4+ subset.[146] The poor BB-DP proliferative response is not due to a generalized defect in proliferation, as BB-DP T cells appear to respond normally to nonspecific stimulation with the T cell mitogen ConA[107] and are also responsive to antibody-mediated stimulation via the T cell receptor.[147] Recent data indicate, however, that signaling via CD4 may be abnormal compared with CD4-mediated signaling in CD4+ T cells from normal donors.[147]

Transplantation of thymus grafts from diabetes-resistant semisyngeneic fetal donors into adult thymectomized BB-DP animals is protective as long as the thymus contains diabetes-resistant thymic macrophages or dendritic cells.[143] The thymic cortex also appears abnormal.[148] The protective effect does not appear to be due to chimerism by the carryover of donor diabetes-resistant thymocytes, is not associated with a reversal of lymphopenia, which was shown not to be influenced by thymus transplantation,[149] and may indicate a role for antigen-presenting cells in influencing the nature of the diabetes-prone T cell repertoire. Whether the recently described low-level expression of class I MHC on NOD macrophages[21] and a suggested defect in human APC function[20,150] are related to this observation requires further study.

Possible Related Mechanisms of Disease

In a comparative analysis of what is known about human versus NOD mouse and BB rat IDDM, the most pronounced difference is the NOD disease bias for females. No sex preference has been observed for BB rat and human disease. The BB rat differs from both mouse and human in the absolute requirement for lymphopenia, which has not been associated with disease in either the mouse or human models. NOD and BB models also may both involve abnormal T cell function and age-related effects that are less clearly defined in humans. Protection from disease in both NOD and BB models can be attributed to thymic antigen presenting cells, and adoptive transfer of disease in both models favors both young recipients and a requirement for both CD4+ and CD8+ T cells. In both models protection can also be gained through treatment with complete Freund's adjuvant or deliberate viral infection. Intensive insulin therapy is also protective.[151] Therefore, even though the only absolute genetic susceptibility locus shared by all three models is class II region of the MHC, it seems likely that all three share a common etiology that can be influenced by various genetic factors. Although several exciting explanations for the way in which the MHC influences disease susceptibility have been presented, the mechanism of MHC involvement remains unknown. It is likely that the commonality of the MHC involvement in all animal models studies thus far is an important key to our understanding of IDDM etiology. The insights gained from the recently solved structure of the MHC class II molecule and the way in which peptides are produced and presented to MHC molecules will be of almost certain value in unraveling the mysteries of this T cell–dependent disease.

References

1. Makino S, Kunimoto D, Muraoka Y, Mizushima Y, Katagiri K, Tochino Y. Breeding of a non-obese, diabetic strain of mice. *Exp Anim* (Tokyo). 1980; 29:1.
2. Kanazawa Y, Komeda K, Sato S, Mori S, Akanuma K, Takaku F. Non-obese-diabetic mice: immune mechanisms of pancreatic B-cell destruction. *Diabetologia.* 1984; 27:113–115.
3. Maruyama T, Takei M, Kataoka K, Matsuki S. Immunological aspect of non-obese diabetic mice: immune islet cell-killing mechanism and cell-mediated immunity. *Diabetologia.* 1984; 27:121–1233.
4. Foulis AK, Liddle CN, Farquharson MA, Richmond JA, Weir RS. The histopathology of the pancreas in type I (insulin dependent) diabetes mellitus: a 25-year review of deaths in patients under 20 years of age in the United Kingdom. *Diabetologia.* 1986; 29:267–274.
5. Maruyama T, Takei I, Yanagawa T, et al. Insulin autoantibodies in non-obese diabetic (NOD) mice and streptozotocin induced diabetic mice. *Diabetes Res.* 1988; 7:93–96.
6. Ziegler AG, Vardi P, Ricker AT, Hattori M, Soeldner JS, Eisenbarth GS. Radioassay determination of insulin autoantibodies in NOD mice: correlation with increased risk of progression to overt diabetes. *Diabetes.* 1989; 38:3358–363.
7. Boitard C, Bach JF. Insulin autoantibodies in non-obese diabetic (NOD) mice. *Clin Exp Immunol.* 1989; 75:457–460.
8. Reddy S, Bibby N, Elliott RB. Longitudinal study of islet cell antibodies and insulin autoantibodies and development of diabetes in non-obese diabetic (NOD) mice. *Clin Exp Immunol.* 1990; 81:400–405.
9. Serreze DV, Leiter EH, Kuff EL, Jardieu P, Ishizaka K. Molecular mimicry between insulin and retroviral antigen p73. Development of cross reactive autoantibodies in sera of NOD and C57BL/KsJ db/db mice. *Diabetes.* 199; 37:351–358.
10. Karounos DG, Thomas JW. Recognition of common islet antigen by autoantibodies from NOD mice and humans with IDDM. *Diabetes.* 1990; 39:1085–1090.
11. Villa M-C, Becourt C, Gia HP, et al. Autoantibodies against pancreatic beta-cells: Characterization by Western blot analysis in the non-obese diabetic (NOD) mouse. *J Autoimmunity.* 1992; 5:47–58.
12. Boitard C, Villa MC, Becourt C, et al. Peripherin: an islet antigen that is cross-reactive with nonobese diabetic mouse class II gene products. *Proc Natl Acad Sci U S A.* 1992; 89:172–176.
13. Elias D, Markovits D, Reshef T, Zee R, Cohen IR. Induction and therapy of autoimmune diabetes in the non-obese diabetic (NOD/Lt) mouse by a 65-kDa heat shock protein. *Proc Natl Acad Sci U S A.* 1990; 87:1576–1580.
14. Reddy S, Liu W, Thompson JM, Bibby NJ, Elliott RB. First phase insulin release in the non-obese diabetic mouse: correlation with insulitis, beta cell number and autoantibodies. *Diabetes Res Clin Pract.* 1992; 17:17–25.

15. Hattori M, Buse JB, Jackson RA, et al. The NOD mouse: recessive diabetogenic gene within the major histocompatibility complex. *Science.* 1986; 231:733–735.
16. Todd JA, Bell JI, McDevitt HO. HLA-DQ beta gene contribution to susceptibility and resistance to insulin dependent diabetes mellitus. *Nature.* 1987; 329:599–604.
17. Wicker LS, Miller BJ, Coker LZ, et al. Genetic control of diabetes and insulitis in the nonobese diabetic (NOD) mouse. *J Exp Med.* 1987; 165:1639–1654.
18. Oldstone MBA. Prevention of type I diabetes in nonobese diabetic mice by virus infection. *Science.* 1988; 239:500–502.
19. Wilberz S, Partke HJ, Dagnaes-Hansen F, Herberg L. Persistent MHV (mouse hepatitis virus) infection reduces the incidence of diabetes mellitus in non-obese diabetic mice. *Diabetologia.* 1991; 34:2–5.
20. Faustman D, Li XX, Lin HY, et al. Linkage of faulty major histocompatibility complex class I to autoimmune diabetes. *Science.* 1991; 254:1756–1761.
21. Serreze DV, Gaskins HR, Leiter EH. Defects in the differentiation and function of antigen presenting cells in NOD/Lt mice. *J Immunol.* 1993; 150:2534–2543.
22. Lund T, O'Reilly L, Hutchings P, et al. Prevention of insulin-dependent mellitus in non-obese diabetic mice by transgenes encoding modified I-A beta chain or normal I-E alpha chain. *Nature.* 1990; 345:727–729.
23. Kay TWH, Campbell IL, Oxbrow L, Harrison LC. Overexpression of class I major histocompatibility complex accompanies insulitis in the non-obese diabetic mouse and is prevented by anti-interferon-gamma antibody. *Diabetologia.* 1991; 34:779–785.
24. McInerney MF, Rath S, Janeway CA Jr. Exclusive expression of MHC class II proteins on CD45+ cells in pancreatic islets of NOD mice. *Diabetes.* 1991; 40:648–651.
25. Leiter E, Christianson G, Serreze D, Ting A, Worthen S. MHC antigen induction by interferon gamma on cultured mouse pancreatic B cells and macrophages. Genetic analysis of strain differences and discovery of an "occult" class I-like antigen in NOD/Lt mice. *J Exp Med.* 1989; 170:1243–1262.
26. Ihm S, Yoon J. Studies on autoimmunity for initiation of B-cell destruction. Macrophages essential for development of B-cell-specific cytotoxic effectors and insulitis in NOD mice. *Diabetes.* 1990; 39:1273–1278.
27. Varey AM, Hutchings P, O'Reilly L, et al. The development of insulin-dependent diabetes mellitus in non obese diabetic mice: the role of CD4+ and CD8+ T cells. *Biochem Soc Trans.* 1991; 19:187–19111.
28. Bendelac A, Carnaud C, Boitard C, Bach JF. Syngeneic transfer of autoimmune diabetes from diabetic NOD mice to healthy neonates. Requirement for both L3T4+ and Lyt 2+ T cells. *J Exp Med.* 1987; 166:823–32.
29. Wicker LS, Miller BJ, Mullen Y. Transfer of autoimmune diabetes mellitus with splenocytes from non-obese diabetic (NOD) mice. *Diabetologia.* 1986; 35(8):855–860.
30. Charlton B, Mandel TE. Progression from insulitis to Beta cell destruction in NOD mouse requires L3T4+T-lymphocytes. *Diabetes.* 1988; 37:1108–1112.
31. Wang Y, Ponteselli RG, Gill RG, LaRosa FG, Lafferty KJ. The role of CD4 and CD8 T cells in the destruction of islet grafts by diabetic NOD mice. *Proc Natl Acad Sci USA.* 1991; 88:527–531.
32. Bradley BJ, Haskins K, La Rosa FG, Lafferty KJ. CD8 T cells are not required for islet destruction induced by a CD4+ islet-specific T-cell clone. *Diabetes.* 1992; 41:1603–1608.

33. Makino S, Kunimoto K, Muraoka Y, Katagiri K. Effect of castration on the appearance of diabetes in the NOD mouse. *Jikken Dobutsu.* 1981; 30:137–140.
34. Shehadeh NN, LaRosa F, Lafferty KJ. Altered cytokine activity in adjuvant inhibition of autoimmune diabetes. *J Autoimmun.* 1993; 6:291–300.
35. Boitard C, Pham-Gia H, Becourt C, Bach JF. Cross-reactivity between major histocompatibility complex class II antigens in mice NOD and an islet antigen with 58 kDa molecular weight. *C R Acad Sci [III].* 1989; 309:229–2344.
36. Baekkeskov S, Aanstoot H, Christgau S, et al. Identification of the 64K autoantigen in insulin dependent diabetes as the GABA-synthesizing enzyme glutamic acid decarboxylase. *Nature.* 1990; 347:151–156.
37. Kaufman DL, Clare-Salzler M, Tian J, et al. Spontaneous loss of T-cell tolerance to glutamic acid decarboxylase in murine insulin-dependent diabetes. *Nature.* 1993; 366:69–72.
38. Tisch R, Yang X-D, Singer SM, Liblau RS, Fugger L, McDevitt HO. Immune response to glutamic acid decarboxylase correlates with insulitis in non-obese diabetic mice. *Nature.* 1993; 366:72–75.
39. Ghosh S, Palmer SM, Rodrigues NR, et al. Polygenic control of autoimmune diabetes in nonobese diabetic mice. *Nature Genetics.* 1993; 4:4044–409.
40. Todd JA, Aitman TJ, Cornall RJ, et al. Genetic analysis of autoimmune type I diabetes mellitus in mice. *Nature.* 1991; 351:542–547.
41. Prins JB, Todd JA, Rodrigues NR, et al. Linkage on chromosome 3 of autoimmune diabetes and defective Fc receptor for IgG in NOD mice. *Science.* 1993; 260:694–698.
42. Nishimoto H, Kikutani H, Yamamura K, Kishimoto T. Prevention of autoimmune insulitis by expression of I-E molecules in NOD mice. *Nature.* 1987; 328:432–4344.
43. Uehira M, Uno M, Kurner T, et al. Development of autoimmune insulitis is prevented in E alpha d but not in A beta K NOD transgenic mice. *Int Immunol.* 1989; 1:209–213.
44. Miyazaki T, Uno M, uehira M, et al. Direct evidence for the contribution of the unique I-ANOD to the development of insulitis in non-obese diabetic mice. *Nature.* 1990; 345:722–724.
45. Acha-Orbea H, McDevitt HO. The first external domain of the nonobese diabetic mouse class II I-A chain is unique. *Proc Natl Acad Sci U S A.* 1987; 84:2435–2439.
46. Nepom GT, Erlich H. MHC class-II molecules and autoimmunity. *Annu Rev Immunol.* 1991; 9:493–525.
47. Ikegami H, Makino S, Harada M, Eisenbarth GS, Hattori M. The CTS mouse, a sister strain of the NOD: similar class II but different class I gene products. *Diabetologia.* 1988; 31:254–258.
48. Ikegami H, Eisenbarth GS, Hattori M. Major histocompatibility complex-linked diabetogenic gene of the NOD mouse: analysis of genomic DNA amplified by polymerase chain reaction. *J Clin Invest.* 1990; 85:18–24.
49. Ikegami H, Makino S, Hattori M. Genetic analysis of the non-obese (NOD) mouise. In: Tsuchiya M, Nagura H, Hibi T, Moro I, eds. *Frontiers of Mucosal Immunology.* Amsterdam, New York, Oxford: Excerpta Medica; 1991: 429–432.
50. Ikegami H, Makino S. Genetic susceptibility to insulin-dependent diabetes mellitus: from NOD mice to humans. In: Shafrir E, ed. *Lessons from Animal Diabetes IV.* 4th ed. Great Britain: Smith-Gordon; 1993:39–50.
51. Ikegami H, Kawaguchi Y, Ueda H, et al. MHC-linked diabetogenic gene of the

NOD mouse: molecular mapping of the 3′ boundary of the diabetogenic region. *Biochem Biophys Res Commun.* 1993; 192:677–682.

52. Monaco JJ. A molecular model of MHC class-I-restricted antigen processing. *Immunol Today.* 1992; 13:173–179.
53. Gaskins HR, Monaco JJ, Leiter EH. Expression of intra-MHC transporter (Ham) genes and class I antigens in diabetes-susceptible NOD mice. *Science.* 1992; 256:1826–1828.
54. Satoh J, Seino H, Abo T, et al. Recombinant human tumor necrosis factor alpha suppresses autoimmune diabetes in nonobese diabetic mice. *J Clin Invest.* 1989; 84:1345–1348.
55. Hattori M, Fukuda M, Ichizawa T, Baumgartl HJ, Katoh H, Makino S. A single recessive non-MHC diabetogenic gene determines the development of insulitis in the presence of an MHC-linked diabetogenic gene in NOD mice. *J Autoimmun.* 1990; 3:1–10.
56. Livingstone A, Edwards CT, Shizura JA, Fathman JA. Genetic analysis of diabetes in the nonobese diabetic mouse. I. MHC and T cell receptor beta gene expression. *J Immunol.* 1991; 146:529–5344.
57. Wicker LS, Miller BJ, Fischer PA, Pressey A, Peterson LB. Genetic control of diabetes and insulitis in the nonobese diabetic mouse: pedigree analysis of a diabetic H-2nod/b heterozygote. *J Immunol.* 1989; 142:781–784.
58. Ikegami H, Jackson RA, Makino S, Watt DE, Eisenbarth GS, Hattori M. Homozygosity for two genes (H-2:chromosome 17 and Thy-1: chromosome 9) linked to development of type I diabetes of the NOD mouse. *Clin Res.* 1986; 34:683A. Abstract.
59. Prochazka M, Leiter EH, Serreze DV, Coleman DL. Three recessive loci required for insulin-dependent diabetes in nonobese diabetic mice. *Science.* 1987; 237:286–289.
60. Heath WR, Allison J, Hoffmann MW, Schonrich G, Arnold B, Miller JF. Autoimmune diabetes as a consequence of locally produced interleukin-2. *Nature.* 1992; 359:547–549.
61. Cornall RJ, Prins JB, Todd JA, et al. Type I diabetes in mice is linked to the interleukin-1 receptor and Lsh/Ity/Bcg genes on chromosome 1. *Nature.* 1991; 353:262–265.
62. Jacob HJ, Pettersson A, Wilson D, Mao Y, Lernmark A, Lander ES. Genetic dissection of autoimmune type I diabetes in the BB rat. *Nature Genetics.* 1992; 2:56–60.
63. Blackwell JM, Roach TI, Atkinson SE, Ajioka JW, Barton CH, Shaw MA. Genetic regulation of macrophage priming activation: the LSH gene story. *Immunol Lett.* 1991; 30(2):241–248.
64. Schurr E, Malo D, Radzioch D, et al. Genetic control of innate resistance to mycobacterial infections. *Immunol Today.* 1991; 12:42–45.
65. Skamene E, Gros P, Forget A, Kongshawn PA, St Charles C, Taylor BA. Genetic regulation of resistance to intracellular pathogens. *Nature.* 1982; 297:506–509.
66. Bowen-Jones D, Fantes J, Gupta R. Diabetes and heat shock protein. *Nature.* 1992; 355:119–120.
67. Garchon HJ, Bedossa P, Eloy L, Bach JF. Identification and mapping to chromosome 1 of a susceptibility locus for periinsulitis in non-obese diabetic mice. *Nature.* 1991; 353:260–262.
68. Julier C, Hyer RN, Davies J, et al. Insulin-IGF2 region encodes a gene implicated in HLA-DR4-dependent diabetes susceptibility. *Nature.* 1991; 354:155–159.

69. Bain SC, Prins JB, Hearne CM, et al. Insulin gene region-encoded susceptibility to type I diabetes is not restricted to HLA-DR4-positive individuals. *Nature Genetics.* 1992; 2:212–215.
70. Lucassen A, Julier C, Beressi J-P, et al. Susceptibility to insulin dependent diabetes mellitus maps to a 4.1 kb segment of DNA spanning the insulin gene and associated VNTR. *Nature Genetics.* 1993; 4:305–310.
71. Van der Auwera BJ, Heimberg H, Schrevens F, Van Waeyenberge C, Flament J, Schuit FC. 5′ insulin gene polymorphism confers risks to IDDM independently of HLA class II susceptibility. *Diabetes.* 1993; 42:851–854.
72. Pugliese A, Bain SC, Todd JA, Awdeh ZL, Alper CA, Eisenbarth GS. INS polymorphisms on chromosome 11 in type 1 diabetes. *Autoimmunity.* 1993; 15 (Suppl):32. Abstract.
73. Hanahan D. Transgenic mice as probes into complex systems. *Science.* 1990; 246:1265–1275.
74. Lipes M, Eisenbarth GS. Transgenic mouse models of type I diabetes. *Diabetes.* 1990; 39:879–884.
75. Bottazzo GF, Pujol-Borrell R, Hanafusa T, Feldmann M. Role of aberrant HLA-DR expression and antigen presentation in induction of endocrine autoimmunity. *Lancet.* 1983; 2:1115–1118.
76. Allison J, Campbell IL, Morahan G, Mandel TE, Harrison LC, Miller JFAP. Diabetes in transgenic mice resulting from over-expression of class I histocompatibility molecules in pancreatic B-cells. *Nature.* 1988; 333:529–533.
77. Lo D, Burkly LC, Widera G, et al. Diabetes and tolerance in transgenic mice expressing class II MHC molecules in pancreatic beta cells. *Cell.* 1988; 53:159–168.
78. Sarvetnick N, Liggitt D, Pitts SL, Hansen SE, Stewart TA. Insulin-dependent diabetes mellitus induced in transgenic mice by ectopic expression of class II MHC and interferon-gamma. *Cell.* 1988; 52:773–782.
79. Parham P. Intolerable secretion in tolerant transgenic mice. *Nature.* 1988; 333:500–503.
80. Bohme J, Haskins K, Stecha P, et al. Transgenic mice with I-A on islet cells are normoglycemic but immunologically intolerant. *Science.* 1989; 244:1179–1183.
81. Markmann J, Lo D, Naji A, Palmiter RD, Brinster RD, Heber-Katz E. Antigen presenting function of class II MHC-expressing pancreatic beta cells. *Nature.* 1988; 336:476–479.
82. Bohme J, Schuhbaur B, Kanagawa O, Benoist C, Mathis D. MHC-linked protection from diabetes dissociated from clonal deletion of T cells. *Science.* 1990; 249:293–295.
83. Lipes MA, Rosenzweig A, Tan KN, et al. Progression to diabetes in nonobese diabetic (NOD) mice with transgenic T cell receptors. *Science.* 1993; 259:1165–1169.
84. Singer SM, Tisch R, Yang XD, McDevitt HO. An Abd transgene prevents diabetes in nonobese diabetic mice by inducing regulatory T cells. *Proc Natl Acad Sci USA.* 1993; 90:9566–9570.
85. Ohashi P, Oehen SH, Buerki K, et al. Ablation of "tolerance" and induction of diabetes by virus infection in viral antigen transgenic mice. *Cell.* 1991; 65:305–317.
86. Oldstone M, Nerenberg M, Southern P, Price J, Lewicki H. Virus infection triggers insulin-dependent diabetes mellitus in a transgenic model: role of anti-self (virus) immune response. *Cell.* 1991; 65:319–331.

87. Laufer TM, von Herrath MG, Grusby MJ, Oldstone MBA, Glimcher LH. Autoimmune diabetes can be induced in transgenic major histocompatibility complex class II-deficient mice. *J Exp Med.* 1993; 178:589–596.
88. Miller JFAP, Heath WR. Self-ignorance in the peripheral T-cell pool. *Immunol Rev.* 1993:133.
89. McInerney Fagan M, Pek Belbez S, Thomas DW. Prevention of insulitis and diabetes onset by treatment with complete Freund's adjuvant in NOD mice. *Diabetes.* 1991; 40:715–725.
90. Reddy S, Bibby NJ, Elliott RB. Early nicotinamide treatment in the NOD mouse: effects on diabetes and insulitis suppression and autoantibody levels. *Diabetes Res.* 1990; 15:95–102.
91. Rabinovitch A, Suarez WL, Power RF. Combination therapy with an antioxidant and a corticosteroid prevents autoimmune diabetes in NOD mice. *Life Sci.* 1992; 51:1937–1943.
92. Hutchings P, O'Reilly L, Parish NM, Waldmann H, Cooke A. The use of a non-depleting anti-CD4 monoclonal antibody to re-establish tolerance to B-cells in NOD mice. *Eur J Immunol.* 1992; 22:1913–1918.
93. Kurasawa K, Sakamoto A, Maeda T, et al. Short-term administration of anti-LsT4 MoAb prevents diametes in NOD mice. *Clin Exp Immunol.* 1993; 39:376–380.
94. Elias D, Reshef T, Birk OS, Zee R, Walker MD, Cohen IR. Vaccination against autoimmune mouse diabetes with a T-cell epitope of the human 65-kDa heat shock protein. *Proc Natl Acad Sci USA.* 1991; 88:3088–3091.
95. Zhang JZ, Davidson L, Eisenbarth GS, Weiner HL. Suppression of diabetes in nonobese diabetic mice by oral administration of porcine insulin. *Proc Natl Acad Sci USA.* 1991; 88:10252–10256.
96. Yang H, Rotter JI, Toyoda H, et al. Ulcerative colitis: a genetically heterogeneous disorder defined by genetic (HLA class II) and subclinical (antineutrophil cytoplasmic antibodies) markers. *J Clin Invest.* 1993; 92:1080–1084.
97. Guytingco R, Quddus J, Richardson B, Pek SB. Single administration of bacillus Calmette-Guerin (BCG) vaccine in nonobese diabetic (NOD) mice results in suppression of in vitro T-lymphocyte proliferation and regression of insulitis. *Diabetes.* 1991; 40:152A. Abstract.
98. Keller RJ, Eisenbarth GS, Jackson RA. Insulin prophylaxis in individuals at high risk of type I diabetes. *Lancet.* 1993; 341:927–928.
99. Posselt AM, Barker CF, Tomaszewski JE, Markmann JF, Choti MA, Naji A. Induction of donor-specific unresponsiveness by intrathymic islet transplantation. *Science.* 1990; 249:1293–1295.
100. Nomura Y, Stein E, Mullen Y. Suppression of diabetes incidence by intrathymic islet isografting in newborn NOD mice. *Transplant Proc.* 1994; 24:2903.
101. Nishimura Y, Iwanaga T, Inamitsu T, et al. Expression of the human MHC, HLA-DQw6 genes alters the immune response in C57BL/6 mice. *J Immunol.* 1990; 145:353–360.
102. Fukui Y, Nishimura Y, Iwanga T, et al. Glycosuria and insulitis in NOD mice expressing the HLA-DQw6 molecule. *J Immunogenet.* 1989; 16:445–453.
103. Nakhooda AF, Like AA, Chappel CI, Murray FT, Marliss EB. The spontaneously diabetic Wistar rat: metabolic and morphologic studies. *Diabetes.* 1976; 26:100–112.
104. Like AA, Rossini AA, Gubreski DK, Appel MC, Williams RM. Spontaneous diabetes mellitus: reversal and prevention in the BB/W rat with antiserum to rat lymphocytes. *Science.* 1979; 206:1421–1423.

105. Colle E, Guttmann RD, Seemayer T. Spontaneous diabetes mellitus syndrome in the rat. I. Association with the major histocompatibility complex. *J Exp Med.* 1981; 154:1237–1242.
106. Guttmannn RD, Colle E, Michel E, Seemayer T. Spontaneous diabetes mellitus syndrome in the rat. II. T lymphopenia and its association with clinical disease and pancreatic lymphocytic infiltration. *J Immunol.* 1983; 130:1731–1735.
107. Bellgrau D, Naji A, Silvers WK, Markmann JF, Barker CF. Spontaneous diabetes in BB rats: evidence for a T cell dependent immune response defect. *Diabetologia.* 1982; 23:359–364.
108. Elder M, Maclaren N. Identification of a profound peripheral T lymphocyte immunodeficiency in the spontaneously diabetic BB rat. *J Immunol.* 1983; 130:1723–1731.
109. Prins JB, Herberg L, Den Bieman M, van Zupthen LF. Genetic variation within and between lines of diabetes-prone and non-diabetes-prone BB rats; allele distribution of 8 protein markers. *Lab Anim.* 1991; 25:207–211.
110. Butler L, Guberski D, Like A. Changes in penetrance and onset of spontaneous diabetes in the BB/Wor rat. In: Shafrir E, ed. *Frontier in Diabetes Research II. Lessons from Animal Diabetes III.* Great Britain: Smith-Gordon, 1990:50–53.
111. Jackson R, Rassi N, Crump A, Haynes BF, Eisenbarth GS. The BB diabetic rat: profound T cell lymphocytopenia. *Diabetes.* 1981; 30:887–889.
112. Like AA, Biron DA, Weringer EJ, Byman K, Sroczynski E, Guberski DL. Prevention of diabetes in BioBreeding/Worcester rats with monoclonal antibodies that recognize T lymphocytes or natural killer cells. *J Exp Med.* 1986; 164(4):1145–1159.
113. Markholst H, Eastman S, Wilson D, Andreasen BE, Lernmark A. Diabetes segregates as a single locus in crosses between inbred BB rats prone or resistant to diabetes. *J Exp Med.* 1991; 174:297–300.
114. Joseph S, Diamond AG, Smith W, Baird JD, Butcher GW. BB-DR/Edinburgh: a lymphopenic, non-diabetic subline of BB-rats. *Immunology.* 1993; 78:318–328.
115. Like AA, Kislauskis E, Williams RM, Rossini AA. Neonatal thymectomy prevents spontaneous diabetes mellitus in the BB rat. *Science.* 1982; 216:644–646.
116. Like AA, Buergski DL, Butler L. Diabetic BioBreeding/Worcester (BB/W) rats need to be lymphopenic. *J Immunol.* 1986; 136:3254–3258.
117. Edouard P, Hiserodt JC, Plamondon C, Poussier P. CD8+ T cells are required for adoptive transfer of the BB rat diabetic syndrome. *Diabetes.* 1993; 42:390–397.
118. Zinkernagel RM, Doherty PC. Restriction of in vitro T cell-mediated cytotoxicity in lymphocytic choriomeningitis within a syngeneic or semiallogenic system. *Nature.* 1974; 248:701–702.
119. Wilson DB. Quantitative studies on the mixed lymphocyte interaction in rats. Conditions and parameters of response. *J Exp Med.* 1967; 126:625–654.
120. Zinkernagel RM, Callahan GN, Althage A, Cooper S, Klein PA, Klein J. On the thymus in the differentiation of "H-2 self-recognition" by T cells; evidence for dual recognition. *J Exp Med.* 1978; 147:882–896.
121. Kisielow P, Teh HS, Bluthman H, von Boehmer H. Positive selection of antigen-specific T cells in thymus by restricting MHC molecules. *Nature.* 1988; 335:730–733.
122. Bjorkman PJ, Saper MA, Samraoui B, Bennett WS, Strominger JL, Wiley DC. The foreign antigen binding site and T cell recognition regions of class I histocompatibility antigens. *Nature.* 1987; 329:512–518.

123. Brown JH, Jardetzky TS, Gorga JC, et al. Three-dimensional structure of the human class II histocompatibility antigen HLA-DR1. *Nature.* 1993; 364:33–39.
124. Ploegh H, Benaroch P. MHC class II dimer of dimers. *Nature.* 1993; 364:16.
125. Ely JM, Greiner DL, Lubaroff DM, Fitch FW. Characterization of monoclonal antibodies that define rat T cell alloantigens. *J Immunol.* 1983; 130:2798–2803.
126. Greiner DL, Handler ES, Nakano K, Mordes JP, Rossini AA. Absence of the RT-6 T cell subset in diabetes-prone BB/W rats. *J Immunol.* 1986; 136:148–151.
127. Groen H, Van Der Berk J, Nieuwenhuis P, Kampinga J. Peripheral T cells in diabetes prone (DP) BB rats are CD45R-negative. *Thymus.* 1989; 14:145–150.
128. Spickett GP, Brandon MR, Mason DW, Williams AF, Woollett GR. MRC OX-22, a monoclonal antibody that labels a new subset of T lymphocytes and reacts with the high molecular weight form of the leukocyte-common antigen. *J Exp Med.* 1983; 158:795–810.
129. McKeever U, Mordes JP, Greiner DL, et al. Adoptive transfer of autoimmune diabetes and thyroiditis to athymic rats. *Proc Natl Acad Sci USA.* 1990; 87:7618–7622.
130. Angelillo M, Grenier DL, Mordes JP, et al. Absence of RT6+ T cells in diabetes prone BioBreeding/Worcester rats is due to genetic and cell development defects. *J Immunol.* 1988; 141:4146–4151.
131. Fangmann J, Schwinzer R, Hedrich H-J, Klotinh I, Wonigeti K. Diabetes-prone BB rats express the RT6 alloantigen on intestinal intraepithelial lymphocytes. *Eur J Immunol.* 1991; 21:2011–2015.
132. Crisa L, Sarkar P, Waite DJ, et al. An RT6 gene is transcribed and translated in lymphopenic diabetes prone BB rats. *Diabetes.* 1993: 42:688–695.
133. Like AA. Depletion of RT6.1+ lymphocytes alone is insufficient to induce diabetes in diabetes-resistant BB/WOR rats. *Am J Pathol.* 1990; 136:5655–574.
134. Greiner DL, Mordes JP, Handler ES, Angelillo M, Nakamura N, Rossini AA. Depletion of RT6.1+ T lymphocytes induces diabetes in resistant biobreeding/Worcester (BB/W) rats. *J Exp Med.* 1987; 166:461–475.
135. Guberski DL, Thomas VA, SSshek WR, et al. Induction of type 1 diabetes by Kilham's rat virus in diabetes-resistant BB/Wor rats. *Science.* 1991; 254:1010–1013.
136. Ewel CH, Sobel DO, Zeligs BJ, Bellanti JA. Poly I:C accelerates development of diabetes mellitus in diabetes-prone BB rat. *Diabetes.* 1992; 41:1016–1021.
137. Woda BA, Like AA, Padden C, McFadden ML. Deficiency of phenotypic cytotoxic-suppressor T lymphocytes in the BB/W rat. *J Immunol.* 1986; 136:856–859.
138. Naji A, Silvers WK, Kimura H, Bellgrau D, Markmann JF, Barker CF. Analytical and functional studies on the T cells of untreated and immunologically tolerant diabetes-prone BB rats. *J Immunol.* 1983; 130:2168–2172.
139. Markmann JF, Naji A, Barker CF, Brayman KL. Immunomodulation of prediabetes in BB rats for prevention of the disease. *Adv Exp Med Biol.* 1988; 246:357–364.
140. Georgiou HM, Lagarde AC, Bellgrau D. T cell dysfunction in the diabetes-prone BB rat: a role for thymic migrants that are not T cell precursors. *J Exp Med.* 1988; 167:132–148.
141. Rossini AA, Mordes JP, Pelletier AM, Like AA. Transfusions of whole blood prevent spontaneous diabetes mellitus in the BB/W rat. *Science.* 1983; 219:975–977.

142. Naji A, silvers WK, Bellgrau D, Anderson A, Plotkin S, Barker CF. Prevention of diabetes in rats by bone marrow transplantation. *Ann Surg.* 1981; 194:328–338.
143. Georgiou HM, Bellgrau D. Thymus transplantation and disease prevention in the diabetes-prone Biobreeding rat. *J Immunol.* 1989; 142:3400–3405.
144. Bellgrau D, Lagarde A-C. Cytotoxic T-cell precursors with low-level CD8 in the diabetes-prone biobreeding rat: implications for the generation of an autoimmune T-cell repertoire. *Proc Natl Acad Sci USA.* 1990; 87:313–317.
145. Plamondon C, Kottis V, Brideau C, Metroz-Dayer M-D, Poussier P. Abnormal thymocyte maturation in spontaneously diabetic BB rats involves deletions of CD4-CD8+ T cells. *J Immunol.* 1990; 144:923–928.
146. Mason DQ, Arthur RP, Dallman MJ, Green JR, Spickett GP, Thomas ML. Function of rat T lymphocyte subsets isolated by means of monoclonal antibodies. *Immunol Rev.* 1983; 74:57–82.
147. Bellgrau D, Redd JM, Sellins KS. Peculiar T cell signalling does not preclude positive selection in the diabetes prone BB rat. *Diabetes.* 1994; 43:47–52.
148. Rozing J, Coolen C, Tielen FJ, et al. Defects in thymic epithelial stroma of diabetes prone BB rats. *Thymus.* 1989; 14:125–135.
149. Francfort JW, Naji A, Silvers WK, Braker CF. The influence of T-lymphocyte precursor cells and thymus grafts on the cellular immunodeficiencies of the BB rat. *Diabetes.* 1985; 34:1134–1138.
150. Faustman D, Schoenfeld D, Ziegler R. T-lymphocyte changes linked to autoantibodies: association of insulin autoantibodies with CD4+ CD4R+ lymphocyte subpopulation in prediabetic subjects. *Diabetes.* 1991; 40:590–597.
151. Gotfredsen CF, Buschard K, Frandsen EK. Reduction of diabetes incidence of BB Wistar rats by early prophylactic insulin treatment of diabetes prone animals. *Diabetologia.* 1985; 28:933–935.

4

The Role of T Cells in Beta Cell Damage in NOD Mice and Humans

D. Wegmann
D. Daniel
J. D. Peterson
K. Haskins

Advancement of our understanding of the role of autoimmunity in diabetes has been greatly facilitated by the availability of animal models of type I diabetes, most notably spontaneous disease models such as the Bio Breeding (BB) rat and the nonobese diabetic (NOD) mouse. Although investigations using each of these models have provided important information on the pathogenesis of insulin-dependent diabetes mellitus (IDDM), this discussion will be restricted to results obtained from the NOD mouse and the limited data available from human subjects.

The NOD mouse

The NOD mouse was established from a subline of CTS (cataract) mice by selective breeding and monitoring for hyperglycemia and was first described in 1980.[1] It was observed that NOD mice spontaneously developed diabetes as a result of destruction of the pancreatic beta cells. This beta cell destruction in NOD mice was associated with heavy cellular infiltrates that surrounded and invaded individual islets beginning at least 7 weeks prior to the onset of overt diabetes.[2,3] Because this disease process appears to closely parallel that observed in humans, the NOD mouse is considered to be a good model for human type I diabetes.

Histology and Effect of T Cell Depletion on IDDM

Among the first indications that disease in the NOD mouse was comparable to that observed in human type I diabetes were the observations of pronounced cellular infiltration of the islets of Langerhans (insulitis) in these animals. Longitudinal histological investigations have indicated that insulitis is first detectable in some mice as early as 4 to 5 weeks of age, whereas individual female NOD mice begin to exhibit overt diabetes at approximately 12 weeks of age.[1] A number of investigators have performed extensive analyses of insulitis in the NOD mouse, using a variety of detection methods, and have detected the presence of T cells at the early stages of infiltration.[2,3] This suggests that T cells selectively infiltrate the pancreatic islets of NOD mice and are involved in beta cell destruction. However, given that the majority of the infiltrating cells have been found to be B cells,[3] the mere presence of T cells in the insulitis is not proof of the role of T cells in diabetes. More direct evidence for involvement of T cells in development of diabetes has been provided by experiments in which T cells were experimentally depleted. For example, neonatal thymectomy[4] and antibody-mediated depletion of T cells[5] in NOD mice was found to reduce the incidence of diabetes. In addition, it has been established in NOD-nude mice that B cells in the absence of T cells do not induce either insulitis or diabetes.[6] Although the results of the above investigations suggest that T cells are required for development of diabetes in NOD mice, these experiments do not provide direct evidence for participation of T cells in beta cell damage.

Adoptive Transfer of Diabetes by T Cells

Evidence for T cell involvement in the development of diabetes in NOD mice has been provided by experiments that demonstrate adoptive transfer of diabetes from diabetic donors to nondiabetic recipients. The first adoptive transfer experiments involved injection of unfractionated spleen cells obtained from newly diabetic NOD mice into sublethally irradiated NOD recipients.[7] Spleen cells transferred from either diabetic mice or older prediabetic mice could accelerate the development of diabetes in recipient mice. In subsequent investigations it was observed that this adoptive transfer of diabetes from diabetic NOD donors to irradiated recipients by T cells did not require recruitment of host B cells.[8] Fractionation of these diabetogenic T cells into CD4+ and CD8+ populations has shown that both subpopulations of T cells were required for induction of diabetes.[9] Although it was clear in these studies that injection of T cells obtained from diabetic donors precipitated diabetes, it was impossible to rule out contributions from the host immune system. Indeed, although sublethal irradiation of the recipients was required for expression of the diabetogenic capacity of the transferred cells,[7] the dose used (775 cGy) was probably not sufficient to deplete all endogenous lymphocytes.

An alternative adoptive transfer system was devised by Bendelac and coworkers.[10] These investigators used neonates as recipients and found that irradiation was not necessary for adoptive transfer of diabetes in mice up to 3 weeks of age. The advantage of this system over the previous one was that transferred diabetes occurred at an age when unmanipulated littermates would have no detectable islet infiltration. This would presumably lessen the potential for contributions from host lymphocytes that may have already been activated and in the process of destroying beta cells. This system of transfer into neonates exhibited the same lack of requirement of B cells,[8] and requirement for both CD4+ and CD8+ cells,[10] that was seen in earlier transfer studies in irradiated adult mice.

Isolation of Islet-Specific T Cell Clones

Perhaps the most compelling evidence for involvement of T cells in the disease process has been provided by the reports of isolation of islet-specific T cell clones.[11–15] The clones that have been described to date have been obtained using three protocols: (1) T cells derived from spleen and lymph nodes of newly diabetic NOD mice, (2) T cells cultured directly from the islet cell infiltrates of prediabetic mice, and (3) T cells cultured from islet cell isografts placed into newly diabetic NOD mice.

The first report of islet-specific T cell clones was described by Haskins and colleagues and has been the most extensively characterized both in vitro and in vivo.[11,12,16,17] These T cell lines were isolated from the spleen and lymph nodes of newly diabetic NOD mice by in vitro stimulation with NOD islet cells as antigen and irradiated sygeneic spleen cells as a source of antigen-presenting cells (APCs). A panel of islet-specific T cell clones was subsequently obtained, the majority of which respond to islet cells from all mouse strains tested, but only in the context of NOD major histocompatibility complex (MHC) class II, I-A^g.[7] All of the T cell clones are CD4+ and secrete the Th1 cytokines interleukin-2 (IL-2) and interferon gamma (IFN-γ). In vivo, the islet-specific T cell clones mediate islet graft destruction[17,18] and accelerate diabetes in young NOD recipients.[16] Additionally, four of the clones were found to transfer insulitis and diabetes to several non–diabetes-susceptible NOD F1 mice.[19] In both the NOD and NOD F1 mice, efficiency of disease transfer was found to be dependent on the age of the recipient, with the highest rate of success occurring in experiments in which recipients were less than 2 weeks old, suggesting a requirement for immunological immaturity.

A second report of islet-specific T cell clones was provided by Reich and coworkers.[13] These cell lines were isolated from the infiltrated islets of newly diabetic female NOD mice by stimulation with syngeneic islets in the presence of recombinant IL-2, but in the absence of splenic APCs. Thus, the islets were used as a source of both antigen and APCs. Not surprisingly, the clones developed by this method responded to islets in in vitro proliferation assays in

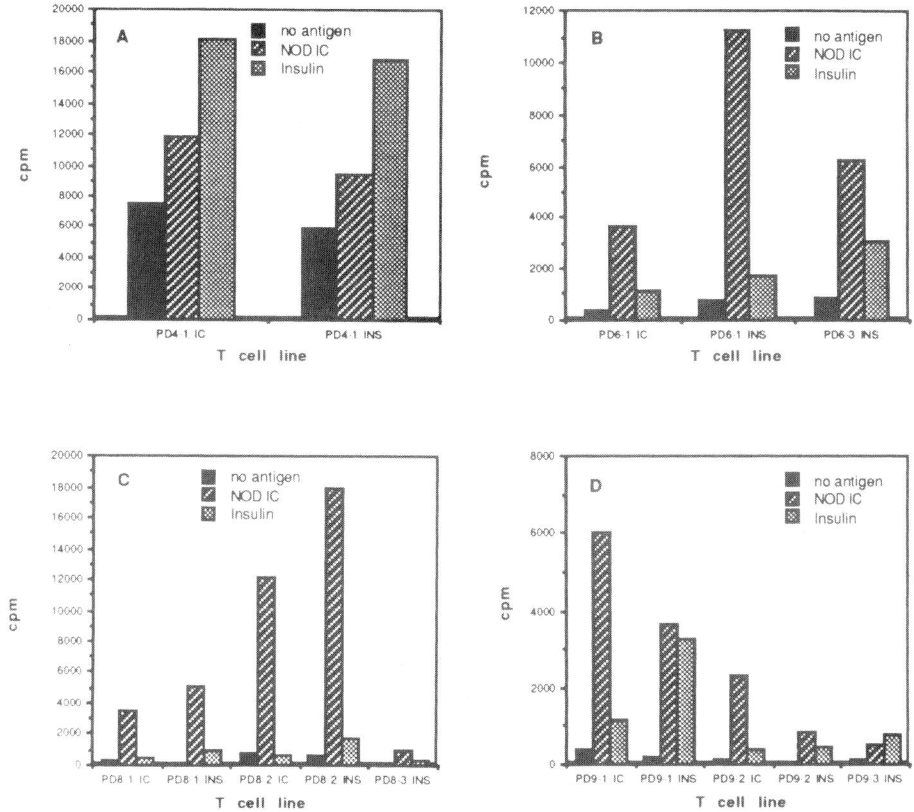

Figure 4.1. Response of islet-specific and insulin-specific T cell lines to either islet cells or insulin. For these experiments, 2.5×10^4 cells from the indicated line were cocultured with 5.0×10^5 irradiated NOD spleen cells and either 100 μg/ml porcine insulin or 1.0×10^4 irradiated NOD islet cells. The cultures were incubated for three days with a pulse of [^{3}H]TdR 6 hours prior to harvest. The lines in panel *A* were established from 4-week-old mice; those in panel *B*, from 6-week-old mice; those in panel *C*, from 8-week-old mice; and those in panel *D*, from 9-week-old mice. The suffix "I" denotes lines that were initiated and propagated using islet cells as antigen. The suffix "INS" denotes lines that were initiated and propagated using porcine insulin as antigen.

the absence of other sources of APCs. These investigators isolated both CD4+ and CD8+ T cells. Adoptive transfer of these T cell clones was performed on sublethally irradiated recipients, and although they did not cause overt diabetes, the clones did mediate extensive insulitis in recipient mice after transfer of a mixture of both CD4+ and CD8+ clones. In addition to islet-specific T cells, some of the clones were defined as "autoreactive" as they proliferated in response to syngeneic splenocytes in the absence of islet cell antigen. In a subsequent report at least one of these autoreactive T cell clones provided some degree of reduction in the incidence of spontaneous diabetes upon adoptive transfer.[20]

Nakano and coworkers[14] isolated T cells from prediabetic NOD mice by culture of infiltrated islets. Over time some of the islet cultures exhibited T cell growth and the resultant T cells were expanded by stimulation with NOD islets as antigen and NOD spleen cells as a source of APCs. All subsequent in vitro propagations were performed using NOD islets and spleen cells and the clones they obtained required both islets and spleen cells for in vitro proliferative responses. These islet-specific T cell clones were all found to be CD4+ and could induce insulitis upon adoptive transfer.

Nagata and Yoon[15] isolated T cells from NOD mice by culturing infiltrated islets in the presence of IL-2 but without added spleen cells as a source of APCs. They obtained both CD4+ and CD8+ T cells by this method and as expected, given that splenic APCs were not used for the isolation, these T cells did not require spleen cells for a response to islets. Of the CD4+ clones tested, four proliferated in vitro to either NOD spleen cells or NOD islet cells while two others responded only to islet cells. The three CD8+ clones responded only to islet cells and were able to mediate direct cytotoxicity of islet cells as determined by ^{51}Cr-release assays.

A different approach for the isolation of islet-specific T cells involved the use of islet isografts placed into spontaneously diabetic mice to recruit islet-specific T cells. The infiltrated graft tissue was subsequently removed and cultured with irradiated NOD islet cells, irradiated syngeneic spleen cells, and IL-2.[21] The kinetics and tissue specificity of the graft rejection implied that the transplanted islet tissue was eliciting a population of "memory" islet-specific T cells that presumably had arisen during the spontaneous disease process. The infiltrates should have been enriched for islet-specific T cells and, thus, could serve as a convenient source for establishment of T cell lines and clones. This was apparently the case, as these investigators observed that the graft infiltrating cells of five of five animals tested yielded T cell lines with potent proliferative responses to islet antigen. All of the derived lines were CD4+, with undetectable levels of CD8+ T cells, and they proliferated only in the presence of antigen and syngeneic spleen cells. The relevance of the T cells obtained from these grafts to the disease process was confirmed by the capacity of clones derived from these lines to induce diabetes upon adoptive transfer into NOD/*scid* mice.[21]

From the results described above, it appears that the culture conditions used for the initial in vitro stimulation and for propagation of T cells may influence the phenotype of T cell clones that are obtained from NOD mice. In the case of the two groups who used spleen cells as a source of APCs and islets as antigen, the clones obtained were uniformly CD4+ and exhibited MHC-restricted responses to islet antigen, reflected by a requirement for syngeneic spleen cells in the response to islet cells. In addition, the majority of these clones were islet-specific in that they did not respond to syngeneic spleen cells in the absence of added islet cells. The majority of these T cell clones appeared to recognize both allogeneic and syngeneic islet cells in the presence of NOD APC. In contrast, the two groups who used only islets or islet cells for in vitro stimulation obtained both CD4+ and CD8+ T cells, and these cells had no requirement for spleen-derived APC in responses to islets. These T cell lines were strain specific in their response to islet antigen and required syngeneic islets for in vitro proliferation. However, CD4+ T cell clones isolated with islets as the only source of accessory cells were often not islet-specific but were autoreactive to syngeneic spleen cells.

The Role of CD4+ Versus CD8+ T Cells in Diabetes

One aspect of the involvement of T cells in induction of diabetes that remains controversial is the contribution of CD4+ versus CD8+ T cells to beta cell destruction. Part of the reason for this controversy is that different experimental systems yield different results with regard to the requirement for CD8+ T cells in development of diabetes. Immunohistochemical analyses have generally revealed the presence of both CD4+ and CD8+ cells in islet infiltrates. Most of the available evidence, which will be summarized below, is consistent with the notion that both CD4+ and CD8+ T cells are involved in the spontaneous development of disease but that populations of islet-specific CD4+ T cells can arise that are capable of transferring diabetes in the absence of CD8+ T cells.

Early studies in both neonates and irradiated adult NOD mice have shown that both CD4+ and CD8+ cells were required for adoptive transfer of diabetes by spleen cells from diabetic NOD mice.[10] On the other hand, destruction of islet isografts in spontaneously diabetic NOD recipients appeared to be mediated primarily by CD4+ cells[22]; depletion of CD8+ cells had no detectable effect, whereas depletion of CD4+ cells prolonged graft survival. Haskins and McDuffie[16] found that two independently derived CD4+ islet-specific T cell clones were sufficient to induce diabetes or insulitis in young recipients, but the results of the clone transfer experiments could not definitively rule out contributions from host cells. Another indication that CD8+ T cells are not required for islet graft destruction was provided by experiments in which it was demonstrated that depletion of CD8+ T cells in recipient mice had no effect on the kinetics of graft destruction mediated by an islet-specific T cell clone.[18] These experiments could not definitively rule out contributions from CD8+ T cells, as it could be argued that CD8+ T cells below the level of detection are sufficient to collaborate with the CD4+ T cell clone.

The recent development of the NOD/*scid* mouse has provided an excellent model for analyzing the cellular requirements for adoptive transfer of diabetes. These mice have no detectable levels of mature, functional B cells and T cells and, thus, develop neither insulitis nor overt diabetes.[23] Christianson and coworkers[24] performed an extensive analysis of adoptive transfer of diabetes to NOD/*scid* mice by spleen cells obtained either from newly diabetic NOD mice or prediabetic mice. They found that there was a qualitative difference in the in vivo activity of CD4+ T cells isolated from prediabetic as opposed to diabetic NOD mice. Unfractionated, B cell–depleted spleen cells isolated from diabetic mice induced disease in 100% of recipients within 30 days after transfer while T cells isolated in the same manner from young prediabetic female donors (6 to 8 weeks old) induced diabetes in only 44% of recipients, with a markedly protracted mean onset time of 85 days. Antibody treatment of recipient animals to remove any contaminating CD8+ T cells in purified CD4+ populations slightly reduced the incidence of transfer by spleen cells obtained from diabetic donors, but completely abrogated disease transfer when cells were obtained from young, prediabetic mice. Thus, it appears from these results that CD8+ T cells are required for adoptive transfer of diabetes when prediabetic mice are used as donors and are not absolutely required, but greatly enhance induction of diabetes, when diabetic mice are used as donors.

Haskins and colleagues have extended the studies of Christianson and coworkers by transferring CD4+, diabetogenic T cell clones into NOD/*scid* mice. Whereas NOD/*scid* recipients of diabetic splenocytes became diabetic 21–28 days following transfer, these investigators found that two to three intravenous (IV) injections of an islet-specific, CD4+ T cell clone, BDC-6.9, were also fully capable of inducing diabetes in a rapid (12–24 days) and efficient (eight out of eight) manner.[19] Histological examination revealed that the insulitis in BDC-6.9 recipients was highly destructive and was indistinguishable from lesions evident in spontaneously diabetic NOD mice, except for the complete absence of CD8+ T cells, as determined by immunohistochemistry. Interestingly, another T cell clone, BDC-2.5, found to be highly diabetogenic in young NOD mice, was unable to transfer diabetes in the NOD/*scid* mice, suggesting that this clone may require host T cell participation in beta cell destruction (Peterson and Haskins, unpublished results). These results clearly show that some, but not all, CD4+ islet-specific T cells can mediate rapid and complete destruction of pancreatic beta cells with no help required from host B cells, CD4+ T cells, or CD8+ T cells.

There are, as yet, no reports to indicate that a CD8+ islet-specific T cell clone is capable of causing diabetes in the absence of CD4+ T cells. Thus far, the proponents of CD8-mediated beta cell destruction have failed to provide compelling direct evidence that CD8+ T cells are capable of destruction of beta cells either in vitro or in vivo.

Candidate Antigens for Nominally Islet-Specific T Cells

Beta Cell–Associated Antigens Other than Insulin. The finding that islet-specific T cells participate in beta cell destruction has led to much interest in the identification of the beta cell–associated T cell antigens in the hope that such identification will lead to the design of specific immunomodulating agents to interfere with the disease pathogenesis. There have been two general approaches to this issue. The first approach has been to determine if bulk populations of T cells obtained from either spleen or lymph node cells of NOD mice respond to defined beta cell–associated antigens. The second approach has been to attempt to isolate and characterize antigens toward which nominally islet-specific T cell clones respond.

There have been a number of investigations in which cells obtained from either spleen or lymph nodes of NOD mice have been used to assess reactivity toward candidate beta cell–associated antigens. Recently, it has been reported that spleen cell responses to a number of well-characterized beta cell–associated antigens increased with increasing age, and that responses to glutamic acid decarboxylase (GAD) were detectable in 4-week-old mice.[25,26] These investigators did not detect significant responses to other antigens such as insulin and heat shock protein (HSP), or to synthetic peptides of HSP in 4-week-old mice. They also observed that administration of GAD to 3-week-old NOD mice either intravenously or into the thymus decreased the incidence of diabetes. When given IV, GAD was found to completely block the development of diabetes and insulitis even up to 37 weeks of age. These authors concluded that GAD is the primary antigen with regard to the T cell response to islets in that a T cell response to GAD is required for initiation of beta cell damage. Another report[27] suggested that a 24-amino acid peptide of HSP 65 (p277) is an important T cell autoantigen recognized during diabetes pathogenesis in NOD mice. The authors found that active immunization to whole HSP 65 triggered acute diabetes and that HSP 65–specific T cells transferred acute diabetes to young prediabetic NOD mice. Vaccination with p277-specific T cells or with p277 peptide induced parallel decreases in both diabetes and immunity to HSP 65. Although it is of interest that these authors observed bulk proliferative responses to GAD or HSP 65 in the spleens of NOD mice, it may be more relevant to characterize antigens recognized by islet-infiltrating cells and established diabetogenic T cell clones.

Bergman and Haskins have made significant progress in characterizing the undefined antigen, or antigens, recognized by a panel of diabetogenic, islet-specific T cell clones.[28] These T cell clones show no reactivity to a number of candidate proteins that have been previously identified by antibody reactivity, including insulin, GAD, heat shock proteins, peripherin, and carboxypeptidase H. The finding that tumor cells derived directly from the NOD/Lt RIP-Tag mouse[29] were highly antigenic for the panel of T cell clones made possible the biochemical localization of islet antigens. Subcellular fractionation of freshly harvested NOD/Lt RIP-Tag islet tumor cells showed that antigen for the T cell clones was highly enriched in the beta granule fraction but could not be detected in cytosol fractions. High and low pH treatments greatly diminished antigenic activity in the beta granules, whereas extraction in low and high salt buffers had little effect, suggesting that the antigen is tightly associated with the granule membrane, possibly as an integral protein.[28] To date, six of six T cell clones tested have been shown to respond to the beta granule antigen. Because each T cell clone was derived from a separate mouse and is diabetogenic in vivo,[16] it would appear that these T cells are not directed to a wide range of proteins but may have been selected by a dominant antigen or antigens present in the membranes of secretory granules.

Insulin as a T Cell Autoantigen in Diabetes. It has been known for some time that during diabetes pathogenesis, in both the NOD mouse and human subjects, circulating insulin autoantibodies (IAAs) arise[29–31,30–32] and that these IAA levels are of good predictive value in identifying individuals at risk for diabetes. This association of IAAs with the development of diabetes has led to the suggestion that development of an immune response to insulin is a rate-limiting step in progression to disease.[33] Indeed, it has been observed that prophylactic insulin treatment[34] or oral administration of insulin[35] in prediabetic NOD mice resulted in a decrease in the incidence and a delay in the onset of diabetes.

Wegmann and coworkers have recently discovered that insulin-specific T cells constitute a major component of nominally islet cell–specific T cell lines and clones established from islet infiltrates of prediabetic female NOD mice.[36] An analysis of 40 nominally islet-specific T cell clones isolated from islet infiltrates obtained from 12-week-old female NOD mice revealed that 22 (55%) were in fact insulin-specific (see Table 4.1). A similar analysis of clones established from 7-week-old mice indicated that 2 of 14 were insulin-specific. These results suggest the insulin-specific component of islet-specific T cells increases with increasing age. An insulin-specific component has been observed in all of approximately 30 nominally islet-specific T cell lines established from individual mice ranging in age from 4 weeks to 13 weeks.[37] Thus it appears that insulin-specific T cells are present in islet infiltrates of most, if not all, mice with significant infiltration. By an independent measure of T cell reactivity using limiting dilution frequency analysis, it was observed that insulin-responsive T cells were approximately 15% of all anti-CD3 activatable T cells isolated from the islet infiltrates of a 9-week-old NOD mouse.[38] Thus, insulin is the first defined antigen toward which nominally islet-specific T cell clones have been demonstrated to respond. In addition a 15-residue B-chain peptide that appears to be the dominant epitope recognized by the insulin-specific T cells has been identified.[38] These results with regard to the prevalence of insulin-specific T cells within islet infiltrates provide a potential mechanism by which oral administration of insulin may inhibit diabetes, namely that

Table 4.1. Frequency of Insulin-Specific T Cell Clones within Nominally Islet-Specific T Cells

Age of Donor	*Number Tested*	*Insulin-Specific*	*Percent Insulin-Specific*
12 weeks	40	22	55%*
7 weeks	14	2	14%*

Frequency of insulin-specific T cell clones as a subset of nominally islet-specific T cells. T cell clones with islet-specificity were tested for responsiveness to porcine insulin by proliferation assays. For the assay 2.5×10^4 cells from the clone of interest were cocultured with 1.0×10^6 irradiated NOD spleen cells in either medium alone or with 16.7 μM porcine insulin (Sigma). The cultures were harvested at 72 hours after a 6-hour pulse with 1.0 μCi ^{3}H Tdr.

*$P = .01$ by Fisher's exact test.

administration of insulin alters the T cell response to insulin in a manner such that beta cell destruction is reduced. This could occur either as a result of induction of unresponsiveness in the insulin-specific component of islet-reactive T cells or as a result of an alteration in the cytokine production profile of insulin-specific T cells present in the islet infiltrates.

Lymphokine Production Profile and Autoimmune Pathology

In 1986 it was reported that T helper cells could be classified into two categories based on profiles of lymphokine production.[39] There have been a number of recent reports, predominantly in experimental autoimmune encephalomyelitis (EAE) models, that indicate the outcome of a T cell response is heavily influenced by the lymphokine profile of the T cells that predominate in that response. Oral tolerance to myelin basic protein (MBP) reduced the incidence of disease and severity of symptoms in a rat model of MBP-induced EAE and that this was associated with release of transforming growth factor–β (TGF-β), IL-4, and prostaglandin E (PGE).[40] Thus, the amelioration of disease by tolerance induction could result from selective induction or expansion of TGF-β– or IL-4–secreting T cells that can regulate the Th1 cells. That a similar mechanism might be operative in the NOD mouse model of diabetes is implied by the results of experiments in which the incidence of diabetes was decreased by oral administration of insulin[35] or prophylactic insulin treatment of NOD mice.[34] It is of interest that while both orally administered and injected insulin result in a decrease in the incidence of diabetes, there was still significant islet infiltration. It appears that the T cells present in islet infiltrates of insulin-treated mice are less aggressive with regard to beta cell damage than T cells in untreated animals. One possible explanation for this effect is that the T cells present in the infiltrates of insulin-treated animals have a predominance of IL-4– or TGF-β–secreting T cells.

Results from Investigations of Human Subjects

Although there is a considerable amount of direct evidence that T cells mediate beta cell destruction in the NOD mouse, there is much less information available with regard to human subjects. The major obstacles to obtaining islet-specific T cells from humans are due to practical and technical problems. The only practical source of starting material from human subjects is peripheral blood. It is likely that the frequency of islet-specific T cells in the peripheral blood of prediabetic or newly diabetic patients is very low and therefore the likelihood of isolating these cells is also low. Although, as will be reviewed below, a number of investigators have obtained evidence that newly diabetic subjects have T cell reactivity to beta cell–associated antigens, evidence that such cells play an active role in beta cell destruction is lacking.

Histological Investigations

The first indication that type I diabetes was an immune-mediated phenomenon was provided by a comprehensive histological examination of pancreata of recently diagnosed diabetics.[41] These investigators observed that most of these subjects had significant infiltration of the islets and loss of beta cell mass. At the time of this report (1965), cellular immunology as we know it today was in its infancy and the observation of these infiltrates provided little insight into the mechanism of beta cell destruction. In a subsequent report published in 1981, it was suggested that these lymphocytic infiltrates accumulated as a result of attraction by antigens present in the beta cells of the islets.[42] The first indication that T cells were involved in beta cell destruction was provided by a detailed immunohistochemical examination of the pancreas from a newly diabetic subject in which it was observed that T cells, particularly CD8+ T cells, were a predominant component of the islet infiltrates present.[43]

Demonstration of In Vitro *T Cell Reactivity to Islets*

The mere presence of T cells in infiltrates is only suggestive of a direct role in development of diabetes, but these histological findings were soon followed by reports of T cell reactivity to beta cell products. The first evidence that T cells reactive to beta cell products were present in the peripheral blood of newly diabetic subjects was provided by Van Vliet and coworkers in 1989.[44] These investigators established T cell lines and clones from the peripheral blood of new-onset diabetics by stimulation with rat insulinoma cells. They found that these cells were CD4+ and restricted to HLA-DR. Of eight clones examined, five appeared to be reactive with the membrane fraction of insulinoma cells. In subsequent reports these investigators have demonstrated that at least some of these T cell clones are specific to a 38-kd component of the beta granule membrane.[45]

Isolation of islet-specific T cell clones from peripheral blood of human subjects is a challenging undertaking, mostly because of technical problems and limited availability of material. This has led a number of investigators to assess T cell reactivity to beta cell products by proliferation assays in which either islet preparations or purified molecules known to be associated with beta cells have been used as antigens.[46–48] Although the results of these investigations are interesting, they provide only a correlation between T cell reactivity to beta cells and type I diabetes. Demonstration of a direct role for islet-specific T cells in human type I diabetes will require evidence that these T cells can destroy islets in vivo. These experiments are obviously not possible in human subjects and will require some sort of animal model, the best candidate perhaps being *scid* mice reconstituted with human lymphocytes[49,50] and transplanted with human islets. The potential use of mice with transplanted human islets as a means of assessing the role of human T cells in beta cell destruction has been reported.[51]

Summary and Conclusions

The NOD mouse has been available to the research community for approximately 10 years and in that time tremendous advances have been made in understanding the role of the immune system in development of type I diabetes. It is clear that beta cell destruction is mediated primarily by T cells, with a dominant role for CD4+ T cells as compared with CD8+ T cells. It should be kept in mind that development of diabetes in the NOD mouse differs from that in humans in several respects, including a marked sex bias in females and very high concordance (80%–90% in NOD female mice) compared with the 30%–50% observed in human identical twins. Nevertheless, the NOD mouse provides a very important model for understanding diabetes pathogenesis in humans.

The data obtained thus far from investigation of human subjects are much less compelling with regard to a direct role for T cells in beta cell destruction than data from the NOD mouse. Nevertheless, it appears that T cells are involved and it is probably only a matter of time before advance in techniques will allow a definitive assessment of the participation of T cells in human type I diabetes.

References

1. Makino S, Kunimoto K, Muraoka Y, Katagiri K, Tochino Y. Breeding of a non-obese, diabetic strain of mice. *Exp Anim.* 1980; 29:1–13.
2. Miyazaki A, Hanafusa T, Yamada K, et al. Predominance of T lymphocytes in pancreatic islets and spleen of pre-diabetic non-obese (NOD) mice: a longitudinal study. *Clin Exp Immunol.* 1985; 60:622–630.
3. Kanazawa Y, Komeda K, Sato S, Mori S, Akanuma K, Takaku F. Non-obese diabetic mice: immune mechanisms of pancreatic β-cell destruction. *Diabetologia.* 1984; 27:113–115.
4. Ogawa M, Maruyama T, Hasegawa T, et al. The inhibitory effect of neonatal thymectomy on the incidence of insulitis in non-obese-diabetic (NOD) mice. *Biomed Res.* 1985; 6:103–105.
5. Koike T, Itoh Y, Ishii T, et al. Preventive effect of monoclonal anti-L3T4 antibody on development of diabetes on NOD mice. *Diabetes.* 1987; 36:539–541.
6. Makino S, Harada M, Kishimoto Y, Hayashi Y. Absence of insulitis and overt diabetes in athymic nude mice with NOD mice with NOD genetic background. *Exp Anim.* 1986; 35:495–498.
7. Wicker LS, Miller BJ, Mullen Y. Transfer of autoimmune diabetes mellitus with splenocytes from nonobese diabatic (NOD) mice. *Diabetes.* 1986; 35:855–860.
8. Bendelac A, Boitard C, Bedossa P, Bazin H, Bach JF, Carnaud C. Adoptive T cell transfer of autoimmune nonobese diabetic mouse diabetes does not require recruitment of host B lymphocytes. *J Immunol.* 1988; 141:2625–2628.
9. Miller BJ, Appel MC, O'Neil JJ, Wicker LS. Both the lyt-2+ and L3T4+ T cell subsets are required for the transfer of diabetes in nonobese diabetic mice. *J Immunol.* 1988; 140:52–58.

10. Bendelac A, Carnaud C, Boitard C, Bach JF. Syngeneic transfer of autoimmune diabetes from diabetic NOD mice to healthy neonates. Requirement for both L3T4+ and lyt-2+ T cells. *J Exp Med.* 1987; 166:823–832.
11. Haskins K, Portas M, Bradley B, Wegmann D, Lafferty KJ. T-lymphocyte clone specific for pancreatic islet antigen. *Diabetes.* 1988; 37: 1444–1448.
12. Haskins K, Portas M, Bergman B, Lafferty K, Bradley B. Pancreatic islet-specific T-cell clones from nonobese diabatic mice. *Proc Natl Acad Sci USA.* 1989; 86:8000–8004.
13. Reich EP, Sherwin RS, Kanagawa O, Janeway CAJ. An explanation for the protective effect of the MHC class II I-E molecule in murine diabetes. *Nature.* 1989; 341:326–328.
14. Nakano N, Kikutani H, Nishinoto H, Kishimoto T. T cell receptor V gene usage of islet β cell-reactive T cells is not restricted in non-obese diabetic mice. *J Exp Med.* 1991; 173:1091–1097.
15. Nagata M, Yoon J. Studies on autoimmunity for T-cell-mediated β-cell destruction: distinct difference in β-cell destruction between CD4+ and CD8+ T-cell clones derived from lymphocytes infiltrating the islets of NOD mice. *Diabetes.* 1992; 41:998–1008.
16. Haskins K, McDuffie M. Acceleration of diabetes in young NOD mice with a CD4+ islet-specific T cell clone. *Science.* 1990; 249:1433–1436.
17. Haskins K, Bradley BJ, Lafferty KJ. Islet-graft destruction by a CD4+ T cell clone is not CD8 T cell dependent. *Diab Nutr Metab.* 1992; 5(Suppl):111–112.
18. Bradley BJ, Haskins K, LaRosa FG, Lafferty KJ. CD8 T cells are not required for islet destruction induced by a CD4+ islet-specific T cell clone. *Diabetes.* 1992; 41:1603–1608.
19. Peterson JD, Pike B, McDuffie M, Haskins K. Islet-specific T cell clones transfer diabetes to nonobese diabetic (NOD) F_1 mice. *J Immunol.* 1994; 153:2800–2806.
20. Reich E-P, Scaringe D, Yagi J, Sherwin RS, Janeway CA Jr. Prevention of diabetes in NOD mice by injection of autoreactive T-lymphocytes. *Diabetes.* 1989; 38:1647–1651.
21. Wegmann DR, Shehadeh N, Lafferty KJ, Norbury-Glaser M, Gill RG, Daniel D. Establishment of islet-specific T-cell lines and clones from islet isografts placed in spontaneously diabetic NOD mice. *J Autoimmun.* 1993; 6:517–527.
22. Wang Y, Pontesilli O, Gill RG, La Rosa FG, Lafferty KJ. The role of CD4 and CD8 T cells in the destruction of islet grafts by spontaneously diabetic mice. *Proc Natl Acad Sci U S A.* 1991; 88:527–531.
23. Prochazka M, Gaskins HR, Shultz LD, Leiter EH. The NOD-*scid* mouse: a model for spontaneous thymomagenesis associated with immunodeficiency. *Proc Natl Acad Sci USA.* 1992; 89:3290–3294.
24. Christianson SW, Shultz LD, Leiter EH. Adoptive transfer of diabetes for immunodeficient NOD-scid/scid mice: relative contributions of CD4+ and CD8+ T lymphocytes from diabetic versus prediabetic NOD.NON-thy-la donors. *Diabetes.* 1993; 42:44–55.
25. Kaufman DL, Clare-Salzer M, Tian J, et al. Spontaneous loss of T-cell tolerance to glutamic acid decarboxylase in murine insulin-dependent diabetes. *Nature.* 1993; 366:69–72.
26. Tisch R, Yang X-D, Singer SM, Liblau RS, Fugger L, McDevitt HO. Immune response to glutamic acid decarboxylase correlates with insulitis in non-obese diabetic mice. *Nature.* 1993: 366:72–75.
27. Elias D, Markovits D, Reshef T, Van Der Zee R, Cohen IR. Induction and therapy

of autoimmune diabetes in the non-obese diabetic (NOD/Lt) mouse by a 65-kDa heat shock protein. *Proc Natl Acad Sci USA.* 1990; 1576–1580.

28. Bergman B, Haskins K. Islet-specific T cell clones from the NOD mouse respond to beta granule antigen. *Diabetes.* 1994; 43:197–203.
29. Hamaguchi K, Gaskins HR; Leiter EH. NIT-1, a pancreatic beta-cell line established from a transgenic NOD/Lt mouse. *Diabetes.* 1991; 40:842–849.
30. Palmer JP, Asplin CM, Clemons P, et al. Insulin antibodies in insulin-dependent diabetics before insulin treatment. *Science.* 1983; 222:1337–1339.
31. Reddy S, Bibby NJ, Elliott RB. Ontogeny of islet cell antibodies, insulin autoantibodies and insulitis in the non-obese diabetic mouse. *Diabetologia.* 1988; 31:322–328.
32. Ziegler AG, Vardi P, Ricker AT, Hattori M, Soeldner JS, Eeisenbarth GS. Radioassay determination of insulin autoantibodies in NOD mice: correlation with increased risk of progression to overt diabetes. *Diabetes.* 1989; 38:358–363.
33. Eisenbarth GS, Jackson RA, Pugliese A. Insulin autoimmunity: the rate limiting factor in pre-type I diabetes. *J Autoimmun.* 1992; 5(Suppl A): 241–246.
34. Atkinson MA, Maclaren NK, Luchetta R. Insulitis and diabetes in NOD mice reduced by prophylactic insulin therapy. *Diabetes.* 1990; 39:933-937.
35. Zhang ZJ, Davidson L, Eisenbarth G, Weiner HL. Suppression of diabetes in nonobese diabetic mice by oral administration of porcine insulin. *Proc Natl Acad Sci USA.* 1991; 88:10252–10256.
36. Wegmann DR, Norbury-Glaser M, Daniel D. Insulin-specific T cells are a predominant component of islet infiltrates in pre-diabetic NOD mice. *Eur J Immunol.* 1994; 24:1853–1857.
37. Wegmann DR, Gill RG, Norbury-Close M, Schloot N, Daniel D. Analysis of the spontaneous T cell response to insulin in NOD mice. *J Autoimmun.* 1994; 7:833–843.
38. Daniel D, Gill RG, Schloot N, Wegmann DR. Epitope specificity, cytokine product on profile and diabetogenic activity of insulin-specific T cell clones isolated from NOD mice. *Eur J Immunol.* 1995; 25:1056–1062.
39. Mosmann TR, Cherwinski H, Bond MW, Giedlin MA, Coffman RL. Two types of murine helper T cell clone. I. Definition according to profiles of lymphokine activities and secreted proteins. *J Immunol.* 1986; 136:2348–2357.
40. Khoury SJ, Hancock WW, Weiner HL. Oral tolerance to myelin basic protein and natural recovery from experimental autoimmune encephalomyelitis are associated with downregulation of inflammatory cytokines and differential upregulation of transforming growth factor beta, interleukin 4, and prostaglandin E expression in the brain. *J Exp Med.* 1992; 176:1355–1364.
41. Gepts W. Pathologic anatomy of the pancreas in juvenile diabetes mellitus. *Diabetes.* 1965; 14;619–633.
42. Gepts W, Lecompte PM. The pancreatic islets in diabetes. *Am J Med.* 1981; 70:105–115.
43. Bottazzo GF, Dean BM, McNally JM, MacKay EH, Swift PGF, Gamble DR. In situ characterization of autoimmune phenomena and expression of HLA molecules in the pancreas in diabetic insulitis. *N Engl J Med.* 1985; 313:353–360.
44. Van Vliet E, Roep BO, Meulenbroek L, Bruining GJ, De Vries RRP. Human T cell clones with specificity for insulinoma cell antigens. *Eur J Immunol.* 1989; 19:213–216.
45. Roep BO, Arden SD, de Vries RRP, Hutton JC. T-cell clones from a type-1 diabetes patient respond to insulin secretory granule proteins. *Nature.* 1990; 345:632–634.

46. Harrison LC, Chu SX, DeAizpurua HJ, Graham M, Honeyman MC, Colman PG. Islet-reactive T cells are a marker of preclinical insulin-dependent diabetes. *J Clin Invest.* 1992; 89:1161–1165.

47. Atkinson MA, Kaufman DL, Campbell L, et al. Response of peripheral-blood mononuclear cells to glutamate decarboxylase in insulin-dependent diabetes. *Lancet.* 1992; 339:458–459.

48. Roep BO, Kallan AA, Hazenbos WLW, et al. T-cell reactivity to 38 kD insulin-secretory-granule protein with recent-onset type 1 diabetes. *Lancet.* 1991; 337: 1439–1441.

49. Mosier DE, Gulizia RJ, Baird SM, Wilson DB. Transfer of a functional human immune system to mice with severe combined immunodeficiency. *Nature.* 1988; 335:256–259.

50. McCune JM, Namikawa H, Shultz LD, Lieberman M, Weissman IL. The SCID-hu mouse: murine model for the analysis of human hematolymphois differentiation and function. *Science.* 1988; 241:1632–1639.

51. Calcinaro F, Hao L, Chase HP, Klingensmith G, Lafferty KJ. Detection of cell-mediated immunity in type I diabetes mellitus. *J Autoimmun.* 1992; 5:137–147.

5

Inflammatory Mediators and Development of Autoimmune Diabetes

F. Calcinaro
K. J. Lafferty
N. N. Shehadeh

Insulin-dependent diabetes mellitus (IDDM) results from damage to the insulin-producing tissue of the pancreas. The process leading to the destruction of the pancreatic islets of Langerhans is thought to be "autoimmune," although the antigen(s) that initiates diabetes has not yet been found. However, there is abundant experimental evidence that IDDM both in human and in animal models is an immune disease. Evidence for the involve-ment of immunity in the pathogenesis of IDDM in man comes from the description of the mononuclear islet filtrate, termed insulitis, in the pancreas of patients who died from early complications of the disease,[1,2] the recurrence of disease in diabetic patients receiving human leukocyte antigen (HLA)–identical[3] or HLA-matched[4] pancreatic grafts, the efficacy of cyclosporin A in preserving residual β-cell function in new-onset diabetic patients,[5] the finding that antibodies to islet cells (ICA),[6] insulin[7] and other β-cell molecules[8,9] can be shown in the serum of diabetics and individuals at risk of developing the disease, even years before the clinical onset of disease.[10–12]

Animal models of IDDM have recently been described that greatly improve our understanding of the pathogenesis of IDDM. The nonobese diabetic (NOD) mouse[13] and the Bio Breeding (BB) rat[14,15] are two inbred rodent strains that develop spontaneous IDDM. Diabetes seen in these animal models, particularly in the NOD mouse, is similar to the human disease.

In clean, pathogen-free colonies, diabetes occurs in female NOD mice at a rate of approximately 80%–85% by the age of 150 days; males have a lower incidence, approximately 30%–40% developing diabetes by the same age. However, the incidence of diabetes drops significantly if microbiological contamination occurs in the colony. Microscopic examination of the pancreas shows the disease to commence as an inflammatory response adjacent to the pancreatic islet; the inflammation is focused primarily in the region adjacent to the islet that carries small pancreatic ducts and blood vessels (Fig. 5.1A). With the passage of time, this inflammation increase and spreads to invade the islet tissue itself. (Fig. 5.1B).

The lesion in the pancreas contains a number of inflammatory cells (T cells, B cells, macrophages) and the destructive process is very specific. Initially, β-cells, which make up the majority of cells in the islet, are intact and α-cells can be seen scattered neatly around the periphery of the islet. As the disease proceeds, β-cells are destroyed while the α-cells, and other minority cells of the islet, remain intact. Eventually the islet collapses into what appears to be an "α-cell islet." That is, the disease process is the result of a specific process leading to β-cell destruction while maintaining the integrity of other cellular components of the pancreatic islet.

The development of diabetes in the NOD mouse is a thymus-dependent process.[16,17] Both cell transfer studies[18–20] and the investigation of disease that develops following cyclophosphamide treatment of disease-prone male animals[21] demonstrates that CD4 and CD8 T lymphocytes are required for the initiation of disease.

The CD4 T cells are thought to be involved in inflammatory reactions and can also exert helper function for both CD8 T cells and B cells. The CD8 T cells are thought to play a role in direct cellular killing. Thus, the requirement for both CD4 and CD8 T cells has been interpreted as indicating that the initiation of disease requires an interaction between CD4 and CD8 T cells and that the CD8 cytotoxic T cell is the effector cell causing islet damage.[18,19,22] This proposal implies a direct attack of the specific CD8 T cell on the islet β-cell (Fig. 5.2) and would provide an explanation for the specificity of the disease process. That is, selective β-cell destruction.

Implications of the Cytotoxic Model

The cytotoxic model (Fig. 5.2) sees diabetes resulting from a direct attack of CD8 cytotoxic T cells on islet β-cells. This model has two implications that can be experimentally examined:

1. The disease process, which involves a direct interaction of T cells with target β-cells, will be dependent on the activity of the CD8 cytotoxic subset.
2. The disease process will be restricted by major histocompatibilty complex (MHC) antigens expressed on the islet tissue (Fig. 5.2). That

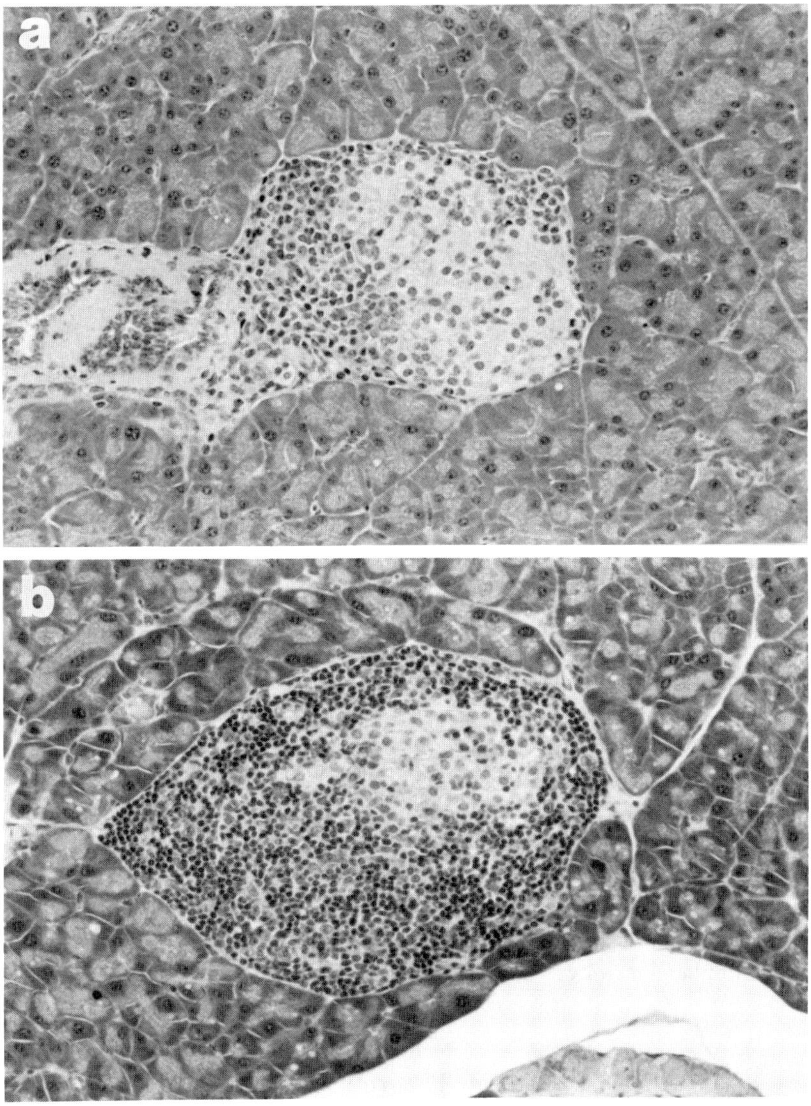

Figure 5.1. *Top:* The early stage of islet inflammation is characterized by the accumulation of mononuclear cells around pancreatic ducts and small blood vessels adjacent to the islet (hematoxylin-eosin). *Bottom:* As the disease progresses the inflammation increases and spreads to invade the pancreatic islet tissue itself (hematoxylin-eosin).

is, allogeneic islet tissue, expressing c1 MHC antigens, will be resistant to autoimmune damage following transplantation to spontaneously diabetic animals of c genotype (Fig. 5.2); the allogeneic tissue will present c1.β on the cell surface while the reactive T cells in the diabetic animals will be specific for c.β, where c1 and c represent MHC antigens

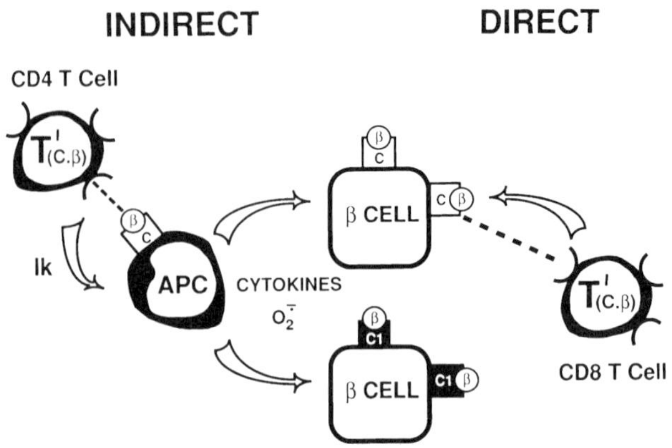

Figure 5.2. Islet destruction may be the result of either an *indirect* or *direct* interaction of the immune system with target beta cells. In the case of the *indirect* reaction, primed T cells [T′(c.β)] interact with an islet-associated peptide [β] on the surface of the animal's antigen-presenting cells (APC). This interaction leads to lymphokine production by the CD4 T cell, activation of the APC and possibly other inflammatory cells, leading to the release of cytokines and oxygen radicals. Either or both of these agents then damage the target β-cell. In the case of the *indirect* reaction both syngeneic and allogeneic islets are equally susceptible to damage.

The *direct* reaction results when a cytotoxic CD8 T cell [T′(c.β)] interacts with the target β-cell expressing c.β on its surface and kills this cell by a cytotoxic mechanism. In the case of the *direct* reaction, the allogeneic islet expressing c1.β on its surface would be resistant to damage because the CD8 T cell is specific for c.β and not c1.β, which is the complex expressed on the surface of the allogeneic β-cell.

expressed on the allogeneic islet or those of the diabetic NOD mouse, respectively, and β designates the β-cell–specific autoantigen(s) (as yet undefined). On the basis of this model the allogeneic islets would be less susceptible to disease than syngeneic NOD islets. Both these implications of the direct cytotoxic model have now been tested.[20]

Testing the Theoretical Models

T Lymphocyte Requirement in the Disease Process

Using an antibody depletion protocol found to be effective in preventing disease transfer, we have examined the T cell requirement for recurrent disease observed when syngeneic (NOD) islets were grafted to spontaneously *diabetic* NOD mice (Fig. 5.3). Depletion of the CD4 subset facilitated graft acceptance, and such islet grafts were unable to reverse diabetes for as long as the CD4 T cells remained absent from the circulation. Depletion of CD8 T cells, on the other hand, did not protect syngeneic islet tissue from disease recurrence.[20] In this latter situation the grafted tissue was heavily infiltrated by inflammatory cells and failed to function. Examination of the lesion following

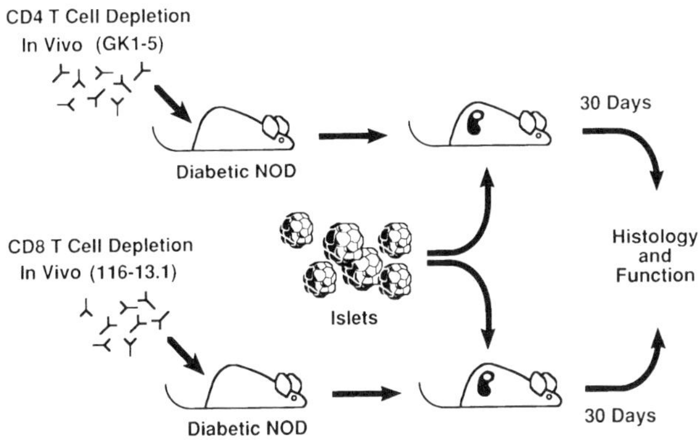

Figure 5.3. Depletion of either CD4 or CD8 T cell subsets was achieved by treating spontaneously diabetic NOD animals with monoclonal antibody reactive to either subset. These animals were then transplanted with islets obtained from nondiabetic NOD animals, and the function of the grafted tissue was followed for 30 days post-transplantation. At the completion of the study, animals were sacrificed and the tissue was examined histologically. Depletion of the CD4 subset protected the grafted tissue from disease recurrence, whereas depletion of the CD8 subset did not prevent disease recurrence and the grafted tissue was destroyed.

CD8 depletion showed large numbers of CD4 T cells to be present in the damaged tissue and the complete absence of CD8 T cells. Thus, although both CD4 and CD8 T cells are required for the *initiation* of disease, the *effector phase* of this disease is not a CD8 T cell–dependent process. In this respect the disease process is distinct from the process of the islet graft rejection, where the effector phase is a CD8 T cell–dependent process.[23–25]

MHC Restriction of the Disease Process

T cell activation is a two-signal event (see Chapter 6); therefore, allograft reactions depend on the presence of antigen-presenting cells (APCs) capable of presenting the alloantigen and delivering a costimulatory signal in conjunction with the engagement of the T cell receptor by alloantigen. As a consequence, a graft depleted of APCs will not elicit an allograft response. Organ culture in 95% oxygen has been shown to effectively remove APCs from endocrine tissues, allowing successful transplantation across major histocomaptibility barriers without the need for immunosuppression.[26–28]

To determine whether the disease process is restricted by the MHC antigens expressed on the islet tissue, nonimmunogenic, O_2-cultured *allogeneic* (SJL) islets were transplanted to the kidney capsule of spontaneously diabetic NOD mice. Graft function was monitored by blood glucose readings, and the grafts were examined histologically at the completion of the study. None of the grafts showed any significant function and histological examination showed complete graft destruction by inflammatory cells. The interpretation of such an experimental study depends on the ability to differentiate between allograft

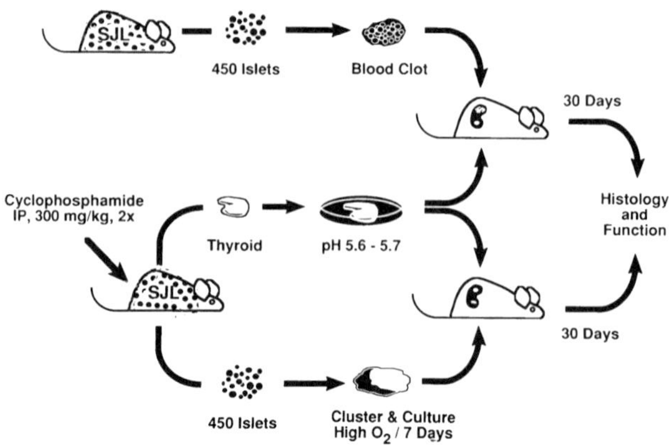

Figure 5.4. Disease recurrence is not restricted by MHC antigens expressed on the islet tissue. In this experiment, both islets and thyroid were taken from allogeneic SJL donor mice, pretreated to eliminate tissue immunogenicity, and then transplanted to spontaneously diabetic NOD animals. The cultured thyroid is used as a sentinel graft to demonstrate any development of an allograft response. In this study the islet tissue was heavily infiltrated and totally destroyed, whereas the thyroid tissue remained intact (see also Fig. 5.5), demonstrating tissue specificity of the disease process. The upper section shows the experimental design in which normal SJL islets, that is islets that were not treated to reduce immunogenicity, were transplanted into diabetic NOD animals along with a precultured sentinel thyroid. In this case, both the islets and the thyroid were totally destroyed, indicating that the thyroid was an adequate monitor of the allograft response in the NOD animal.

immunity and disease recurrence as the cause of islet destruction. Unlike allograft immunity, the recurrence of spontaneous diabetes in an islet graft will be (a) *tissue specific;* islet tissue but not some other tissue, such as thyroid, would be destroyed by disease recurrence, and (b) *disease associated;* that is, disease-dependent islet graft destruction would only be observed when tissue is transplanted to diabetic NOD mice; the same tissue would survive in nondiabetic animals.

To test tissue specificity of the destructive process, cultured allogeneic islets *and* cultured thyroid tissue were transplanted to diabetic NOD mice (Fig. 5.4). In this study, the thyroid graft acted as a sentinel to demonstrate any activation of the allograft response. Graft survival was determined by blood sugar control, in the case of the islet graft, or by labelled iodine uptake by the thyroid. These measures of graft function were confirmed by microscopic examination of the tissues. The results of this study were clearcut. All cultured islet allografts were heavily infiltrated and damaged when transplanted to diabetic NOD mice (Fig. 5.5A), whereas the thyroid grafts transplanted at the same time remained intact in all recipients some 3–4 weeks after grafting (Fig. 5.5B). Functional analysis showed the allogeneic thyroid grafts had the capacity to incorporate iodine at levels similar to control tissues.[20] Control studies demonstrated the acute destruction of cultured allogeneic thyroid tissue following the grafting of cultured thyroid and uncultured (immunogenic) islet

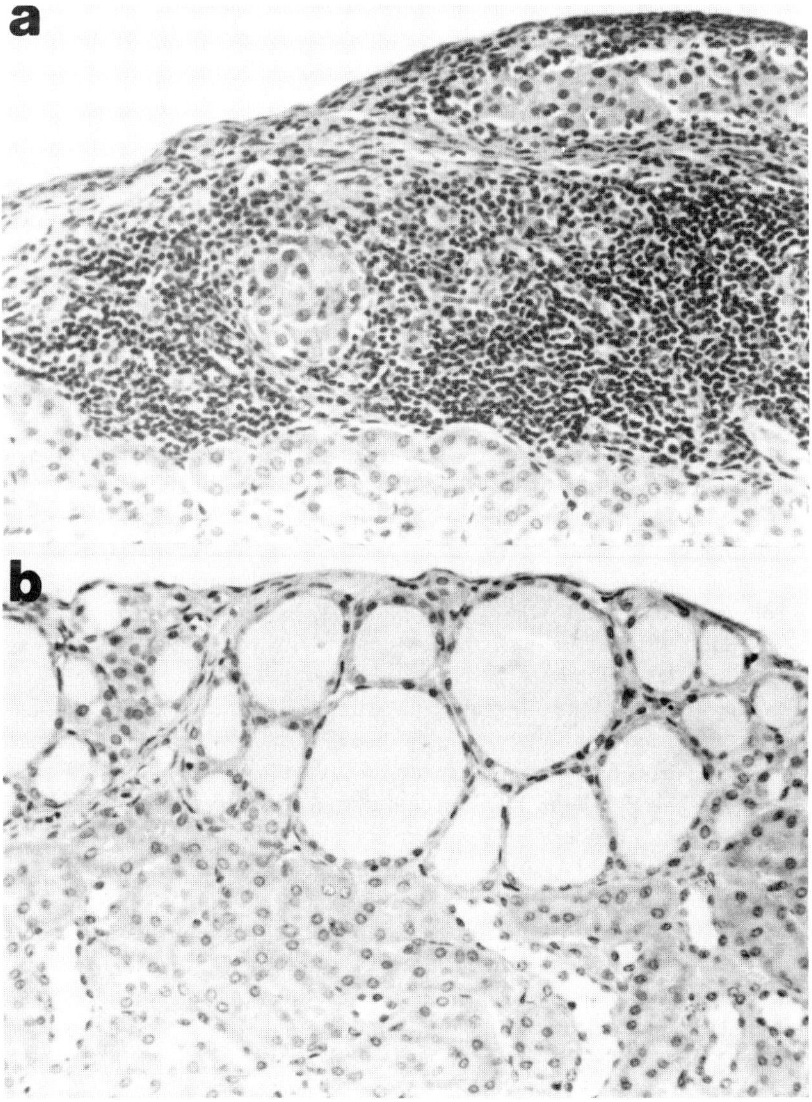

Figure 5.5. Histological appearance of APC-depleted islets and thyroid tissue (SJL) transplanted to spontaneously diabetic NOD mice. *a.* Note the heavy infiltration and damage to the islet graft. *b.* Note the normal appearance of thyroid tissue transplanted under the same kidney capsule of the NOD mouse. The tissue specificity of this reaction indicates that we are not dealing with an allograft response. Thus, we conclude that disease recurrence occurs in allogeneic islets and therefore the disease process is not restricted by MHC antigens expressed on the islets.

tissue from the same donor, thus demonstrating the capacity of the cultured thyroid graft to act as a sentinel for the detection of the allograft response. The comparison of allogeneic (SJL) islet tissue transplanted to nondiabetic and diabetic NOD animals showed that this destructive process was disease associated.[20]

These studies demonstrate clearly that disease recurrence in islet tissue grafted to spontaneously diabetic animals *is not restricted* by MHC antigens expressed on the grafted tissues. This lack of MHC restriction of the disease process by islet MHC antigens is not consistent with the direct killing hypothesis (Fig. 5.2).

T Cell Cloning Studies

The experiments described above suggest that CD4 T cells are sufficient to mediate the islet graft destruction observed in disease recurrence. If this is the case one would expect islet-specific CD4 T cell clones to be capable of in vivo destruction of β-cells.

Work from the Barbara Davis Center involving the cloning of islet-reactive T cells from the NOD mouse (see Chapter 4) has demonstrated that islet-specific CD4 T cell clones have the capacity to destroy NOD islet tissue in the absence of CD8 T lymphocytes, and to induce disease in both young NOD mice and in NOD/*scid* recipients (mice with NOD genetic background, but lacking both B and T cells).[29–33] Thus, although both CD4 and CD8 T cells are required for the activation of the disease process in the NOD mouse, the CD4 T cell is the only T cell that has been demonstrated to express effector function. Moreover, this function is expressed in the absence of CD8 T cells.[34] This would indicate that the CD8 T cell plays a facilitating role in the initiation of the disease process and is not the immunological effector cell. The precise function of the CD8 T cell in this process requires further elucidation.

The dependence of the actual disease process on the CD4 T cell leads us to propose that autoimmune diabetes is the result of CD4 T cell–dependent inflammatory tissue damage (the *indirect* process; Fig. 5.2): a β-cell–associated antigen is processed by an APC and presented, in association with the correct MHC antigen, to a CD4 T cell. This interaction would trigger cytokine release and oxygen radical production, which in turn would generate an inflammatory focus at the site of the graft. According to this model, both syngeneic and nonsyngeneic islets would be equally sensitive to the deleterious inflammatory mediators, explaining why the disease process is not restricted by the MHC expressed on the islet tissue.

One problem with this notion is the cellular specificity of the disease process. If damage is simply the result of inflammatory mediators, how do we account for specific β-cell destruction in this disease? An answer to the question can be found in the following section in which the role of inflammatory mediators in diabetes is reviewed.

Islet Sensitivity to Mediators of Inflammatory Tissue Damage

Role of Cytokines

Cytokines are proteins produced by lymphoid cells to control and regulate immune responses, hemopoiesis, and inflammation. More than 20 different cytokines have been described so far, and most of them have several actions that may produce local or general effects. Cytokines are mainly produced by lymphoid cells (lymphokines and monokines). However, other cells, such as endothelial cells and fibroblasts, can also produce cytokines.

Cytokines that are important as the mediators of inflammation are interferon γ (IFN-γ), interleukin-1 (IL-1), and tumor necrosis factor–α (TNF-α). IFN-γ is a T cell product with antiproliferative and antiviral activities. IL-1 and TNF-α are mainly produced by macrophages and monocytes. They both promote local pro-inflammatory actions, such as phagocyte stimulation, increased vascular permeability, chemotaxis, and free radical production. IL-1 and TNF-α are also responsible for general, endocrine-like activities such as the induction of fever and the release of corticosteroids via activation of the hypothalamic-hypophyseal-adrenal axis. Positive and negative feedback loops between cytokines regulate the magnitude of the inflammatory response. IFN-γ induces synthesis of TNF receptors and also enhances the production of IL-1 and TNF-α by macrophages, which in turn will induce the release of IL-2 and IFN-γ from T cells. Cytokines play a major role in regulating the immune response. IFN-γ increases MHC class I antigen expression on cells, facilitating cytotoxic T cell killing of target cells. This effect is important in islet allograft destruction.[35,36] It also induces expression of MHC class II antigens on macrophages and adhesion molecules on endothelial cells and APCs.

CD4 T cells have recently been divided into two subsets, termed Th1 and Th2, based on the cytokine secretion patterns.[37] Th1 cells produce IL-2, IFN-γ, and TNF-β (lymphotoxin); Th2 cells secrete IL-4, IL-5, IL-6, and IL-10. These two types of CD4 T cells mediate different immunological responses. The Th1 subset is mainly involved in delayed-type hypersensitivity (DTH) reactions, whereas Th2 cells are responsible for B-cell helper function and antibody production.[38] The balance between the two responses appears to regulate the pathogenesis of several diseases in addition to the expression of clinical diabetes in disease-prone individuals (see "Regulation of Autoimmune Diabetes").

In Vitro Effects of Cytokines on β-cells. There is evidence that crude cytokine preparations can either stimulate insulin secretion or cause inhibition of secretion and islet cell death.[39] These effects were dose dependent and it has been proposed that IL-1 is the cytokine responsible for these effects.[40–43] Studies from several laboratories have demonstrated, in different model systems, that IL-1β, TNF (α or β) and IFN-γ are all capable of reversibly impairing β-cell function in vitro when tested singly. These agents can exert a synergistic cytotoxic effect when present in combination.[44] This in vitro toxicity has also been observed with human islet cells in monolayer cultures.[45] It should be noted that the in vitro cytotoxic effects of IL-1β, TNF, and IFN-γ are not β-cell specific; other islet cell lineages were also damaged when whole islets were tested. However, selective inhibition of β-cell function and preservation of glucagon production have been demonstrated using purified preparations of β- and α-cells[46] or tumor cell lines.[47] The ability of IFN-γ to increase the density of cellular MHC antigen expression has already been mentioned. Combined in vitro treatment of islet tissue with IFN-γ and TNF can induce de novo synthesis of MHC class II molecules on β-cells.[48] Because aberrant MHC class II antigen expression on β-cells has been observed in NOD mice[49] as well as in patients with new-onset diabetes,[50] a pathogenetic role for aberrant presentation of islet autoantigens in spontaneous diabetes has been suggested. Although fascinating, this hypothesis has not been supported by more recent studies. Transgenic mice expressing MHC class II molecules on their β-cells do not develop diabetes.[51] In addition, no aberrant MHC class II antigen expression on β-cells has been found in pancreatic specimens obtained from patients with recent-onset diabetes[52] or with recurrent disease after pancreas transplantation.[4] It should also be noted that if aberrant MHC class II antigen expression on β-cells had a pathogenetic role, cultured (nonimmunogenetic) allogeneic islets transplanted to diabetic NOD mice should not be destroyed by recurrent disease. Under these conditions, even if aberrant expression of MHC class II antigen occurred, the grafted islet cells would display on their surface allogeneic MHC class II molecules, and the islet-reactive T cells of the diabetic host would not be able to recognize the supposed trigger antigen presented in such an allogeneic MHC contest. Our data show that in the NOD mouse this is not the case, and cultured islet allografts are regularly destroyed when trans-planted to diabetic animals (Fig. 5.5A).[20]

Both in situ immunofluorescence and mRNA hybridization techniques have detected cytokines (IFN-γ, TNF, IL-1, IL-4), or their specific mRNA, in the cells infiltrating the islets of diabetic rodents[53–55] and new-onset diabetic patients.[56] The recombinant DNA technology has provided new insights into the role cytokines play in the development of diabetes.

In Vivo Effects of Cytokines. In vivo administration of recombinant cytokines can protect diabetes-prone animals from progressing to overt disease. Short-term administration of IL-1 has been shown to interfere with glucose-stimulated insulin release in the NOD mouse.[57] However, chronic IL-1 therapy significantly decreases insulitis and incidence of diabetes in the same animal model.[58] IL-1β administration in the BB rat modulates the "autoimmune" diabetogenic process in a dose-dependent manner: low doses (0.5 μg/kg) of IL-1β significantly reduce the frequency of insulin-dependent diabetes, whereas high doses (10 μg/kg) of the same agent accelerate the onset of diabetes in this animal model.[59] TNF-α also consistently reduces insulitis and diabetes in animal models of IDDM when administered in vivo,[58,60,61] probably because of its ability to suppress Th1-dependent immune reactions.[62]

TNF-β has also been shown to protect the NOD mouse from insulitis and IDDM.[63]

A recent report shows that long-term recombinant IL-4 treatment in vivo can protect prediabetic NOD mice from the clinical disease.[64] The cellular basis for these cytokine effects is discussed below (see "Regulation of Autoimmune Diabetes").

Lessons from Transgenic Animals. It is now possible to combine gene sequences coding for cytokines with regulatory elements of the gene coding for insulin promotion (insulin promoter). The DNA construct resulting from the fusion (transgene) can artificially be inserted in fertilized mouse eggs, so that the islet β-cells of the mice generated will produce the cytokine coded by the transgene. This technique allows the definition of the role cytokine production has in the development of insulitis and diabetes in otherwise non–diabetes-prone mouse strains.

Mice transgenic for IFN-γ develop severe insulitis leading to islet destruction and diabetes.[65,66] No insulitis or diabetes develops when the transgene is expressed in mice with severe combined immunodeficiency. Thus, the IFN-γ appears to act via cells of the lymphoid system in mediating β-cell destruction.

Transgenic mice bearing the gene coding for TNF-α[67,68] or TNF-β[68] have also been generated. These animals develop progressive insulitis, but they never become diabetic; insulitis per se is not diabetogenic.

IL-10 production in pancreatic islets of mice transgenic for its gene causes pancreatic extravasation of leukocytes, but the process is not focused on the islets and does not lead to diabetes.[69] In these animals, small-vessel endothelial cells become activated and hyperexpress both MHC class II antigens and adhesion molecules. Thus, IL-10 provides a powerful recruitment signal for leukocyte migration in vivo, but this effect alone is not sufficient to initiate islet destruction.

A recent report provides evidence that IFN-α may also be involved in the pathogenetic process leading to diabetes.[70] The authors have generated transgenic mice expressing IFN-α in the islet β-cells. These animals develop pancreatic pathology characterized by progressive islet infiltration, β-cell destruction, persistence of α- and δ-cells, and final islet atrophy resulting in insulin deficiency and clinical diabetes in 50% of the animals by age 180 days. Moreover, the administration of a specific neutralizing monoclonal antibody anti–IFN-α can protect the transgenic mice from disease. IFN-α is known to activate macrophages and natural killer (NK) cells and to induce IL-2 production by activated T cells. Thus, local production of IFN-α may generate a powerful inflammatory reaction involving several cell lineages and leading to β-cell destruction. Since IFN-α expression has been reported in diabetic patients[71] and viral infections induce transient IFN-α expression,[71,72] this cytokine could play a critical role in the pathogenesis of IDDM.

Taken together, these findings indicate that several cytokines may be involved in the pathogenetic process leading to IDDM. Some of them, such as

IFN-γ, are consistently associated with the development of autoimmune diabetes. The role of other cytokines, namely IL-1 and TNF, remains controversial because their in vivo effects are not consistent with the in vitro data. Most interesting is the notion that some cytokines, such as IL-4 and IL-10, protect from the disease (see below).

Regulation of Autoimmune Diabetes

Because IFN-γ is mainly produced by the Th1 subset of T cells and IL-4 and IL-10 are products of the Th2 subset, it has been suggested that autoimmune diabetes develops in genetically prone individuals when Th1 and Th2 T cell–dependent effects are unbalanced. This interpretation is consistent with decreased productions of IL-2 and IL-4 observed in the NOD mouse[64,73] and the protective effects of in vivo IL-4 administration in this animal model.[64] Both IL-4 and IL-10 suppress IFN-γ production in vivo,[74–76] and because IFN-γ appears to be important in the initiation and expression of β-cell damage, cytokine regulation may be of central importance in the pathogenesis of autoimmune diabetes.

Recently, complete Freund's adjuvant (CFA), a suspension of *Mycobacterium tuberculosis* fragments in oil, has been shown to block the development of diabetes in both NOD mice and BB rats.[55,77–81] In the NOD mouse, CFA is also effective in preventing diabetes when given late in the disease process.[81–84] Our data demonstrate that administration of CFA as late as 84 days of age, that is, approximately 5 days before the first animals in the colony develop clinical disease, is effective in completely inhibiting the development of clinical diabetes (Fig. 5.6).[84] In our own studies, bacillus Calmette-Guérin (BCG) vaccine, commonly used to vaccinate against tuberculosis in humans, was also administered to a group of 15 female NOD animals at 84 days of age.[84] Only one animal became diabetic during the follow-up period of approximately 120

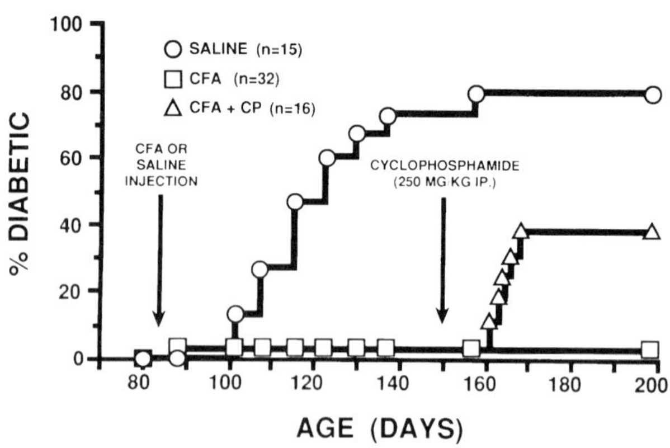

Figure 5.6. The development of diabetes in female NOD mice treated either with CFA (test group) or saline (control group). At 150 days nondiabetic animals in the test group were given cyclophosphamide (250 mg/kg, i.p.). Approximately 40% of these animals became diabetic within 17 days.

days ($P < .0001$ BCG vs saline, Fisher's test). CFA- and BCG-treated groups were not statistically different. Although CFA- and BCG-treated animals fail to develop clinical disease, adjuvant therapy does not block the development of autoimmunity; the proportion of pancreatic islets showing an accumulation of mononuclear cells in the peri-islet area is comparable in vaccinated and untreated control animals.[55] However, the infiltrate that develops after CFA or BCG treatment is qualitatively different from the one that develops in control animals. It does not invade and destroy the islet tissue. This "nondestructive insulitis" is morphologically and phenotypically different from the "destructive insulitis" responsible for islet destruction in the development of spontaneous diabetes.

We have recently studied the cytokine secretion patterns of T cells infiltrating syngeneic islets transplanted to the kidney capsule of either CFA-treated (nondiabetic) or spontaneously diabetic NOD mice. In these experiments the syngeneic islet graft acts as a sentinel for the ongoing disease process, and the inflammatory process that develops around the graft mirrors the process taking place in the pancreas of the animal. Our studies demonstrate that CFA-regulated lesions show a predominant population of IL-4–producing T cells.[55] In contrast, the majority of the cells found in the destructive lesions were shown to produce IFN-γ.[55] Further evidence for cytokine involvement in CFA-mediated protection from diabetes in the NOD mouse comes from data recently gained in our laboratory showing that combined anti–IL-4 and anti–IL-10 antibody treatment can partially reverse the protective adjuvant effect (F. Calcinaro, paper submitted). It should be emphasized that CFA- and BCG-treated mice remain disease prone. Thus, when cyclophosphamide was administered to CFA- or BCG-treated animals, approximately 50% became acutely diabetic within 17 days (Fig. 5.6).[84] These data indicate that adjuvant therapy does not inhibit the development of autoimmunity, but diverts the autoimmune response from a destructive to a nondestructive process.

The picture that emerges is one in which cytokines, IFN-γ and IFN-α, play an important role in the activation and development of clinical disease. The expression of autoimmunity as overt diabetes is regulated by IL-4 and IL-10 producing T cells, and the balance of the counteracting cytokine-dependent effects is tipped toward nondestructive autoimmunity following stimulation of the immune system with CFA or by BCG vaccination. This capacity for autoimmunity to be expressed either as a destructive or as a nondestructive response can explain characteristics of both the human and the animal disease.

In animals such as the NOD mouse or the BB rat (animals inbred to genetic homogeneity), not all individuals develop clinical disease, and disease incidence is influenced by the microbiological exposure of the colony. In humans, identical twins have a relatively low concordance for the development of IDDM. The key to understanding this phenomenon is the fact that all animals of the disease-prone genotype develop insulitis, but it is only those that develop destructive insulitis that go on to IDDM, and the proportion developing the destructive autoimmune response is inversely related to exposure to environmental antigenic challenge.

Role of Free Radicals

Cytokines, such as IL-1 and IFN-γ, may act directly on the islet β-cell. Il-1 has been reported to activate plasma membrane phospholipase A_2, resulting in arachidonic acid production and consequent prostaglandin E_2 (PGE_2) formation in several target cells,[85] including islet cells.[86,87] Although IL-1–induced inhibition of insulin release has not been prevented by cyclo/lipoxygenase inhibitors,[88] cytotoxic effects of combined exposure of β-cell tissue to TNF and IFN-γ have in fact been prevented by such inhibitors.[45]

Cytokines can also exert their effect by activating free radical production. Free radicals are metabolites displaying an unpaired electron on their outer orbitol ($O_2^{\cdot}$, $OH^{\cdot}$). This unique electronic configuration makes them highly reactive, unstable molecules, capable of damaging DNA, enzymes, and biological membranes.[89–91] The cell continuously neutralizes oxygen free radical production by the activities of various enzymes such as superoxide dismutase, catalase, and glutathione peroxidase. Il-1 and IFN-γ have been shown to induce free radical formation in a variety of cell types.[92] The Okamoto model of islet damage (Fig. 5.7) sees free radical production as a final common pathway in β-cell damage.[89,91] On the basis of this model, superoxide production at the inflammatory site would be the source of islet toxicity. Superoxide $O_2^{\cdot}$ can be converted to the reactive hydroxyl radical within the cell.[93] This radical can cause DNA breaks, and DNA damage activates the repair enzyme poly-(ADP-ribose)-synthetase, which uses cellular adenosine diphosphate (ADP) as a source of adenine. Thus, the repair process depletes the cell's nicotine adenine dinucleotide (NAD) and in this way shuts off protein synthesis.[89,91] Because NAD is also involved in the electron transport system required for radical scavenging, the damaged cell becomes more susceptible to radical attack, the ultimate result of this process being death of the cell. This

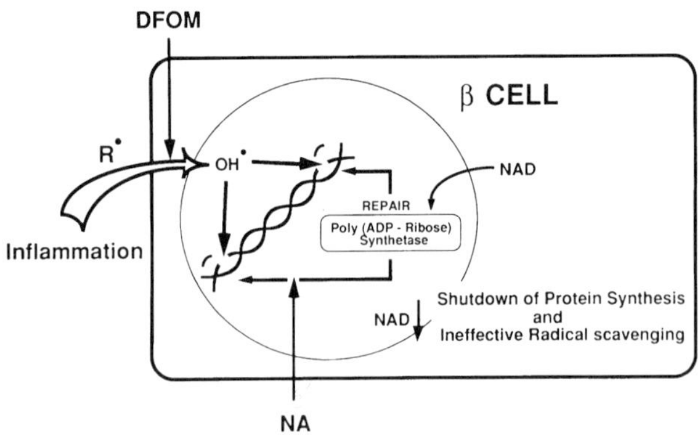

Figure 5.7. Okamoto model (see text). Desferrioxamine (DFOM) could interfere with the process by blocking the production of hydroxyl radicals. Nicotinamide (NA) would be protective by inhibiting the DNA-repair enzyme and thus maintaining cellular NAD levels required for efficient radical scavenging. The model predicts that these two agents will be synergistic.

general process applies particularly to the β-cells, because they are highly sensitive to oxygen free radical injury as a result of their high metabolic rate and the relative low activity of some cellular scavenging enzymatic systems such as mitochondrial manganese superoxide dismutase (MnSOD)[94] and glutathione peroxidase.[95] Oxygen free radicals have been detected in islets by means of resonance spectroscopy.[96] Nitric oxide production in response to IL-1 could also be involved in radical damage to islet β-cells (see below).

According to this model, it is theoretically possible to interfere with the process. The chelating agent desferrioxamine (DFOM) could be used to remove iron from the system; the conversion of superoxide to the reactive hydroxyl radical is catalyzed by iron. It is also possible to block the DNA repair process with nicotinamide (NA), which inhibits poly-(ADP-ribose)-synthetase. Such a blockade would reduce the degree of DNA depletion and so protect the cell from radical damage. NA has been shown to protect islet tissue from streptozotocin-induced damage.[97,98] NA has also been shown to inhibit the development of diabetes in NOD mice.[99]

We have investigated these implications of the Okamoto model using both NA and DFOM in an attempt to control disease recurrence in tissue grafted to spontaneously diabetic NOD mice.[100,101] In these studies, recipient animals were treated with DFOM or NA or a combination of the two. The animals were then transplanted with cultured allogeneic (BALB/c) islet tissue. All grafted animals receiving no prior therapy showed no evidence of graft function.[100,101] However, animals treated with either DFOM or NA became normoglycemic within a few days of grafting and remained so for approximately 7 days. More striking results were obtained when animals were treated with both DFOM and NA. These animals became normoglycemic following islet grafting and remained in a normal gylcemic condition for extended periods of time.[100.101] These studies demonstrate that DFOM and NA afford some protection from inflammatory tissue damage and that these agents act synergistically as would be expected on the basis of the Okamoto model. Further evidence for the involvement of oxygen radicals in the "autoimmune" diabetogenic process was obtained by examining the capacity of polythelene glycol–modified superoxide dismutase (PEG-SOD) to protect grafted islet tissue from damage in the diabetic animal (Fig. 5.8). In these studies, grafting of spontaneously diabetic NOD animals was effective in reversing diabetes only when the diabetic animals were treated with PEG-SOD for 10 days from the time of islet grafting.[102] The use of PEG-modified enzyme in these studies is required to reduce the immunogenicity of the bovine enzyme and to provide enzymatic activity with a prolonged half-life (approximately 36 hours) in the recipient animal.

Nitric oxide (NO˙) has been identified as a molecule that, in addition to several specific functions (neurotransmitter, platelet aggregation inhibitor), is the principal means by which immune cells, such as macrophages, kill parasites and intracellular bacteria. NO˙ is produced from L-arginine by NO˙synthase. Two isoforms of the enzyme have been described. The *constitutive* isoform is Ca^{2+}-dependent and produces limited quantities of NO˙, which account for the physiological functions of this mediator. The second isoform, also

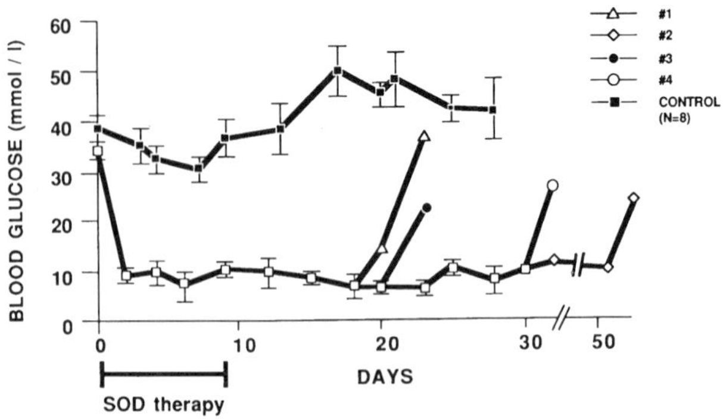

Figure 5.8. Superoxide dismutase (SOD) therapy protects the islet allograft from disease recurrence following transplantation to spontaneously diabetic NOD mice. In the control study, APC-depleted BALB/c islets were transplanted to spontaneously diabetic animals. All animals remained hyperglycemic for the length of the experimental study. Test animals were treated with SOD for seven days following transplantation of APC-depleted BALB/c islet tissue. All animals became normoglycemic within 24–48 hours and remained normoglycemic for an extended period following cessation of SOD therapy. Disease recurrence was eventually seen in all animals following the cessation of SOD therapy. These studies show that islet damage in the disease process is oxygen radical dependent.

Ca^{2+}-dependent, is *inducible* by endotoxins and cytokines, namely IL-1, TNF, and IFN-γ. The inducible form of NO˙ synthase is able to produce large amounts of NO˙, which can activate iron and thiol groups of cellular enzymes leading to impaired glycolysis,[103] inefficient oxidative phosphorylation,[104] and DNA strand breakages.[105]

NO˙ has been shown to play a major role in IL-1–mediated inhibition of insulin secretion by β-cells.[106,107] Inhibitors of NO˙ synthase, such as analogues of L-arginine, protect β-cells from IL-1–dependent inhibition of insulin release.[108,109] The inducible isoform of NO˙ synthase is present in purified rat β-cells, but not in α-cells.[110] The activation of the inducible isoform of NO˙ synthase in the β-cell could explain why inflammatory tissue damage, which is nonspecific, can result in specific β-cell destruction within the islets. Selective β-cell destruction observed in IDDM may also be accounted for by the peculiar sensitivity of the insulin-producing tissue to inflammatory mediators, such as NO˙, produced by activated macrophages.[111–113] It is still under debate whether NO˙ is produced by the macrophages present in the islet infiltrates or by the β-cells themselves.[114] IL-1–induced NO˙ production from either rat or human macrophages still awaits formal demonstration. However, cytokines have been shown to induce the synthesis of large amounts of NO˙ in human islets with a concomitant reduction in insulin secretion.[115] Further investigation is needed to determine the cellular source of NO˙ and the relative contribution of NO˙ and other oxygen free radical molecules to β-cell damage in IDDM.

The Disease Process in Man

The data discussed above have been obtained from in vitro studies and from animal studies carried out mostly in the NOD mouse. Although this mouse develops spontaneous insulin-dependent diabetes that is similar to the human disease, we have to keep in mind that what applies to this animal model may not apply to the human disease.

Little information is available on the pathogenesis of type I diabetes in man due to several obvious limitations: heterogeneous genetic background, variations in environmental role, unavailability of pancreatic tissue for histology studies. But, if the disease in humans also results from inflammatory tissue damage and not a direct attack of cytotoxic T cells on target islets, it should be possible to detect and study cell-mediated immunity (CMI) in type I diabetes by using xenogeneic islets as a target: this involves transferring unpurified mononuclear blood cells (MBCs) from diabetic patients into immunodeficient mice unable to reject the inoculum. Under those conditions, human APCs (mainly monocytes and B cells) could process an islet-associated, human/murine cross-reactive antigen and display it in the correct HLA context to an islet-reactive CD4 T cell from the same donor. This interaction would trigger the release of cytokines, the generation of oxygen free radicals, and, eventually, inflammation around the islet tissue, leading to islet-specific damage. Such a reaction would be dependent on the use of crude white cell preparations as a source of APCs and HLA-compatible T cells.

In light of our animal studies, we therefore set out to test the hypothesis that islet-specific damage can be transferred from IDDM subjects to the athymic nude mouse, a strain that lacks T cells and T cell–mediated immunity.[116]

Briefly, MBCs from 10 new-onset diabetic patients (six tested positive for anti-islet cell antibodies, ICA) and from 10 control healthy subjects were injected intraperitoneally (*IP*) into groups of two to four nude mice. Plasma from the same individuals was also injected into additional groups of animals. Nonfasting blood glucose was monitored twice a week in all the test mice and oral glucose tolerance tests were carried out at weekly intervals. At the completion of the study, 4 weeks after cell transfer, the pancreata were harvested for histological examination.

Even though we could not show any modification of the glycemic control of the mice that received injection, irrespective of the cell source, we were able to demonstrate that it is possible to transfer islet-reactive CMI from type I diabetic patients to the nude mouse. In fact, MBCs, and not plasma, from 6 out of 10 newly diagnosed patients induced significant damage in the pancreas of recipient nude mice (Fig. 5.9A,B,C); no damage was seen when mononuclear cells from 10 normal control subjects were injected into nude mice under the same conditions ($P = .005$) (Fig. 5.9D). In all cases a mononuclear cell filtrate, of variable extent, was found focused on the islet tissue. Different degrees of insulitis and islet damage, ranging from β-cell degranulation to islet disruption, were observed (Fig. 5.9A,B,C). Immunostaining for glucagon showed an unusual α-cell concentration among infiltrating mononuclear cells in many

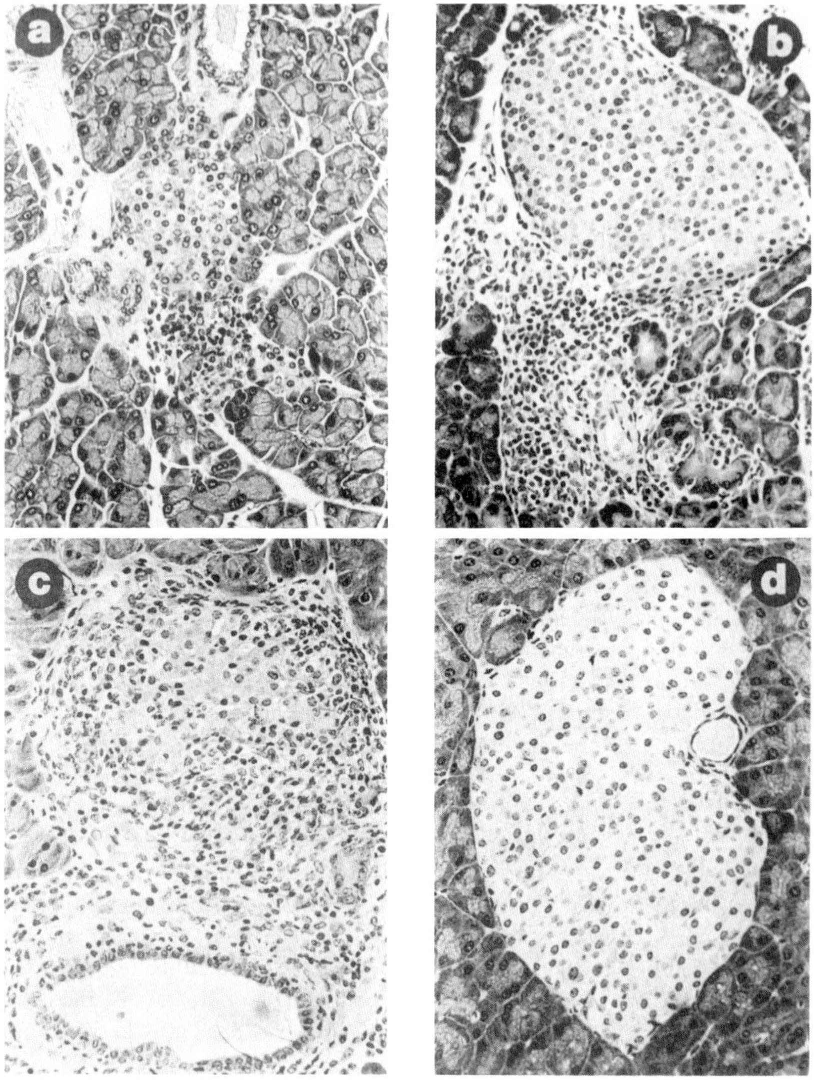

Figure 5.9. Transfer of human mononuclear blood cells (MBCs) to the nude mouse: pancreatic histology (hematoxylin-eosin). *a, b, c*: MBCs from diabetic patients; *d*: MBCs from control subject. *a*. Bouin's fixative. Accumulation of infiltrating MBCs at a pole of the pancreatic islet. Note the absence of any infiltrating cells among the pancreatic exocrine cells. *b*. Formalin fixative. Periductular mononuclear cell infiltrate in the process of surrounding a pancreatic islet which still appears relatively well preserved. *c*. Formalin fixative. Impressive periductular mononuclear infiltrate that has filled the peri-islet space and is causing islet disruption. *d*. Formalin fixative. Normal pancreatic islet appearance. No signs of inflammation.

cases, suggesting β-cell death and islet collapse. Indirect immunofluorescence studies showed rare human leukocytes among the filtrating cells. No inflammation was found in tissues other than islets, strongly suggesting the tissue specificity of the process.

The finding that no animals in either the test or control group showed any impairment of blood glucose homeostasis probably results from the fact that only a fraction of the islets in the pancreas of recipient mice showed evidence of inflammation and only a proportion of the inflamed islets were damaged to the extent shown in Fig. 5.9C.

The failure to consistently induce islet lesions in recipient mice and the variability in the extent of damage seen in different islets were probably due to recirculation defects of the human blood cells in a murine environment.

The data presented here clearly show that pathology detected in this model system is islet specific and disease associated, providing us with a way to study human IDDM outside of human subjects. Moreover, this finding is consistent with the notion that the human disease is also the result of inflammatory tissue damage. New experimental model systems are being developed to better characterize the disease process in human subjects.

Implications for Therapy

Evidence from animal models demonstrates that "autoimmune" diabetes is dependent on T cell function. In humans, suppression of T cell activity with cyclosporine has been shown to arrest the development of this disease.[5] However, treatment of type I diabetics with immunosuppressive agents such as cyclosporine carries too many demonstrable and theoretical side effects to be useful as lifelong therapy. The demonstrated effectiveness of superoxide dismutase and other oxygen free radical scavengers in preventing the development of disease recurrence in transplanted pancreatic tissue suggests that agents directed at blocking inflammatory mediators, such as interleukins and oxygen radicals, may be effective in preventing damage to susceptible pancreatic β-cells.

Another approach could be to identify, by cloning procedures, the specific human CD4 T cell subsets that are involved in pancreatic islet damage. Having identified such cells and the diversity of their expressed receptor, it may be possible to design specific immunosuppressive therapies that "surgically" remove just those cells from the repertoire, so providing what is in effect antigen-specific immunosuppression that would not carry with it the same lifetime risks of pan-immunosuppressive agents such as cyclosporine. However, the T cell repertoire utilized in islet-specific autoimmunity may not be all that restricted (see Chapter 4).

BCG vaccination may enable us to regulate the disease process in humans. In a pilot study we have demonstrated that BCG significantly prolongs clinical remission when administered to new-onset diabetic patients.[84]

Table 5.1. Clinical Data of Test and Control Patients

		BCG Treated (*n=17*)	*Untreated* (*n=29*)	*P Value*
Age (years, mean ± SD)		12.6 ± 5.7	10 ± 4.1	NS*
Male/female ratio		9/8	15/14	NS
Insulin requirement at onset (U/kg/day, mean ± SD)		0.56 ± 0.29	0.67 ± 0.24	NS
Insulin injections:	n = 2	8	17	NS
	n = 3	9	12	NS
HbA1c at diagnosis (%, mean ± SD)		14.8 ± 3.6	15.9 ± 5	NS
Ketoacidosis at diagnosis		6/17 (35%)	10/29 (34%)	NS

*NS = not significant.

Table 5.2 Clinical Remission Onset in Test and Control Patients

	Patients in Clinical Remission (%)				
Weeks after Diagnosis	*4*	*8*	*12*	*Total*	*P Value*
BCG treated (n = 17)	6 (35%)	4 (23%)	1 (6%)	11 (65%)	< .0001
Untreated (n = 29)	1 (3.5%)	—	1 (3.5%)	2 (7%)	

We have studied 17 newly diagnosed type I diabetic patients with no acute or chronic dermatologic inflammatory diseases, no natural or acquired immunodeficiency conditions, and a negative tuberculin skin test. Twenty-nine new-onset diabetic patients admitted to the clinic for insulin treatment in the past 2 years served as historical controls. Table 5.1 shows the clinical data of test and control subjects. A single intracutaneous injection of 0.1 ml of freeze-dried BCG vaccine reconstituted with buffered saline to a final concentration of 1 mg/ml was administered to the test subjects within 1 month of diagnosis. Clinical remission was defined in both test and control groups as fasting and postprandial blood glucose levels less than 150 and 200 mg/dl, respectively, and subcutaneous exogenous insulin requirement less than 0.2 U/kg/day for more than 4 weeks.

Table 5.2 shows the data obtained in this pilot study, which has now been in progress for a period of approximately 1 year. In the BCG-treated group, clinical remission was achieved in 11 patients out of 17 (65%). Six patients out of 17 (35%) have met the criteria for remission within 4 weeks of diagnosis, 4 patients (23%) 8 weeks after diagnosis, and 1 patient (6%) 12 weeks after the onset of the disease. Two BCG-treated patients are still in remission (duration range 1–6 months). No side effects were reported. In the untreated control group, only 2 patients in 29 (7%) achieved clinical remission, one at 4 weeks after diagnosis and the other at 12. In this group the first patient met the criteria for remission for 10 months and the second for 3 months. We conclude from these data that BCG vaccination can significantly alter the pathogenesis of IDDM in newly diagnosed type I diabetic patients ($P < .0001$ BCG vs control group, Fisher's test).

This report is consistent with the animal data and provides evidence that BCG vaccination could be effective in modifying the pathogenesis of diabetes in humans. The value of this promising and benign procedure requires further careful study, but a safe immunomodulatory intervention for diabetes may be at hand.

Acknowledgments

This work was supported in part by grant DK46621 from the U.S. Public Health Service.

References

1. Gepts W. Pathologic anatomy of the pancreas in juvenile diabetes mellitus. *Diabetes.* 1965; 14:619–633.
2. Gepts W, Lecompte PM. The pancreatic islets in diabetes. *Am J Med.* 1981; 70:105–115.
3. Sibley RK, Sutherland DER, Goetz F, Michael AF. Recurrent diabetes mellitus in the pancreas iso- and allograft; a light and electron microscopic and immunohistochemical analysis of four cases. *Lab Invest.* 1985; 53:132–144.
4. Santamaria P, Nakhleh RE, Sutherland DE, Barbosa JJ. Characterization of T lymphocytes infiltrating human pancreas allograft affected by isletitis and recurrent diabetes. *Diabetes.* 1992; 41:53–61.
5. Dupre J, Stiller CR, Gent M, Donner A, von Graffenried B, Heinrichs D, Jenner M, Keown P, Mahon J, Martell R, Momah CI, Murphy G, Rodger NW, Wolfe BM. Clinical trials of cyclosporin in IDDM. *Diabetes Care.* 1988; 11(Suppl. 1):37–44.
6. Bottazzo GF, Florin-Christensen A, Doniach D. Islet cell antibodies in diabetes mellitus with autoimmune polyendocrine deficiencies. *Lancet.* 1974; 2:1279–1282.
7. Palmer JP, Asplin CM, Clemons P, Lyen K, Tatpati O, Raghu PK, Paquette TL. Insulin antibodies in insulin-dependent diabetes before insulin treatment. *Science.* 1983; 222:1337–1339.
8. Baekkeskov S, Aanstoot HJ, Christgau S, Reetz A, Solimena M, Cascalho M, Folli F, Richter-Olesen H, De Camilli P. Identification of the 64K autoantigen in insulin-dependent diabetes as the GABA-synthesizing enzyme glutamic acid decarboxylase. *Nature.* 1990; 347:151–156.
9. Pietropaolo M, Castano L, Babu S, Buelow R, Kuo Y-LS, Martin S, Martin A, Powers AC, Prochazka M, Naggert J, Leiter EH, Eisenbarth GS. Islet cell autoantigen 69 kD (ICA69) molecular cloning and characterization of a novel diabetes-associated autoantigen. *J Clin Invest.* 1993; 92:359–371.
10. Eisenbarth GS. Type I diabetes mellitus: a chronic autoimmune disease. *N Engl J Med.* 1986; 314:1360–1368.
11. Dotta F, Eisenbarth GS. Type I diabetes mellitus: a predictable autoimmune disease with interindividual variation in the rate of β cell destruction. *Clin Immunol Immunopathol.* 1989; 50:585–595.

12. Ziegler AG, Herskowitz RD, Jackson RA, Soeldner JS, Eisenbarth GS. Predicting type I diabetes. *Diabetes Care.* 1990; 13:762–775.
13. Makino S, Kunimoto K, Muraoka Y, Mizushima Y, Katagiri K, Tochino Y. Breeding of a non-obese, diabetic strain of mice. *Exp Anim.* 1980; 29:1–13.
14. Like A, Rossini A, Guberski D, Appel M. Spontaneous diabetes mellitus: reversal and prevention in the BB/W rat with antiserum to rat lymphocytes. *Science.* 1979; 206:1421–1423.
15. Koevary S, Rossini A, Stoller W, Chick W. Passive transfer of diabetes in the BB/W rat. *Science.* 1983; 220:727–728.
16. Ogawa M, Maruyama T, Hasegawa T, Kanaya T, Kobayashi F, Tochino Y, Uda H. The inhibitory effect of neonatal thymectomy on the incidence of insulitis in non-obese-diabetic (NOD) mice. *Biomed Res.* 1985; 6:103–105.
17. Makino S, Harada M, Kishimoto Y, Hayashi Y. Absence of insulitis and overt diabetes in athymic nude mice with NOD genetic background. *Exp Anim.* 1986; 35:495–498.
18. Bendelac A, Carnaud C, Boitard C, Bach JF. Syngeneic transfer of autoimmune diabetes from diabetic NOD mice to healthy neonates. Requirement for both L3T4+ and lyt-2+ T cells. *J Exp Med.* 1987; 166:823–832.
19. Miller BJ, Appel MC, O'Neil JJ, Wicker LS. Both the lyt-2+ and L3T4+ T cell subsets are required for the transfer of diabetes in nonobese diabetic mice. *J Immunol.* 1988; 140:52–58.
20 Wang Y, Pontesilli O, Gill RG, La Rosa FG, Lafferty KJ. The role of CD4+ and CD8+ T cells in the destruction of islet grafts by spontaneously diabetic mice. *Proc Natl Acad Sci USA.* 1991; 88:527–531.
21. Charlton B, Mandel TE. Progression from insulitis to β-cell destruction in NOD mouse requires L3T4+ T lymphocytes. *Diabetes.* 1988; 37:1108–1112.
22. Nagata M, Yokono K, Hayakawa M, Kawase Y, Hatamori N, Ogawa W, Yonezawa K, Shii K, Baba S. Destruction of pancreatic islet cells by cytotoxic T lymphocytes in nonobese diabetic mice. *J Immunol.* 1989; 143:1155–1162.
23. Lafferty KJ, Prowse SJ, Simeonovic CJ, Warren HS. Immunobiology of tissue transplantation: a return to the passenger leukocyte concept. *Annu Rev Immunol.* 1983; 1:143–173.
24. Rosenberg AS, Mizuochi T, Singer A. Analysis of T-cell subsets in rejection of K^b mutant skin allografts differing at class I MHC. *Nature.* 1986; 322:829–831.
25. Hao L, Wang Y, Gill RG, Lafferty KJ. CD4 T cells and allograft rejection. *Transplant Proc.* 1988; 20:56–60.
26. Lafferty KJ, Cooley MA, Woolnough F, Walker KZ. Thyroid allograft immunogenicity is reduced after a period in organ culture. *Science.* 1975; 188:259–261.
27. Lafferty KJ, Bootes A, Dart G, Talmage DW. Effect of organ culture on the survival of thyroid allografts in mice. *Transplantation.* 1976; 22:138–149.
28. Prowse SJ, Steele EJ, Lafferty KJ. Islet allografting without immunosuppression: Reversal of insulitis-associated diabetes and a case of spontaneous juvenile onset diabetes in mice. *Aust J Exp Biol Med Sci.* 1982; 60:619–627.
29. Haskins K, Portas M, Bradley B, Wegmann D, Lafferty K. T-lymphocyte clone specific for pancreatic islet antigen. *Diabetes.* 1988; 37:1444–1448.
30. Haskins K, Portas M, Bergman B, Lafferty K, Bradley B. Pancreatic islet-specific T-cell clones from nonobese diabetic mice. *Proc Natl Acad Sci USA.* 1989; 86:8000–8004.
31. Haskins K, McDuffie M. Acceleration of diabetes in young NOD mice with a CD4+ islet-specific T cell clone. *Science.* 1990; 249:1433–1436.

32. Bradley BJ, Wang Y, Lafferty KJ, Haskins K. In vivo activity of an islet-reactive T-cell clone. *J Autoimmun.* 1990; 3:449–456.
33. Wegmann DR, Shehadeh N, Lafferty KJ, Norbury-Glaser M, Gill RG, Daniel D. Establishment of islet-specific T-cell lines and clones from islet isografts placed in spontaneously diabetic NOD mice. *J Autoimmun.* 1993; 6:517–527.
34. Bradley BJ, Haskins K, La Rosa FG, Lafferty KJ. CD8 T cells are not required for islet destruction induced by a CD4+ islet-specific T cell clone. *Diabetes.* 1992; 41:1603–1608.
35. Hao L, Wang Y, Gill RG, La Rosa FG, Talmage DW, Lafferty KJ. Role of γ-interferon in islet allograft rejection: class I MHC antigen induction. *Transplant Proc.* 1989; 21:2697–2699.
36. Hao L, Wang Y, Gill RG, La Rosa FG, Talmage DW, Lafferty KJ. Role of lymphokine in islet allograft rejection. *Transplantation.* 1990; 49:609–614.
37. Mosmann TR, Cherwinski H, Bond MW, Giedlin MA, Coffman RL. Two types of murine helper T cell clones. I. Definition according to profiles of lymphokine activities and secreted proteins. *J Immunol.* 1986; 136:2348–2357.
38. Mosmann TR, Coffman RL. TH1 and TH2 cells: different patterns of lymphokine secretion lead to different functional properties. *Annu Rev Immunol.* 1989; 7:145–173.
39. Mandrup-Poulsen T, Bendtzen K, Nielsen J, Bendixen G, Nerup J. Cytokines cause functional and structural damage to isolated islets of Langerhans. *Allergy.* 1985; 538:1–6.
40. Bendtzen K, Mandrup-Poulsen T, Nerup J, Nielsen JH, Dinarello CA, Svenson M. Cytotoxicity of human p17 interleukin-1 for pancreatic islets of Langerhans. *Science.* 1986; 232:1545–1547.
41. Mandrup-Poulsen T, Spinas GA, Prowse SJ, Hansen BS, Jorgensen DW, Bendtzen K, Nielsen JH, Nerup J. Islet cytotoxicity of interleukin 1: Influence of culture conditions and islet donor characteristics. *Diabetes.* 1987; 36:641–647.
42. Mandrup-Poulsen T, Egeberg J, Nerup J, Bendtzen K, Nielsen JH, Dinarello CA. Ultrastructural studies of time-course and cellular specificity of interleukin-1 mediated islet cytotoxicity. *Acta Pathol Microbiol Immunol Scand.* 1987; 95:55–63.
43. Wogensen L, Nerup J, Helqvist S, Pociot F, Johannesen J, Mandrup-Poulsen T. Intra-peritoneal administration of interleukin-1β induces impaired insulin release from the perfused rat pancreas. *J Autoimmun.* 1990; 7:1–12.
44. Pukel C, Baquerizo H, Rabinovitch A. Destruction of rat islet cell monolayers by cytokines. Synergistic interactions of interferon-γ, tumor necrosis factor, lymphotoxin, and interleukin-1. *Diabetes.* 1988; 37:133–136.
45. Rabinovitch A, Sumoski W, Rajotte RV, Warnock GL. Cytotoxic effects of cytokines on human pancreatic islet cells in monolayer culture. *J Clin Endocrinol Metab.* 1990; 71:152–156.
46. Ling Z, In't Veld PA, Pipeleers DG. Interaction of interleukin-1 with islet β-cells. *Diabetes.* 1993; 42:56–65.
47. Hamaguchi K, Leiter EH. Comparison of cytokine effects on mouse pancreatic α-cell and β-cell lines: viability, secretory function, and MHC antigen expression. *Diabetes.* 1990; 39: 415–425.
48. Pujol-Borrell R, Todd I, Doshi M, Bottazzo GF, Sutton R, Gray D, Adolf GR, Feldman M. HLA class II induction in human islet cells by interferon-gamma plus tumor necrosis or lymphotoxin. *Nature.* 1987; 326:304–306.
49. Hanafusa T, Fujino-Kurihara H, Miyazaki A, Yamada K, Nakajima H, Miyagawa J, Kono N, Tarui S. Expression of class II major histocompatibility complex antigens on pancreatic β cells in the NOD mouse. *Diabetologia.* 1987; 30:104–108.

50. Bottazzo GF, Pujol-Borrell R, Hanafusa T. Role of aberrant HLA-DR expression and antigen presentation in induction of endocrine autoimmunity. *Lancet.* 1983; 2:1115–1118.

51. Markmann J, Lo D, Naji A, Palmiter RD, Brinster RL, Heber-Katz E. Antigen presenting function of class II MHC expressing pancreatic beta cells. *Nature.* 1988; 336:476–479.

52. Hanninen A, Jalkanen S, Salmi M, Toikkanen S, Nikolakaros G, Simell O. Macrophages, T cell receptor usage, and endothelial cell activation in the pancreas at the onset of insulin-dependent diabetes mellitus. *J Clin Invest.* 1992; 90:1901–1910.

53. Jarpe AJ, Hickman MR, Anderson JT, Winter WE, Peck AB. Flow cytometric enumeration of mononuclear cell populations infiltrating the islets of Langerhans in prediabetic NOD mice: Development of a model of autoimmune insulitis for type I diabetes. *Reg Immunol.* 1991; 3:305–317.

54. Jiang Z, Woda BA. Cytokine gene expression in the islets of the diabetic BioBreeding/Worcester rat. *J Immunol.* 1991; 146:2990–2994.

55. Shehadeh NN, LaRosa F, Lafferty KJ. Altered cytokine activity in adjuvant inhibition of autoimmune diabetes. *J Autoimmun.* 1993; 6:291–300.

56. Foulis AK, McGill M, Farquharson MA. Insulitis in type I (insulin-dependent) diabetes mellitus in man—macrophages, lymphocytes, and interferon-γ containing cells. *J Pathol.* 1991; 165:97–103.

57. Wang Y, Goodman M, Lumerman J, Sussman KE, Dahl R, Lafferty KJ, Draznin B. In vivo administration of interleukin-1 inhibits glucose-stimulated insulin release. *Diabetes Res Clin Prac.* 1989; 7:205–211.

58. Jacob CO, Asiso S, Michie SA, McDevitt HO, Acha-Orbea H. Prevention of diabetes in nonobese diabetic mice by tumor necrosis factor (TNF): similarities between TNF-α and interleukin-1. *Proc Natl Acad Sci USA.* 1990; 87:968–972.

59. Wilson CA, Jacobs C, Baker P, Baskin DG, Dower S, Lernmark A, Toivola B, Vertrees S, Wilson D. IL-1β modulation of spontaneous autoimmune diabetes and thyroiditis in the BB rat. *J Immunol.* 1990; 144:3784–3788.

60 Satoh J, Seino H, Abo T, Tanaka S, Shintani S, Ohta S, Tamura K, Sawai T, Nobunaga T, Oteki T, Kumagai K, Toyota T. Recombinant human tumor necrosis factor α suppresses autoimmune diabetes in nonobese diabetic mice. *J Clin Invest.* 1989; 84:1345–1348.

61. Satoh J, Seino H, Shintani S, Tanaka S-I, Ohteki T, Masuda T, Nobunaga T, Toyota T. Inhibition of type I diabetes in BB rats with recombinant human tumor necrosis factor-alpha. *J Immunol.* 1990; 145:1395–1399.

62. Gordon C, Wofsy D. Effects of recombinant murine tumor necrosis factor-α on immune function. *J Immunol.* 1990; 144:1753–1758.

63. Seino H, Takahashi K, Satoh J, Zhu XP, Sagara M, Masuda T, Nobunaga T, Funahashi I, Kajikawa T, Toyota T. Prevention of autoimmune diabetes with lymphotoxin in NOD mice. *Diabetes.* 1993; 42:398–404.

64. Rapoport MJ, Jaramillo A, Zipris D, Lazarus AH, Serreze DV, Leiter EH, Cyopick P, Danska JS, Delovitch TL. Interleukin 4 reverses T cell proliferative unresponsiveness and prevents the onset of diabetes in nonobese diabetic mice. *J Exp Med.* 1993; 178:87–99.

65. Sarvetnick N, Liggitt D, Pitts SL, Hansen SE, Stewart TA. Insulin-dependent diabetes mellitus induced in transgenic mice by ectopic expression of class II MHC and interferon-gamma. *Cell.* 1988; 52:773–782.

66. Sarvetnick N, Shizuru J, Liggitt D, Martin L, McIntyre B, Gregory A, Parslow T,

Stewart T. Loss of pancreatic islet tolerance induced by β-cell expression of interferon-γ. *Nature.* 1990; 346:844–847.

67. Higuchi Y, Herrera P, Muniesa P, Huarte J, Belin D, Ohashi P, Aichele P, Orci L, Vassalli JD, Vassalli P. Expression of a tumor necrosis factor α transgene in murine pancreatic β cells results in severe and permanent insulitis without evolution towards diabetes. *J Exp Med.* 1992; 176:1719–1731.
68. Picarella D, Kratz A, Li CB, Ruddle N, Flavell RA. The expression of TNFα and TNFβ in the pancreas of transgenic mice results in an islet-specific inflammatory response. *Diabetes.* 1992; 41(Suppl. 1):96A.
69. Wogensen L, Huang X, Sarvetnick N. Leukocyte extravasation into the pancreatic tissue in transgenic mice expressing interleukin 10 in the islets of Langerhans. *J Exp Med.* 1993; 178:175–185.
70. Stewart TA, Hultgren B, Huang X, Pitts-Meek S, Hully J, MacLachlan NJ. Induction of type I diabetes by interferon-γ in transgenic mice. *Science.* 1993; 260:1942–1946.
71. Foulis AK, Farquharson MA, Meager A. Immunoreactive α-interferon in insulin-secreting β cells in type 1 diabetes mellitus. *Lancet.* 1987; 2:1423–1427.
72. Gendelman HE, Baca LM, Kubrak CA, Genis P, Burrous S, Friedman RM, Jacobs D, Meltzer MS. Induction of IFN-α in peripheral blood mononuclear cells by HIV-infected monocytes. Restricted antiviral activity of the HIV-induced IFN. *J Immunol.* 1992; 148:422–429.
73. Serreze DV, Leiter DH. Defective activation of T supressor cell function in nonobese diabetic mice. *J Immunol.* 1988; 11: 3801–3807.
74. Sadick MD, Heinzel FP, Holaday BJ, Pu RT, Dawkins RS, Locksley RM. Cure of murine leishmaniasis with anti-interleukin 4 monoclonal antibody. *J Exp Med.* 1990; 171:115–127.
75. Chatelain R, Varkila K, Coffman RL. IL-4 Induces a Th2 response in Leishmania major-infected mice. *J Immunol.* 1992; 148:1182–1187.
76. Silva JS, Morrissey PJ, Grabstein KH, Mohler KM, Anderson D, Reed SG. Interleukin 10 and interferon γ regulation of experimental *Trypanosoma cruzi* infection. *J Exp Med.* 1992; 175:169–174.
77. Sadelain MWJ, Qin H-Y, Lauzon J, Singh B. Prevention of type 1 diabetes in NOD mice by adjuvant immunotherapy. *Diabetes.* 1990; 39:583–589.
78. Sadelain MWJ, Qin H-Y, Sumoski W, Parfrey N, Singh B, Rabinovitch A. Prevention of diabetes in the BB rat by early immunotherapy using Freund's adjuvant. *J Autoimmun.* 1990; 3:671–680.
79. McInerney MF, Pek SB, Thomas DW. Prevention of insultitis and diabetes onset by treatment with complete Freund's adjuvant in NOD mice. *Diabetes.* 1991; 40:715–725.
80. Ulaeto D, Lacy PE, Kipnis DM, Kanagawa O, Unanue ER. A T-cell dormant state in the autoimmune process of nonobese diabetic mice treated with complete Freund's adjuvant. *Proc Natl Acad Sci USA.* 1992; 89:3927–3931.
81. Qin H-Y, Sadelain MWJ, Hitchon C, Lauzon J, Singh B. Complete Freund's adjuvant-induced T cells prevent the development and adoptive transfer of diabetes in nonobese diabetic mice. *J Immunol.* 1993; 150:2072–2080.
82. Lakey JRT, Wang T, Warnock GL, Singh B, Rajotte RV. Prevention of recurrence of insulin-dependent diabetes mellitus in islet cell–transplanted diabetic NOD mice using adjuvant therapy. *Transplant Proc.* 1992; 24:2848.
83. Wang T, Singh B, Warnock GL, Rajotte RV. Prevention of recurrence of IDDM in islet-transplanted diabetic NOD mice by adjuvant immunotherapy. *Diabetes.* 1992; 41:114–117.

84. Shehadeh NN, Calcinaro F, Bradley B, Bruchlim I, Vardi P, Lafferty KJ. Effect of adjuvant therapy on development of diabetes in mouse and man. *Lancet.* 1994; 343:706–707.
85. Smith RJ, Epps DE, Justen JM, Sam LM, Wynalda MA, Fitzpatrick FA, Yein FS. Human neutrophil activation with interleukin-1: a role for intracellular calcium and arachidonic acid lipoxygenation. *Biochem Pharmacol.* 1987; 36:3851–3858.
86. McDaniel ML, Hughes JH, Wolf BA, Easom RA, Turk JW. Descriptive and mechanistic considerations of interleukin 1 and insulin secretion. *Diabetes.* 1988; 37:1311–1315.
87. Dayer-Metroz MD, Wollheim CB, Seckinger P, Deyer JM. A natural interleukin-1 (IL-1) inhibitor counteracts the inhibitory effect of IL-1 on insulin production in cultured rat pancreatic islets. *J Autoimmun.* 1989; 2:163–171.
88. Sandler S, Bendtzen K, Hakan-Borg LA, Eizirik DL, Strandell E, Welsh N. Studies on the mechanisms causing inhibition of insulin secretion in rat pancreatic islets exposed to human interleukin-1β indicate a perturbation in the mitochondrial function. *Endocrinology.* 1989; 124:1492–1501.
89. Okamoto H. Regulation of proinsulin synthesis in pancreatic islets and a new aspect to insulin-dependent diabetes. *Mol Cell Biochem.* 1981; 37:43–61.
90. Halliwell B. Oxygen is poisonous: the nature and medical importance of oxygen radicals. *Med Lab Sci.* 1984; 41:1–15.
91. Okamoto H. The role of poly (ADP-ribose) synthetase in the development of insulin-dependent diabetes and islet β-cell regeneration. *Biomed Biochim Acta.* 1985; 44:15–20.
92. Marklund SL. Regulation by cytokines of extracellular superoxide dismutase and other superoxide dismutase isoenzymes in fibroblasts. *J Biol Chem.* 1992; 6696–6701.
93. Fantone JC, Ward PA. Role of oxygen-derived free radicals and metabolites in leukocyte-dependent inflammatory reactions. *Am J Pathol.* 1982; 107:397–418.
94. Asayama K, Kooy NW, Burr IM. Effect of vitamin E deficiency and selenium deficiency on insulin secretory reserve and free radical scavenging systems in islets: decrease of islet manganosuperoxide dismutase. *J Lab Clin Med.* 1986; 107:459–464.
95. Malaisse WJ, Malaisse-Lagae F, Sener A, Pipeleers DG. Determinants of the selective toxicity of alloxan to the pancreatic β cell. *Proc Natl Acad Sci USA.* 1982; 79:927–930.
96. Pieper GM, Turk M, Roza AM, Felix CC, Kalyanaraman B. Detection and characterization by electron spin resonance (ESR) spectroscopy of DMPO-hydroxyl adduct formation in fresh and cultured islets. *Diabetes.* 1992; 41(Suppl. 1):158A.
97. Lazarus SS, Shapiro SH. Influence of nicotinamide and pyridine nucleotides on streptozotocin and alloxan-induced pancreatic β cell cytotoxicity. *Diabetes.* 1973; 22:499–506.
98. Uchigata Y, Yamamoto H, Nagai H, Okamoto H. Effect of poly (ADP-ribose) synthetase inhibitor administration to rats before and after injection of alloxan and streptozotocin on islet proinsulin synthesis. *Diabetes.* 1983; 32:316–318.
99. Yamada K, Nonaka K, Hanafusa T, Miyazaki A, Toyoshima H, Tarui S. Preventive and theraputic effects of large-dose nicotinamide injections on diabetes associated with insulitis: an observation in nonobese diabetic (NOD) mice. *Diabetes.* 1982; 31:749–753.
100. Prowse SJ, Lafferty KJ, Nomikos IN, Carotenuto P. The pathogenesis of spontaneous diabetes. *Ann Inst Pasteur Immunol.* 1986; 137D:459–462.
101. Nokimos IN, Prowse SJ, Carotenuto P, Lafferty KJ. Combined treatment with

nicotinamide and desferrioxamine prevents islet allograft destruction in NOD mice. *Diabetes.* 1986; 35:1302–1304.

102. Nokimos IN, Wang Y, Lafferty KJ. Involvement of O_2 radicals in "autoimmune" diabetes. *Immunol Cell Biol.* 1989; 67:85–87.
103. Dimmeler S, Lottspeich BB. Nitric oxide causes ADP-ribosylation and inhibition of glyceraldehyde-3-phosphate dehydrogenase. *J Biol Chem.* 1992; 267:16771–16774.
104. Moncada S, Palmer RMJ, Higgs EA. Nitric oxide: physiology, pathophysiology, and pharmacology. *Pharmacol Rev.* 1991; 43:109–142.
105. Nguyen T, Brunson D, Crespi CL, Penman BW, Wishnok JS, Tannenbaum SR. DNA damage and mutation in human cells exposed to nitric oxide in vitro. *Proc Natl Acad Sci USA.* 1992; 89:3030–3034.
106. Corbett JA, Wang JL, Hughes JH, Wolf BA, Sweetland MA, Lancaster JR, Jr., McDaniel ML. Nitric oxide and cyclic GMP formation induced by interleukin 1β in islets of Langerhans—evidence for an effector role of nitric oxide in islet dysfunction. *Biochem J.* 1992; 286:1–7.
107. Corbett JA, McDaniel ML. Perspectives in diabetes: does nitric oxide mediate autoimmune destruction of β-cells? Possible therapeutic interventions in IDDM. *Diabetes.* 1992; 41:897–903.
108. Southern C, Schulster D, Green IC. Inhibition of insulin secretion by interleukin-1β and tumor necrosis factor-α via an L-arginine-dependent nitric oxide generation mechanism. *FEBS Lett.* 1990; 276:42–44.
109. Laychock SG, Modica ME, Cavanaugh CT. L-arginine stimulates cyclic guanosine 3′,5′-monophosphate formation in rat islets of Langerhans and RINm5F insulinoma cells: evidence for L-arginine:nitric oxide synthase. *Endocrinology.* 1991; 129:3043–3052.
110. Corbett JA, Wang JL, Sweetland MA, Lancaster JR Jr., McDaniel ML. Interleukin-1β induces the formation of nitric oxide by β-cells purified from rodent islets of Langerhans. Evidence for the β-cell as a source and site of action of nitric acid. *J Clin Invest.* 1992; 90:2384–2391.
111. Kronke K, Kolb-Bachofen V, Berschick B, Bukart V, Kolb H. Activated macrophages kill pancreatic syngeneic islet cells via arginine-dependent nitric oxide generation. *Biochem Biophys Res Commun.* 1991; 175:752–758.
112. Kolb H, Kolb-Bachofen V. Nitric oxide: a pathogenic factor in autoimmunity. *Immunol Today.* 1992; 13:157–160.
113. Feshel K, Jalowy A, Qi S, Burkart V, Hartmann B, Kolb H. Islet cell DNA is a target of inflammatory attack by nitric oxide. *Diabetes.* 1993; 42:496–500.
114. Mandrup-Poulsen T, Corbett JA, McDaniel ML, Nerup J. What are the types and cellular sources of free radicals in the pathogenesis of type I (insulin-dependent) diabetes mellitus? *Diabetologia.* 1993; 36:470–473.
115. Corbett JA, Sweetland MA, Wang JL, Lancaster JRJ, McDaniel ML. Nitric oxide mediates cytokine-induced inhibition of insulin secretion by human islets of Langerhans. *Proc Natl Acad Sci USA.* 1993; 90:1731–1735.
116. Calcinaro F, Hao L, Chase HP, Klingensmith G, Lafferty KJ. Detection of cell-mediated immunity in type I diabetes mellitus. *J Immunol.* 1992; 5:137–147.

6

The Immunobiology of Pancreatic Islet Transplantation

R. G. Gill

Insulin-dependent diabetes mellitus is the result of autoimmune destruction of pancreatic islet beta cells.[1] As such, the only actual cure for this irreversible loss of islet tissue is through the replacement of insulin-producing capacity. Presently, this can be accomplished by the transplantation of either the whole pancreas organ or isolated pancreatic islets. Currently, there is controversy over the relative utility of whole pancreas versus islet transplantation in insulin-dependent diabetes. As a clinical practice, pancreas grafting has a current advantage over islet transplantation in terms of the proportion of recipients achieving a significant period of insulin independence.[2,3] However, islet transplantation has shown increasing evidence of clinical success.[4–7] Further, there are important future advantages to islet transplantation such as the potential for modifying tissue immunogenicity (immunomodulation), the application of various forms of tissue encapsulation to avoid immune recognition (immunoisolation), the establishment of cryopreserved tissue banks, and the potential for grafting in immune-privileged sites. Islet grafting would also provide for the application of xenografting, thus overcoming the shortage of available allogeneic tissue.

Type I diabetes represents a unique problem for the field of transplantation. The rationale for pancreatic islet grafting is to prevent the debilitating complications associated with the disease process. Indeed, islet transplantation has been shown to prevent or arrest diabetic complications.[8–10] However, unlike other conditions of end-stage organ failure where transplantation is required to sustain life, diabetes is not immediately life-threatening as a result of the advent of exogenous insulin therapy. Thus, for type I diabetes, the risks associated with current regimens of immunosuppression used in transplantation, such as nephrotoxicity, opportunistic infections, and neoplasia, certainly rival the consequences of disease-associated complications. Therefore, the criteria for islet transplantation in diabetic recipients prior to the manifestations of disease complications must be more stringent than those for patients with other forms of organ failure. This problem is reflected by the current status of clinical islet transplantation, where islet grafts are usually performed in diabetic patients receiving simultaneous solid organ grafts (usually kidney) with concomitant immunosuppression.[11] The future goal of islet transplantation, however, must be the grafting of islets in the diabetic recipient prior to the onset of disease complications, using minimal host immunosuppression. As such, the purpose of this chapter is to examine the immunological problems encountered in islet transplantation.

Three important obstacles hamper the routine use of islet grafting in diabetes. Two of these barriers are due to immune-mediated damage to the graft: (1) *transplantation immunity*, resulting in graft rejection, and (2) *disease recurrence*, the re-enactment of the underlying autoimmune pathogenesis that can destroy transplanted islet tissue both in humans[12] and animal models of autoimmune diabetes, the nonobese diabetic (NOD) mouse[13] and the Bio Breeding (BB) rat.[14] The nature of disease pathogenesis in islet transplants is a focus of another contribution to this volume and so will not be primarily addressed here. A third, more logistical problem in islet transplantation results from the shortage of available clinical tissue for transplantation. This problem requires the consideration of tissue from other species (xenografts) as a potential source of donor material. Understanding of the processes resulting in islet allograft or xenograft destruction will be crucial for developing future strategies to circumvent these responses.

Pancreatic Islet Allografting: The Allograft Paradox

The Two-Signal Hypothesis for T Cell Activation

According to the classic view of allograft immunity, major histocompatibility complex (MHC) antigens were inherently strong immunogens; that is, binding of the MHC molecule by the antigen-specific receptor directly triggered T cell activation.[15] Although allograft rejection clearly represents a response to transplantation antigens, especially MHC antigens, there has been a persistent problem with this classic view. Early attempts to isolate and characterize transplantation antigens found them to be quite weak immunogens.[16] Later studies of Batchelor and coworkers[17] demonstrated that MHC antigens, either class I or class II, isolated from the cell surface were poor immunogens. These observations lead us to a *transplantation paradox*: allograft immunity represents a violent response to antigens that are inherently weak immunogens.

The solution to this paradox was provided by the proposition of Lafferty and Cunningham that two signals were required for T cell activation,[18] a concept derived from the original two-signal model for self-nonself discrimination

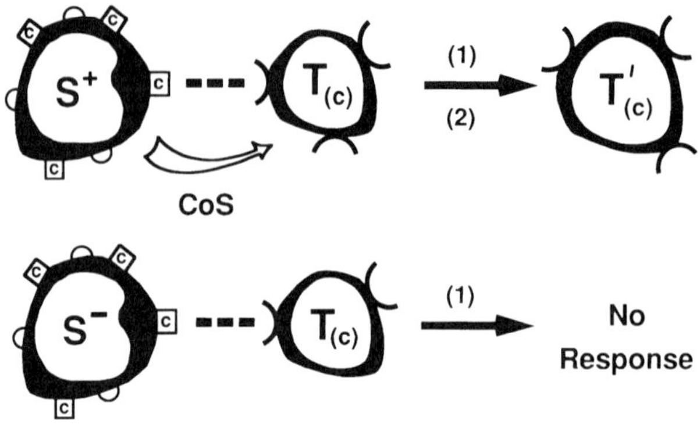

Figure 6.1. The stimulator cell model. Alloantigens presented by an S^+ cell will provide a source of both signals (antigen and costimulator) required for T cell activation (T cell specificity indicated by the parentheses). Alloantigen presented on the surface of an S^- cell will not be directly immunogenic because these cells cannot provide a source of the second signal. According to this model, costimulator activity is triggered by engagement of a control structure ('C') on the surface of the S^+ cell.

developed by the Bretscher and Cohn model.[19] According to the Lafferty/Cunningham model, signal one (antigen) was provided by binding of the T cell receptor, and signal two was provided by an inductive molecule, or *costimulator* (CoS), produced by a metabolically active antigen-presenting cell (APC), or *stimulator* cell (Fig. 6.1). Although previous studies show that cytokines can demonstrate CoS activity in vitro,[20] recent work has brought attention to the role of accessory molecule interactions between T cells and APC involved in providing costimulatory signals required for T cell activation. Key cell-surface molecules involved in this process are CD28[21] and CTLA-4[22] expressed by T cells interacting with the B7/BB1 molecule expressed by APCs and activated B cells.[23] Other accessory molecules expressed by APCs, such as ICAM-1 and LFA-3,[24] may also have important costimulatory functions. Regardless of the exact nature of costimulatory signals, cells capable of exhibiting CoS activity will have a stimulatory (S^+) phenotype, whereas other cells, such as tissue parenchymal cells, that express the same antigens but do not produce CoS activity, will have a nonstimulatory phenotype (S^-).

The role of MHC in this process is that of a *control* structure; that is, CoS activity is triggered by engagement of MHC on the surface of an S^+ cell. Experimental evidence supporting the role of MHC as a control molecule comes from a study by Nabavi and coworkers that indicates that class II MHC signaling triggers the surface expression of the costimulatory molecule B7.[25] This two-signal model provides a solution to the transplantation paradox. The immunogenicity of MHC antigen is not due to its inherent antigenic properties but rather to its *functional* role as a control structure for the expression of CoS activity. This model predicts that MHC antigens will only be immunogenic while on the surface of metabolically active S^+ cells; isolated MHC antigens or MHC antigens on the surface of S^- cells will not be immunogenic. The significant contribution of this two-signal hypothesis to transplantation biology is the concept that alloantigen alone is not the barrier to allografting. Rather, tissue immunogenicity will be a function of S^+ cells, or "passenger leukocytes," resident within the graft.[26]

Alteration of Tissue Immunogenicity

The notion that alloantigen presentation between S^+ and S^- cells within the graft represent qualitatively different forms of antigen presentation led back to an early concept that graft immunogenicity can be reduced by appropriate tissue pretreatment.[16] That is, selective depletion of S^+ cells within the graft should lead to prolonged graft acceptance. Tissue pretreatment has been strikingly successful for facilitating allograft acceptance of endocrine tissues. Early work indicated that pretreatment of thyroid tissues in 95% O_2 culture would facilitate long-term graft acceptance in non-immunosuppressed, allogeneic recipient mice.[27] This technique later was applied for the modification of pancreatic islet allograft immunogenicity.[28] Grafting experimentally induced diabetic mice with untreated islet allografts results in initial return to euglycemia followed by a rapid return to hyperglycemia due to graft rejection. Following organ culture in 95% O_2 for 7 days, islet allografts survive and function indefinitely in recipient mice.[28] Application of 95% O_2 culture has also allowed successful islet allografting in rats[29] and in outbred mice,[30] though short-term immunosuppression with cyclosporin A was necessary for long-term graft survival in this later study.

A variety of other tissue pretreatment techniques have likewise led to long-term islet allograft acceptance. Graft pretreatment with low-temperature culture,[31] anti-Ia or dendritic cell antibodies,[32–34] ultraviolet irradiation,[35] and low pH media[36] have all facilitated islet allograft acceptance. Hegre and coworkers[37] have shown that perinatal rat islets isolated by in vitro cultivation are accepted in nonimmunosuppressed, allogeneic recipients. Further, appropriate graft pretreatment techniques have led to prolonged graft acceptance of a variety of tissues including thyroid and parathyroid,[27,38,39] ovarian tissue,[40] and keratinocytes.[41] Taken together, a wide range of techniques with a variety of donor-recipient strain combinations indicate that allograft acceptance can be facilitated by appropriate pretreatment of the graft.

Antigenicity versus Immunogenicity of MHC Alloantigens

A key question centers on the mechanism whereby pretreated tissues survive in immunocompetent, allogeneic recipients. Is the immunogenicity of cultured grafts altered due to the modulation of graft antigens, or by the elimination/inactivation of passenger leukocytes (S^+ cells)? This issue is important in light of the finding that hyperbaric oxygen culture of thyroid tissue leads to reduced antigen expression of the graft.[38,42] Studies by Hullet and coworkers[38] show that thyroid grafts cultured in hyperbaric oxygen survive even in recipient mice primed against donor antigens. These results indicated that the regulation of graft antigen expression may play a role in subsequent graft survival. Although antigen modulation may occur during some forms of organ culture, a number of studies indicate that this modulation is not *necessary* for allograft acceptance. That is, loss of immunogenicity does not require a loss of antigenicity in the graft.

In the late 1970s Batchelor's laboratory addressed this issue of graft immunogenicity versus antigenicity by examining the role of donor antigen expression in long-term kidney allograft survival. These investigators demonstrated that kidney grafts would survive in allogeneic recipients that had been tolerized by a regimen of donor-specific antibody administration.[43] When such long-surviving kidney allografts were transplanted from the primary recipient to a secondary recipient of the same haplotype, the kidney did not elicit a rejection response in the untreated, secondary recipient.[43] The failure of long-surviving kidney grafts to activate a rejection response could not be attributed to a lack of either class I or class II antigen expression in the graft,[44] leading these investigators to conclude that the effect resulted from a gradual replacement of donor-derived passenger leukocytes in the graft with host-derived APC while residing in the primary recipient. Importantly, they showed that immunization with donor strain dendritic cells (a source of S^+ cells) in very low numbers would trigger rejection of the established kidney graft.[44] Clearly, the antigens of the grafted kidney could not elicit alloimmunity but could serve as a target of immune destruction once the animal was primed.

Islet allografts cultured in 95% O_2 also are vulnerable to rejection by active immunization of the recipient.[45] Challenge of the recipient animal with donor-type S^+ cells during the immediate post-transplant period triggers acute rejection of the established islet graft. Active immunization of the host also triggers the rejection of established cultured thyroid[46] and keratinocyte[41] allografts. These results illustrate the distinction between graft antigenicity and immunogenicity; the cultured graft cannot trigger allograft immunity but can serve as a target for immune destruction.

The issue of class II MHC immunogenicity was elegantly examined by Markmann and coworkers.[47] These investigators studied the response to fetal pancreas grafts from transgenic mice expressing a class II MHC alloantigen (I-E) under control of the insulin promoter (ins-I-E), leading to tissue-specific, ectopic expression of the I-E molecule on the surface of pancreatic islet β cells. Importantly, the I-E class II MHC molecule was expressed on islet parenchymal cells and not on hematopoietic (S^+) cells.[48] Despite a high level of expression of the transgene product on the β cell surface, such fetal pancreas grafts did not trigger alloimmunity in I-E^- parental strain mice. However, immunizing recipient mice with I-E^+ spleen cells (a source of S^+ cells) triggered a prompt rejection response to the ins-I-E graft, indicating that the ins-I-E fetal pancreas could serve as a target for immune destruction. What these experiments clearly demonstrated was that the class II MHC antigen was not inherently immunogenic and so was not sufficient to trigger allograft immunity.

LaRosa and Talmage[42] later tested the relationship between donor antigen expression and the survival of cultured thyroid allografts. In these experiments thyroid grafts were cultured in 95% O_2 to reduce tissue immunogenicity. These cultured thyroid grafts were then grafted directly or were pretreated with interferon gamma (IFN-γ) to induce high levels of class I MHC antigen expression on the graft. Whereas fresh (uncultured) thyroid grafts were uniformly rejected, the acceptance of cultured grafts was not altered by IFN-γ treatment of the graft. That is, acceptance of the cultured graft was not due simply to the alteration of antigen expression. Our own experiments using IFN-γ–treated cultured islet allografts also indicate that the enhanced expression of class I MHC molecules on islet tissue does not increase the rejection response (unpublished observations).

Taken together, these varied studies indicate that neither class I nor class II MHC alloantigens are the primary barrier to allografting. Given that the goal of islet transplantation is to eliminate or reduce the immunosuppression of the recipient, tissue pretreatment aimed at eliminating S^+ cells from the graft may, at least in part, be a useful tool in future clinical islet allografting.

Pancreatic Islet Xenografting: the Xenograft Paradox

A major dilemma facing clinical organ and tissue grafting is the shortage of donor tissue for transplantation. This problem requires the consideration of tissues from other species (xenografts) as a potential source of donor material. The classification by Calne[49] denoted xenografts as discordant or concordant based on the presence or absence, respectively, of preformed or natural antibodies against the donor. The presence of such natural antibodies roughly correlates with the phylogenetic disparity between species and is thought to be responsible for the initiation of hyperacute rejection that occurs between discordant species combinations.[50,51] A major target of such natural antibodies appears to be carbohydrate moieties expressed on the xenogeneic vascular endothelium.[52] Although hyperacture rejection presents a major barrier to the survival of anastomosed solid-organ xenografts, neovascularized xenografts—such as skin and cellular transplants—generally do not appear as sensitive to hyperacute rejection but rather involve cellular immunity.[50,53] The relative lack of vulnerability of cellular xenografts to hyperacute rejection is likely due to the fact that the graft vasculature is of *host* rather than donor origin, thus eliminating the vascular target of antibody-mediated hyperacute rejection.[50,51]

Understanding of the cellular immune response to xenogeneic tissues is less clear than is understanding of the allograft response, as illustrated by an important paradox concerning xenoreactivity: Although cellular xenograft immunity in vivo—apart from hyperacute rejection—is generally more vigorous than allograft rejection,[50,53,54] the intensity of the T cell–dependent response to xenogeneic antigen-presenting cells in vitro tends to *decrease* as the phylogenetic disparity between stimulating and responding species increases.[53–57] This hyporeactivity of the interspecies T cell–APC interaction in vitro could be attributed to three primary defects in the response.

1. *Low precursor frequency.* The view that the T cell receptor (TcR) repertoire is positively selected in the thymus using the MHC of the species as a template[58] would leave the possibility that the frequency of xenoreactive T cells might be quite low relative to the high precursor frequency of alloreactive T cells. This possibility would account for the low xenoreactive precursor frequency on a quantitative basis.
2. *Species-specific accessory/co-receptor molecule interactions.* A number of cell-surface molecules, in addition to the antigen-specific TcR, facilitate T cell activation. For example, the CD4 and CD8 co-receptor molecules, which characterize T cell subsets, interact with conserved regions of class I and class II MHC molecules, respectively.[59] Importantly, the interaction of these accessory/co-receptor molecules with their respective ligands can display species specificity. The interaction of CD4 and CD8 with MHC molecules from different species can be quite weak. Although human CD4 is capable of functionally associating with mouse class II,[60] the reciprocal binding of mouse CD4 to human class II is quite weak.[61,62] Further, the association of CD8 with the $\alpha3$ domain of class I MHC also displays species specificity between human and mouse.[63,64]
3. *Species specificity of cytokines required for T cell activation.* A number of cytokines exhibit species specificity/preference such that cytokines necessary for T cell activation may not function across particular species barriers.[55,56] Studies addressing these issues have found that reconstitution of xenoreactivity in vitro can occur through restoring appropriate accessory/co-receptor molecule interactions[62–65] or by the addition of the relevant responder-type cytokines.[55,56] Such studies indicate that the potential frequency of xeno-specific T cells may be fairly high, with the lack of reactivity being due to species-specific interactions that are secondary to the TcR repertoire.

'Direct' Versus 'Indirect' Antigen Presentation

In light of these deficiencies in the xenogeneic T cell–APC interaction, a key question is: how does a low reactivity in vitro account for the violent reactivity in vivo? One solution to this paradox can be inferred by considering the consequence of two pathways of host sensitization by the graft, *direct* (donor APC–dependent) and *indirect* (host APC–dependent) presentation (Fig. 6.2). Direct antigen presentation would be the result of host T cell recognition and activation by donor-derived APC. It is this pathway of activation that is expected to be sensitive to the species-specific interactions required for T cell activation mentioned above. The indirect pathway would involve the processing and presentation of graft antigens by host APCs. Although this indirect (responder APC–dependant) pathway can occur in allorecognition,[66]

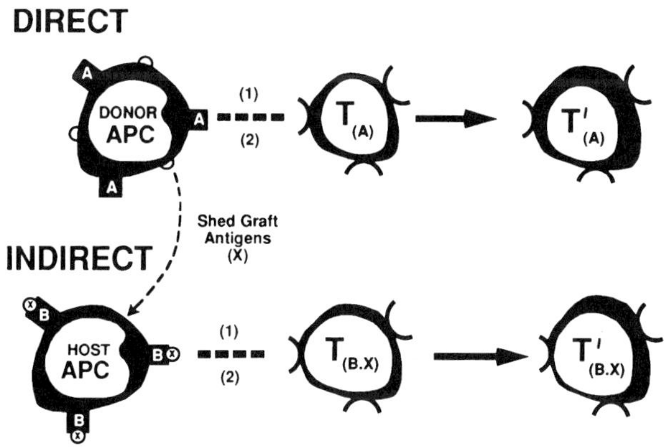

Figure 6.2. Direct versus indirect antigen presentation. *Direct*: Donor-type APCs present antigen ('A') to T cells along with an appropriate second signal (costimulator) required for T cell activation (T cell specificity indicated by the parentheses). Such a T cell will be specific for graft antigens directly on the surface of donor cells. *Indirect*: Graft antigens, generically termed 'x', will be processed by host-type APC of genotype 'B' and presented in association with class II MHC. Responsive T cells will not be directly graft specific but rather specific for graft antigens in association with host class II MHC (specificity 'B.x').

some xenogeneic combinations may depend on this pathway for T cell activation. The operation of the indirect pathway in xenoreactivity is shown by the observation that primary mouse anti-human[67] and human anti-mouse[68] responses in vitro require responder-type APCs. Allogeneic responses, or some xenogeneic combinations such as mouse anti-rat, do not require responder-type APCs.[54]

The function of the indirect (host APC-dependent) pathway may solve the xenograft paradox: Although the xenogeneic APC cannot activate responding T cells via the direct pathway, the antigenic disparity of the xenograft relative to the host might favor a strong response to antigens processed by host APC. This form of xeno-presentation would be expected to activate host CD4 T cells specific for xenogeneic antigens in the context of self class II MHC. The function of this indirect pathway may explain why xenograft rejection is more dependent on CD4 T cells than is allograft rejection in some cases.[69–71]

Role of T Cell Subsets in Islet Graft Rejection: A Central Role for CD4 T Cells

It is clear that both islet allograft[72,73] and xenograft[70,71,74,75] rejection are heavily dependent on the function of CD4 T cells. However, this does not mean that the role of the CD4 cell is the same in each case. Three possible functions for the CD4 T cell can be envisioned in the rejection process (Fig. 6.3): (1) a helper cell for the activation of CD8 T cells, which in turn mediate graft destruction; (2) a helper cell for antibody-producing B cells, leading to a graft-specific antibody response; or (3) an effector cell mediating islet graft

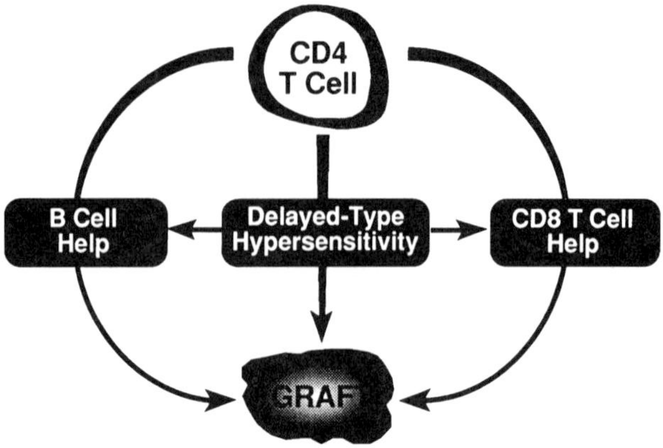

Figure 6.3. Possible roles for class II MHC-restricted CD4 T cells in the rejection response.

destruction by direct interaction with the graft and/or through inflammatory tissue damage.[76,77]

A difference in the role of CD4 T cells in islet xenograft versus allograft immunity is demonstrated by examining the requirement for other lymphocyte subpopulations in these responses. Unlike islet allograft immunity, xenograft immunity does not appear to require class I MHC-restricted CD8 T cells.[71] Our cell transfer studies into severe-combined-immune-deficient C.B.17*scid* mice show that although CD4 T cells are both necessary and sufficient to reconstitute these animals for islet xenograft immunity, islet allograft immunity requires both CD4 and CD8 T cells (Wolf et al, in preparation). B cells were not required for either response. Furthermore, other studies show that islet allografts from transgenic mice that are deficient in class I MHC expression enjoy prolonged survival as allografts but are acutely rejected as xenografts.[78] Taken together, these results indicate that neither CD8 T cells nor their corresponding class I MHC target antigens are required for islet xenograft rejection. From these findings we form the hypothesis that a major pathway for islet xenograft immunity is through indirect antigen presentation of xenoantigens, which elicits a CD4-dependent inflammatory response. Interestingly, such a response has been suggested as a model for CD4-dependent inflammatory islet damage in spontaneous diabetes.[76]

The Role of Donor APCs in Allograft versus Xenograft Immunity

The difference in the nature of allogeneic versus xenogeneic responses has important implication concerning the role of donor-type APC (passenger leukocytes) in triggering rejection responses. In the discussion of the allograft response above, the case was made for improving graft survival by eliminating/inactivating the S^+ APCs within the graft that were responsible for triggering host immunity. Implicit in this approach is the assumption that the indirect pathway, the presentation of graft antigens by host-type APC, is not a major pathway for eliciting a graft-destructive response (Fig. 6.2). Empirically, the observation that APC-depleted islet allografts survive in nonimmunosuppressed recipients is consistent with this concept. The xenograft, however, represents a different situation. If the xenograft response is primarily a function of the indirect pathway of antigen presentation (Fig. 6.2), then the host response should be dependent on host-type, and not donor-type, APC. This predicts that removal of APCs from islet xenografts should have little influence on the rejection response. This issue remains controversial in that our studies suggest that APC-depleted xenografts are readily rejected,[54] while other studies have shown a benefit to islet xenograft survival through tissue pretreatment.[74,75] Thus, a potential role for pretreating xenogeneic tissues to reduce immunogenicity remains to be clarified.

Islet Xenografting in Autoimmune Diabetes

An important goal for islet xenotransplantation will be grafting in spontaneous, autoimmune diabetes. Previous studies show that the recurrence of disease in islet grafts in NOD mice is CD4 T cell dependent.[77] Combined with the finding that islet xenograft immunity is CD4 T cell dependent, anti-CD4 therapy should facilitate xenograft survival in diabetic autoimmune NOD mice. This has been shown to be the case for fetal pig pancreas xenografts.[79,80] An important aspect of these results was that xenografts actually showed superior survival relative to allografts in anti-CD4–treated NOD mice. We have generated similar results whereby rat islet xenografts show prolonged function relative to BALB/c islet allografts in anti-CD4–treated diabetic NOD mice[81] (Table 6.1). On one hand, such results may reflect the fact that xenograft

Table 6.1. Allograft versus Xenograft Survival in Anti-CD4–Treated NOD Mice

*Donor**	*Anti-CD4 Treatment*	*n*	*Graft Function (days)*	*MST† ±SEM*
BALB/c mouse	–	12	0, 0, 0, 0, 0, 2, 5, 6, 7, 8, 9, 11	4.0 ± 1.2
BALB/c mouse	+	12	0, 0, 2, 2, 5, 7, 14, 21, 30, 33, 37, 70	18.4 ± 6.1
DA rat	–	11	2, 2, 3, 4, 4, 5, 6, 6, 6, 7, 7	4.7 ± 0.6
DA rat	+	15	0, 13, 21, 30, 31, 33, 40, 42, 43, 45, 46, 47, 54, 66, 69	38.6 ± 4.7

*Spontaneously diabetic nonobese diabetic (NOD) mice were treated with the anti-CD4 monoclonal antibody GK1.5 (10 mg/kg/day) days −7, −1, 0, 1, 2, 7, 14, 21, 28 relative to transplantation. Recipients were grafted with 450 untreated pancreatic allografts (BALB/c mouse) or xenografts (DA rat) beneath the kidney capsule. Graft function was indicated by restoration of euglycemia; graft failure was indicated by the first of consecutive blood glucose values above normal range. Rat xenograft survival was significantly longer ($P<.05$) than BALB/c allograft survival.

†Mean survival time; SEM= standard error of the mean.

immunity is more exquisitely CD4 dependent than is allograft immunity. Indeed, CD8 T cells may play a greater role in allograft rejection than in xenograft rejection.[71] However, another hypothesis is that the autoimmune disease process displays a degree of species specificity; that is, islet-reactive T cells from NOD mice may preferentially recognize murine islet-associated antigens. This concept is supported by the findings by Haskins and coworkers that a panel of islet-reactive T cell clones derived from NOD mice show little cross-reactivity with islet antigens from differing species.[82] The key rationale for considering islet xenotransplantation has generally been to fill the shortage of available allogeneic tissues. However, if autoimmune diabetes indeed is species specific, then islet xenografts may have an additional benefit by being relatively resistant to the disease process. A clear definition of the degree of cross-species recognition of autoimmune T cells will require identifying the relevant autoantigens that are targeted by the disease process.

Future Direction: Donor-Specific Tolerance Induction

Widespread application of pancreatic islet grafting in type I diabetes will require minimal recipient manipulation. Therefore, the ultimate goal of islet grafting, as in transplantation generally, is the induction of host tolerance induction via some form of transient induction regimen. Long-term graft acceptance and sometimes donor-specific tolerance of islet allografts have been achieved through a variety of approaches, such as short-term drug treatment with cyclosporin A[83] or mycophenolic mofetil[84] as well as with treatments such as anti-CD4 monoclonal antibodies[72,73] or anti-lymphocyte serum.[85] Whether similar approaches will be applicable for the induction of xenogeneic tolerance remains to be clarified. Differences in the nature of the rejection responses to allografts versus xenografts raises the possibility that the nature of tolerance induction to these sources of tissue may differ as well. The induction of donor hematopoietic chimerism has been shown to be an effective tolerogenic protocol for both allografting and xenografting.[86,87] Also, as in islet allografting, anti-CD4 monoclonal antibody treatment has resulted in long-term acceptance and even tolerance induction to islet xenografts.[74,75,80] Interestingly, other forms of recipient treatment, such as administration of the hybrid molecule CTLA4Ig (which interferes with the CTLA-4/B7 interaction),[88] cytokine intervention,[89,90] and donor-specific antibody treatment[91] have all resulted in marked prolongation of islet xenografts. In most cases, the mechanism of graft prolongation/tolerance induction induced by these varied approaches remains in need of clarification. However, the potential for tissue pretreatment, along with an increasing variety of tolerogenic regimens and the prospect of immunoisolation technology, provide the foundation for clinically relevant approaches to islet transplantation in the future. The introduction of protective molecules into islets via gene transfer is a new, promising area of study. Regulatory molecules such as Fas ligand[92] may be candidate molecules for such an approach.

Acknowledgments

This work was supported in part by PHS grants R01 #DK45773 and DK33470.

References

1. Eisenbarth GS. Type 1 diabetes mellitus: a chronic autoimmune disease. *N Engl J Med.* 1986; 314:1360–1368.
2. Browatzki CC, Schultz A, Bretzel RG, Federlin KF. Clinical islet transplantation—registry report, accomplishment in the past and future needs. *Cell Transplant.* 1993; 2:269–282.
3. Sutherland DER. Report from the international panceas transplant registry. *Diabetologia.* 1991; 134(suppl 1):S28–S39.
4. Scharp DW, Lacy PE, Santiago JV, et al. Results of our first nine intraporal islet allografts in type I, insulin-dependent diabetic patients. *Transplantation.* 1991; 51:71–85.
5. Ricordi C, Tzakis AG, Carroll PB, et al. Human isolation and allotransplantation in 22 consecutive cases. *Transplantation.* 1992; 53:407–414.
6. Warnock GL, Kneteman NM, Ryan EA, Rabinovitch A, Rajotte RV. Long-term follow-up after transplantation of insulin-producing pancreatic islets into patients with type I (insulin dependent) diabetes mellitus. *Diabetologia.* 1992; 35:89–95.
7. Gores PF, Stephanian E, Kelley SL, Najarian JS, Lloveras JJ, Sutherland DER. Insulin independence in type I diabetics after transplantation of unpurified islets from single donor with 15-deoxyspergualin. *Lancet.* 1993; 341;19–21.
8. Gray BN, Watkins E. Prevention of vascular complications of diabetes by pancreatic islet transplantation. *Arch Surg.* 1976; 111:254–257.
9. Federlin KF, Bretzel RG. The effect of islet transplantation on complications in experimental diabetes of the rat. *World J Surg.* 1984; 8:169–178.
10. Woehrle M, Spitzer D, Linn T, Federlin K, Bretzel RG. The effect of early islet transplantation on prevention of nephropathy in the spontaneously diabetic RR rat. *Transplant Proc.* 1990; 22:819–820.
11. Warnock GL, Rajotte RV. Human pancreatic islet transplantation. *Transplant Rev.* 1992; 6(4):195–208.
12. Sutherland DER, Sibley R, Xu, XZ, Srikanta MS, Taub F, Najarian J, Goetz FC. Twin-to-twin pancreas transplantation: reversal and reenactment of the pathogenesis of type I diabetes. *Trans Assoc Am Physicians.* 1984; 97:80–87.
13. Terada M, Lennartz K, Mullen Y. Allogeneic and syngeneic pancreas transplantation in non-obese diabetic mice. *Transplant Proc* 1987; 19:960–961.
14. Naji A, Silvers WK, Kimura H, Anderson AO, Barker CF. Influence of islet and bone marrow transplantation on the diabetes and immunodeficiency of BB rats. *Metabolism.* 1983; 32(suppl 1):62–68.
15. Medawa PB. *The Uniqueness of the Individual.* 2nd rev. ed. New York: Dover Publications, 1957:1–155.
16. Snell GD. The homograft reaction. *Ann Rev Microbiol.* 1957; 11:439–458.
17. Batchelor JR, Welsh K, Burgos H. Transplantation antigens per se are poor immunogens within a species. *Nature.* 1978; 273:54–56.

18. Lafferty KJ, Cunningham AJ. A new analysis of allogeneic interactions. *Aust J Exp Biol Med Sci.* 1975; 53:27–42.
19. Bretscher P, Cohn M. A theory of self-nonself discrimination. *Science.* 1970; 169:1042–1049.
20. Talmage DW, Woolnough JA, Hemmingsen H, Lopez L, Lafferty KJ. Activation of cytotoxic T cells by nonstimulating tumor cells and spleen cell factor(s). *Proc Natl Acad Sci USA.* 1977; 74:1610–1614.
21. June CH, Ledbetter JA, Linsley PS, Thompson CB. Role of the CD28 receptor in T-cell activation. *Immunol Today.* 1990; 11:211–216.
22. Linsley PS, Brady W, Urnes M, Grosmarie LS, Damle NK, Ledbetter JA. CTLA-4 is a second receptor for the B cell activation antigen B7. *J Exp Med.* 1991; 174:561–569.
23. Schwartz RH. Costimulation of T lymphocytes: the role of CD28, CTLA-4, and B7/BB1 in interleukin-2 production and immunotherapy. *Cell.* 1992; 71:1065–1068.
24. Kamle NK, Klussman K, Linsley PS, Aruffo A. Differential costimulatory effects of adhesion molecules B7, ICAM-1, LFA-3, and VCAM-1 on resting and antigen-primed CD4+ T lymphocytes. *J Immunol.* 1992; 148:1985–1992.
25. Nabavi N, Freeman GJ, Gault A, Godfrey D, Nadler LM, Glimcher LH. Signalling through the MHC class II cytoplasmic domain is required for antigen presentation and induces B7 expression. *Nature.* 1992; 360:266–268.
26. Lafferty KJ, Prowse SJ, Simeonovic CJ. Immunology of tissue transplantation: a return to the passenger leukocyte concept. *Annu Rev Immunol.* 1983; 1:143–173.
27. Lafferty KJ, Bootes A, Dart G, Talmage DW. Effect of organ culture on the survival on thyroid allografts in mice. *Transplantation.* 1976; 22:138–149.
28. Bowen KM, Andrus L, Lafferty KJ. Successful allotransplantation of mouse pancreatic islets to nonimmunosuppressed recipients. *Diabetes.* 1980; 29:98–104.
29. Haug CE, Gill RG, Babcock SK, Lafferty KJ, Bellgrau D, Weil R III. Cyclosporin-induced tolerance requires antigens capable of initiating an immune response. *J Immunol.* 1987; 139:2947–2949.
30. Simeonovic CJ, Prowse SJ, Lafferty KJ. Survival and function of islet allografts in outbred mice. *Transplant Proc.* 1986; 18:316–318.
31. Lacy PE, Davie JM, Finke EH, Scharp DW. Prolongation of islet allograft survival. *Transplantation.* 1979; 27:171–174.
32. Faustman D, Hauptfeld V, Lacy P, Davie J. Prolongation of murine islet allograft survival by pretreatment of islets with antibody directed to Ia determinants. *Proc Natl Acad Sci USA.* 1981; 78:5156–5159.
33. Morrow CE, Sutherland DER, Steffes MW, Najarian JS, Bach FH. Lack of donor-specific tolerance in mice with established anti-Ia-treated islet allografts. *Transplantation.* 1983; 36:691–694.
34. Faustman DL, Steinman RM, Gebel HM, Hauptfeld V, Davie JM, Lacy PE. Prevention of rejection of murine islet allografts by pretreatment with anti-dendritic cell antibody. *Proc Natl Acad Sci USA.* 1984; 81:3864–3868.
35. Lau H, Reemtsma K, Hardy MA. Prolongation of rat islet allograft survival by direct ultraviolet irradiation of the graft. *Science.* 1984; 223:607–608.
36. La Rosa FG. Abrogation of mouse pancreatic islet allograft rejection by a four-day culture. *Transplantation.* 1988; 46:330–333.
37. Hegre OD, Hickey Ge, Marshall S, Serie JR. Modification of allograft immunogenicity in perinatal islets isolated and purified in vitro. *Transplantation.* 1984; 37:227–233.

38. Hullett DA, Landry AS, Leonard DK, Sollinger HW. Enhancement of thyroid allograft survival following organ culture. *Transplantation.* 1989; 47:24–27.
39. La Rosa FG, Talmage DW. The abrogation of thyroid allograft rejection by culture in acid medium. *Transplantation.* 1987; 44:592.
40. Jacobs BB. Ovarian allograft survival. *Transplantation.* 1974; 18:454–457.
41. Ramrakha PS, Sharp RJ, Yeoman H, Stanley MA. The influence of MHC-compatible and MHC-incompatible antigen-presenting cells on the survival of MHC-incompatible cultured murine keratinocyte allografts. *Transplantation.* 1989; 48:676–680.
42. La Rosa FG, Talmage DW. Major histocompatibility complex antigen expression on parenchymal cells of thyroid allografts is not by itself sufficient to induce rejection. *Transplantation.* 1990; 49:605–609.
43. Batchelor J, Welsh K, Maynard A, Burgos H. Failure of long surviving, passively enhanced kidney allografts to provoke T-dependent alloimmunity. I. Retransplantation of (AS X AUG)F_1 kidneys into secondary AS recipients. *J Exp Med.* 1979; 150:455–464.
44. Lechler RI, Batchelor JR. Restoration of immunogenicity to passenger cell-depleted kidney allografts by the addition of donor strain dendritic cells. *J Exp Med.* 1982; 155:31–41.
45. Bowen KM, Prowse SJ, Lafferty KJ. Reversal of diabetes by islet transplantation: vulnerability of the established allograft. *Science.* 1981; 213:1261–1262.
46. Vesole DH, Dart GA, Talmage Dw. Rejection of stable cultured allografts by active or passive (adoptive) immunization. *Proc Natl Acad SCI USA.* 1982; 79:1626–1628.
47. Markmann J, Lo D, Naji A, Palmiter RD, Brinster RL, Heber-Katz E. Antigen presenting function of class II MHC expressing pancreatic beta cells. *Nature.* 1988; 336:476–479.
48. Lo D, Burkly LC, Widera G, Cowling C, Flavell RA, Palmiter RD, Brinster RL. Diabetes and tolerance in transgenic mice expressing class II MHC molecules in pancreatic beta cells. *Cell.* 1988; 53:159–168.
49. Calne RY. Organ transplantation between widely disparate species. *Transplant Proc.* 1970; 2:550.
50. Auchincloss HJ. Xenogeneic transplantation: a review. *Transplantation.* 1988; 46:1–20.
51. Platt Jl, Bach FH. The barrier to xenotransplantation. *Transplantation.* 1991; 52:937–947.
52. Galili U. Interaction of the natural anti-Gal antibody with α-glactosyl epitopes; a major obstacle for xenotransplantation in humans. *Immunol Today.* 1993; 14:480.
53. Sachs DH, Bach FH. Immunology of xenograft rejection. *Hum Immunol.* 1990; 28:245–251.
54. Gill RG. The role of direct and indirect antigen presentation in the response to islet xenografts. *Transplant Proc.* 1992; 24:642–643.
55. Lafferty KJ, Warren HS, Woolnough JA, Talmage DW. Immunological induction of T lymphocytes: role of antigen and the costimulator. *Blood Cells.* 1978; 4:395.
56. Alter BJ, Bach FH. Cellular basis of the proliferative response of human T cells to mouse xenoantigens. *J Exp Med.* 1990; 171:333–338.
57. Moses R, Winn HJ, Auchincloss H Jr. Evidence that multiple defects in cell-surface molecule interactions across species differences are responsible for diminished xenogeneic T cell responses. *Transplantation.* 1992; 203–209.
58. Sprent J. The thymus and T cell tolerance. *Today's Life Sci.* 1991; 3:14–20.

59. Swain SL. T cell subsets and the recognition of MHC class. *Immunol Rev.* 1983; 74:129–142.
60. von Hoegen P, Miceli MC, Tourvieille B, Schilham M, Parnes JR. Equivalence of human and mouse CD4 in enhancing antigen responses by a mouse class II-restricted T cell hybridoma. *J Exp Med.* 1089; 170:1879–1886.
61. Clayton LK, Sieh M, Pious DA, Reinherz EL. Identification of residues affecting class II versus HIV-1 gp120 binding. *Nature.* 1989; 339:548.
62. Barzaga-Gilbert E, Grass D, Lawrence SK, Peterson PA, Lacy E, Engelhard VH. Species specificity and augmentation of responses to class II major histocompatibility complex molecules in human CD4 transgenic mice. *J Exp Med.* 1992; 175:1707–1715.
63. Irwin MJ, Heath WR, Sherman LA. Species-restricted interactions between CD8 and the $\alpha 3$ domain of class I influence the magnitude of the xenogeneic response. *J Exp Med.* 1989; 170:1091–1101.
64. Kalinke U, Arnold B, Hammerling GJ. Strong xenogeneic HLA response in transgenic mice after introducing an $\alpha 3$ domain into HLA B27. *Nature.* 1990; 348:642–644.
65. Greenstein JL, Foran JA, Gorga JC, Burakoff SJ. The role of T cell accessory molecules in the generation of class II-specific xenogeneic cytolytic T cells. *J Immunol.* 1986; 136:2358–2363.
66. Golding H, Singer A. Role of accessory cell processing and presentation of shed H-2 alloantigens in allospecific cytotoxic T lymphocyte responses. *J Immunol.* 1984; 133:597.
67. Yoshizawa K, Yano A. Mouse T lymphocytes proliferative responses specific for human MHC products in mouse anti-human xenogeneic MLR. *J Immunol.* 1984; 132:2820–2829.
68. Brunswick M, Lake P. Functional interactions of human and murine lymphoid cells. *Cell Immunol.* 1986; 103:441.
69. Pearson RN III, Winn HJ, Russell Ps, Auchincloss H. Xenogeneic skin graft rejection is especially dependent on CD4+ T cells. *J Exp Med.* 1989; 170:991–996.
70. Mandel TE, Koulmanda M, Loudovaris T, Bacelj A. Islet grafts in NOD mice: a comparison of iso-, allo-, and pig xenografts. *Transplant Proc.* 1989; 21:3813.
71. Gill RG, Coulombe M. Rejection of pancreatic islet xenografts does not require CD8+ T-lymphocytes. *Transplant Proc.* 1992; 24:2877–2878.
72. Shizuru JA, Gregory AK, Chao CTB, Fathman CG. Islet allograft survival after a single course of treatment of recipient with antibody to L3T4. *Science.* 1987; 237:278–280.
73. Hao L, Wang Y, Gill RG, Lafferty KJ. Role of the L3T4+ T cell in allograft rejection. *J Immunol.* 1987; 139:4022.
74. Lacy PE, Ricordi C, Finke EH. Effect of transplantation site and αL3T4 treatment on survival of rat, hamster, and rabbit islet xenografts in mice. *Transplantation.* 1989; 47:761–766.
75. Ricordi C, Lacy PE, Sterbenz K, Davie JM. Low-temperature culture of human islets or in vivo treatment with L3T4 antibody produces a marked prolongation of islet human-to-mouse xenograft survival. *Proc Natl Acad Sci USA.* 1987; 84:8080–8084.
76. Gill RG, Lafferty KJ. The role of islet transplantation in the treatment of insulin-dependent diabetes mellitus. *Imm Aller Clin N Am.* 1989; 9:165–186.
77. Wang Y, Pontesili O, Gill RG, LaRosa FG, Lafferty KJ. The role of CD4+ and

CD8+ T cells in the destruction of islet grafts by spontaneously diabetic mice. *Proc Natl Acad Sci USA.* 1991; 88:527–531.

78. Desai NM, Bassiri H, Odorico JS, Koller BH, Smithies O, Naji A, Barker CF, Markmann JF. Pancreatic islet allograft and xenograft survival in CD8+ T-lymphocyte-deficient recipients. *Transplant Proc.* 1993; 25:961–962.
79. Mandel TE, Koulmanda M. The survival of xeno-, allo- and isografts in NOD mice and xenografts in other strains, after immunosuppression with anti-CD4 monoclonal antibody. *Diabetes Nutr Metab.* 1992; 5(suppl 1):91–96.
80. Simeonovic CJ, Wilson JD. CD4+ T-cell depletion in mice facilitates induction of tolerance to pig proislet xenografts: a comparison of NOD and CBA/H recipient models. *Diabetes Nutr Metab.* 1992; 5(suppl 1):133–138.
81. Gill RG, Coulombe M. Islet xenografting in autoimmune diabetes. *Transplant Proc.* 1994; 26:1140.
82. Haskins K, Portas M, Bergman B, Lafferty K, Bradley B. Pancreatic islet-specific T-cell clones from nonobese diabetic mice. *Proc Natl Acad Sci USA.* 1989; 86:8000–8004.
84. Haug CE, Gill RG, Babcock SK, Lafferty KJ, Bellgrau D, Weil R III. Cyclosporin-induced tolerance requires antigens capable of initiating an immune response. *J Immunol.* 1987; 139:2947.
84. Hao L, Calcinaro F, Gill RG, Eugui EM, Allison AC, Lafferty KJ. Facilitation of specific tolerance induction in adult mice by RS-61443. *Transplantation.* 1992; 53:590.
85. Gotoh M, Porter J, Monaco AP, Maki T. Induction of antigen-specific unresponsiveness to pancreatic islet allografts by antilymphocyte serum. *Transplantation.* 1988; 45:429.
86. Ildstad ST, Sachs DH. Reconstitution with syngeneic plus allogeneic or xenogeneic bone marrow leads to specific acceptance of allografts or xenografts. *Nature.* 1984; 307:168.
87. Zeng Y, Ricordi C, Tzakis A, Rilo HLR, Carroll PB, Starzl TE, Ildstad ST. Long-term survival of donor-specific pancreatic islet xenografts in fully xenogeneic chimeras (WF rat → B10 mouse). *Transplantation.* 1992; 53:277.
88. Lenschow DJ, Zeng Y, Thistlethwaite JR, Montag A, Brady W, Gibson MG, Linsley PS, Bluestone JA. Long-term survival of xenogeneic pancreatic islet grafts induced by CTLA4Ig. *Science.* 1992; 257:789.
89. Carel J-C, Schreiber RD, Falqui L, Lacy PE. Transforming growth factor β decreases the immunogenicity of rat islet xenografts (rat to mouse) and prevents rejection in association with treatment of the recipient with a monoclonal antibody to interferon g. *Proc Natl Acad Sci USA.* 1990; 87:1591–1595.
90. Gerasimidi A, Sheehan KCF, Schreiber Rd, Lacy PE. Tumor necrosis factor-a prevents rejection of islet xenografts (rat to mouse). *Diabetes.* 1993; 42:651.
91. Faustman D, Coe C. Prevention of xenograft rejection by masking donor HLA class I antigens. *Science.* 1991; 252:1700–1702.
92. Bellgrau D, Gold D, Selawry H, Moore J, Franzusoff A, Duke RC. A role for Fas ligand in preventing graft rejection. *Nature* (in press).

7

Human Type I Diabetes Mellitus: Genetic Susceptibility and Resistance

A. Pugliese
G. S. Eisenbarth

The autoimmune process leading to the onset of type I diabetes (insulin-dependent diabetes mellitus, IDDM) mainly occurs in genetically susceptible individuals.[1–5] The genetic background is thought to have a predisposing effect and, since the concordance for the disease is usually less than 50% even in identical twins,[6–14] still unknown factors other than inherited alleles must play a role in determining development of IDDM. The identification of IDDM susceptibility genes could dramatically improve our ability to predict and prevent the disease, allowing the earliest recognition of individuals at high IDDM risk by a combination of genetic and immunological testing.

Previous epidemiological studies within multiplex IDDM families have shown that the risk of developing IDDM has a nonlinear correlation with the number of alleles shared with the proband. Monozygotic twins have the highest risk (100% sharing), followed by first-degree (50% sharing), second-degree (25% sharing), and third-degree relatives (12.5% sharing). The low concordance rate observed for monozygotic twins that may approximate 70% with long-term follow-up[124] indicates that susceptibility genes do not have a 100% penetrance. Based on estimates of the observed risk, it has been proposed that IDDM susceptibility is linked to a major locus with higher penetrance than other several minor loci contributing to IDDM risk in an epistatic way. This model generates the risk curve that is most similar to the observed risk.[15]

A major IDDM susceptibility gene is very likely localized in the major histocompatibility complex (MHC), because it has been estimated that the MHC provides approximately 60%–70% of the genetic susceptibility[16] and it has a central role also in the nonobese diabetic (NOD) mouse[1,17,18] and Bio Breeding (BB) rat[19–24] animal models of diabetes. As regards the minor contributing loci, a large number of additional loci have recently been implicated both for human IDDM[25–28] and the above animal models, for which the complex genetics of the disease is being unravelled and is extensively reviewed in Chapter 3.[29–31] In recent genome-wide analysis of sibling pairs no locus outside of the MHC showed major distortion of sharing,[27,32] while multiple loci with potential small effects were implicated.

Even if the development of new research strategies has significantly improved the ability to identify disease or susceptibility genes for several disorders,[33] our effort of mapping diabetes genes is complicated by the small potential individual effect of the contributing loci outside the MHC and by their relative abundance in the general population. These factors make the contribution of these loci less apparent, and therefore their identification requires analysis of a very large number of patients.

On the other hand, some alleles appear to be very rare in IDDM patients and therefore they are considered protective or associated with resistance to IDDM. The identification of such protective genes and the understanding of the mechanisms by which their protective effects are exerted are equally important, considering their hypothetical utilization for gene therapy–based preventive strategies.

This chapter will summarize the current knowledge on both genetic susceptibility and resistance to type I diabetes.

MHC Susceptibility

In man, genes coding for molecules controlling the immune response are clustered on the short arm of chromosome 6 within the major histocompatibility complex (MHC).[34,35] The majority of MHC genes are very polymorphic, and this polymorphism is thought to be essential to generate a wide variety of physiological immune responses. However, several studies have shown that many autoimmune diseases are associated with MHC alleles, and this is true also for IDDM.[36,37]

Initial studies based on serological typing techniques indicated that several class I human leukocyte antigens (HLA) such as HLA-B8, B18, and B15 were increased in frequency in IDDM.[38–40] However, with the development and refinement of typing techniques, many other MHC loci have been identified and later studies have shown that class II antigens are more closely related to IDDM susceptibility than class I antigens.

The great majority of patients with IDDM have the HLA-DR3 or -DR4 class II antigens and approximately 30% are DR3/DR4 heterozygous.[41–44] The combination of DR3 and DR4 confers the highest IDDM risk as a result of a synergistic mode of action.[42,44] DR4 homozygosity confers IDDM risk of a slightly lesser magnitude than DR3/DR4 heterozygosity and DR4 is thought to act in a dominant-like fashion. In contrast, DR3 homozygosity is associated with a lower risk and its mode of inheritance is believed to be recessive.[43–45] However, as a whole, HLA alleles confer recessive susceptibility and, as discussed subsequently, HLA protection associated with DQB1*0602 is dominant over susceptibility.

Because of the strong linkage disequilibrium existing on the short arm of chromosome 6, alleles at several loci tend to occur together with a higher frequency than expected by chance. This phenomenon has led to the identification of several HLA extended haplotypes. For instance, the [HLA-B8, DR3, SC01], [HLA-B18, DR3, F1C30], [HLA-B15, DR4, SC33], and [HLA-BW38, DR4, SC21] haplotypes are found with increased frequency in IDDM,[46] but the identification of the true susceptibility gene in their context is not an easy task.

The development of DNA sequencing and typing technology has dramatically improved our ability to identify polymorphic variants, increasing the probability of mapping disease genes. Recent studies with such improved technology have allowed susceptibility alleles to be more precisely identified at least on DR4 haplotypes, where genetic risk is strongly associated with the class II HLA-DQ locus.[47-50] This locus encodes for several variants of the HLA-DQ antigen, whose heterodimeric structure is typically formed by two glycoprotein chains (α,β). HLA-DQ molecules function (similar to DR and DP molecules) on antigen-presenting cells such as macrophages to bind short peptides and present them to the T cell receptor on CD4-positive T cells. Of note, unlike the DR locus whose α-chain is invariant, both the α- and β-chain of the DQ locus are highly polymorphic, giving origin to numerous $\alpha\beta$ combinations.[35,51] Among whites DQ typing has allowed the identification of two common DR4 haplotypes carrying the DQB1*0302 or DQB1*0301 allele. Most (95%) of the DR4 haplotypes found in patients with IDDM carry the allele DQB1*0302, in contrast to the general population, where the two haplotypes are more evenly distributed.[47,48] The DQB1*0302 allele differs from the DQB1*0301 allele in that it lacks an aspartic acid residue at position 57 of its second exon (similar to the I-A molecule of the NOD mouse, reviewed in Chapter 3). Since the DQB1*0201 allele found on DR3 haplotypes also lacks aspartic acid at position 57, this has been proposed as the molecular explanation for IDDM genetic susceptibility and for the increased risk conferred by DR4, DQB1*0302/DR3, DQB1*0201 heterozygosity.[47,52,53] However, this theory has been disputed by transracial studies,[54–56] including analysis of Japanese,[18,57,58] Chinese,[59] Mexican-American,[60] and black patients with IDDM.[61] For instance, the DQB1 alleles found with increased frequency in Japanese patients have aspartic acid at position 57, and also in whites there have been reports of IDDM in patients carrying similar alleles.[62] Moreover, other DQB1 genotypes lacking aspartic acid at position 57, such as DQB1*0302 (DR4)/DQB1*0201 (DR7), DQB1*0201 (DR3)/DQB1*0201 (DR3), and DQB1*0201 (DR3)/DQB1*0201

(DR7), are associated with a much lower IDDM risk.[63] In addition, because among whites most DR3 haplotypes carry the DQB1*0201 allele, an independent contribution of DQB1*0201 to IDDM susceptibility has not been directly demonstrated, and DQB1*0201 is also carried on DR7 and DR9 haplotypes associated with low IDDM risk. However, based on indirect evidence derived from calculating the relative risks for different DQ genotypes, it has been postulated that DQB1*0201 also may contribute to IDDM susceptibility in the context of the DQA1*0501/DQB1*0201 heterodimer. In fact, alleles at the DQA1 locus, and in particular an arginine residue at position 52 of the DQα chain, have also been associated with IDDM susceptibility.[64,65] Therefore, the different IDDM risk conferred by DQB1*0201 on DR3 and DR7 haplotypes may be explained by the different DQA1 alleles (*0501 on DR3, *0201 on DR7) linked to DQB1*0201 on such haplotypes.

In addition, transcomplementation of DQ α- and β-chains from opposite haplotypes has been recently demonstrated, and this significantly increases the diversity of class II antigens participating in the immune response and the potential for HLA-DQ contribution to IDDM susceptibility. A transcomplementating DQ$\alpha\beta$ heterodimer would be unique to a heterozygous individual and usually it would not be expressed in his parents. Thus, this phenomenon has been proposed as an explanation for the increased IDDM risk observed in DR4, DQB1*0302/DR3, DQB1*0201 heterozygotes.[66,67]

More recent studies have indicated that alleles at the DRB1 locus also affect IDDM susceptibility, with different relative risks reported for DR4, DQB1*0302 haplotypes differing at the DRB1 and DRB4 loci[37,49,68] (Table 7.1).

It is controversial whether the TAP2 locus may confer susceptibility and resistance to IDDM in an epistatic way with the DQ loci. The TAP2 locus encodes for the synthesis of peptide transporters associated with antigen processing and it is localized centromeric to the DQ loci on the short arm of chromosome 6.[69,70] Homozygosity for the TAP2*0101 allele was associated with increased IDDM risk independent of HLA-DQ susceptibility in a French study,[71] although other studies have failed to show such independent effect and suggested linkage disequilibrium between the HLA-DQ and TAP2 loci.[72,73] Of note, a mutation at the same locus has been implicated as the cause of the class I deficiency associated with IDDM in recent studies in man and the NOD mouse.[74–76]

Finally, it has been suggested that susceptibility genes may also lie in the central MHC between the class I and complement regions both in humans[77] and in the NOD mouse.[78]

Therefore, the DQB1 locus is likely to have a major role in IDDM susceptibility but several other MHC loci may contribute to IDDM risk. Although the extent and significance of their contribution is presently under investigation, typing for class II alleles with DNA-based techniques is likely to improve identification of individuals at increased diabetes risk within the general population.

Table 7.1 HLA Class II DR-DQ Linkage Patterns and IDDM Susceptibility in Whites

	DQA1	*DQB1*	*DRB1*	*Susceptibility*
DR2	0102	0602	1501	Protective
DR2	0102	0502 (AZH)	1601	Susceptible
DR2	0103	0601	1502	Neutral
DR3	0501	0201	0301	Susceptible
DR4	0301	0302	0401	Susceptible
DR4	0301	0302	0402	Susceptible
DR4	0301	0302	0403	Protective
DR4	0301	0302	0404	Neutral
DR4	0301	0302	0405	Neutral
DR4	0301	0301	0401	Neutral
DR4	0301	0301	0403	Neutral

MHC and Clinical Immunogenetic Heterogeneity of IDDM

A different distribution of HLA haplotypes among patients with IDDM onset at different ages has been recently reported and may reflect phenotypic variation of the disease.[56,79] Caillat-Zucman and coworkers have found a decreased frequency of DR3 and DR4 haplotypes and of DR3/DR4 heterozygosity among patients who had developed diabetes after age 15.[77–80] In our analysis of 297 patients (Pugliese A, personal observation), we have observed a significantly reduced frequency of DR3/DR4 heterozygotes only in patients with IDDM onset after age 30. In the same group we have found an increased frequency of DR3 homozygosity, which seems to correlate with a slower rate of the disease process. The immunogenetic analysis of islet cell antibody (ICA)–positive first-degree relatives from our family study has confirmed that DR3 (in the absence of DR4/DQB1*0302) is associated with a slower rate of progression to diabetes. This slower rate may be in part explained by a recessive lack of humoral response to insulin during the prediabetic period that we have recently noted in a subset of first-degree relatives at increased IDDM risk. This lack of humoral anti-insulin autoimmunity is mostly associated with DR3 homozygosity, but we could observe it also in relatives with DR5 or DR8 haplotypes. All these haplotypes carry DQA1 alleles from the evolutionary lineage 4[81,82] sharing glutamic acid and phenylalanine amino acid residues at position 40 and 51 of the second exon (GL alleles), suggesting that low responsiveness to insulin during the prediabetic period maybe associated with this particular subset of DQA1 alleles rather than with DR3 itself.[83] As shown in Figure 7.1, relatives homozygous for DQA1 GL alleles are characterized by lack or very low levels of insulin autoantibodies in contrast to relatives with

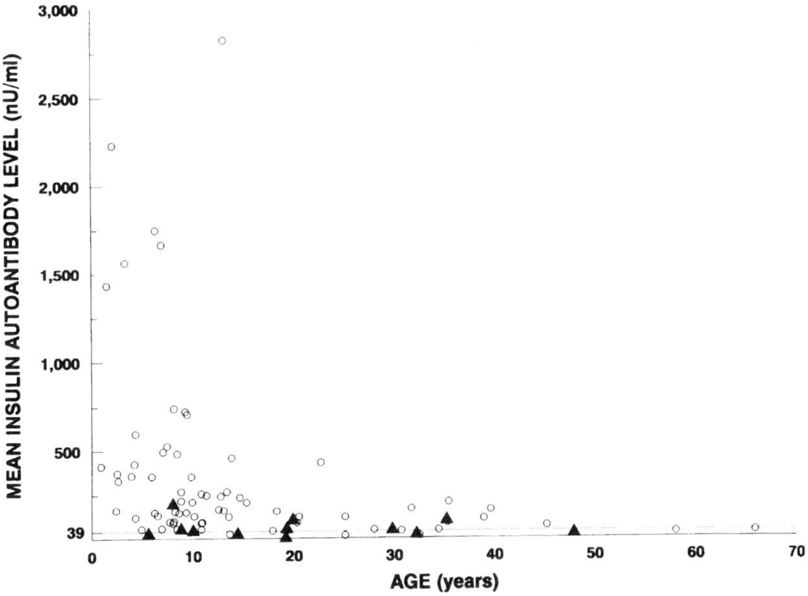

Figure 7.1. Mean insulin autoantibody levels versus age for at-risk first-degree relatives with DQA1 GL or DQA1 EF alleles. Relatives homozygous for DQA1 GL alleles (*solid triangles*) have low levels or completely lack insulin autoantibodies during the prediabetic period and show no correlation with age. Relatives with DQA1 EF alleles (*open circles*) have higher insulin autoantibody levels and show a clear inverse correlation with age. Upper limit of normal for insulin autoantibodies is 39 nU/ml.

DQA1 alleles from evolutionary lineages 1–3 (EF alleles, because of the presence of glutamic acid and phenylalanine at positions 40 and 51).

MHC Protective Genes

It was initially noticed that HLA-DR2 haplotypes have a reduced frequency among patients with IDDM.[44,45] Further characterization of the DR-DQ linkage pattern of DR2 haplotypes has indicated that genetic protection maps more closely to the DQB1 locus (Table 7.1). In fact, of the three DQB1 alleles usually linked to DR2 in whites (DQB1*0601, DQB1*0602, DQB1*0502), only DQB1*0602 is negatively associated with IDDM. The allele DQB1*0601 is rare in whites and has been reported as neutral for IDDM risk.[56,63] The allele DQB1*0502 is frequently found associated with IDDM, especially in Sardinia and other Mediterranean areas. It basically accounts for most cases of DR2-associated IDDM in whites (so-called DR2 AZH haplotype), although its effect on IDDM susceptibility is more likely neutral.[47,84] Moreover, a few patients with IDDM and DR2 have been reported carrying recombinant haplotypes with other DQB1 alleles (eg DQB1*0402, *0201, *0301, *0503) rather than

DQB1*0602.[62,85] Although DBQ1*0602 is found in approximately 20%–25% of white controls, DBQ1*0602 is very rarely seen (<1%) in patients with IDDM among white, black, and Japanese patients.[56,63] In our family study of 182 white patients with IDDM, only one carried DQB1*0602 (Pugliese A, personal observation). Other alleles such as DQB1*0603 and DQB1*0605 have a very similar sequence to DQB1*0602 and they also are rarely observed in IDDM patients (Pugliese A, personal observation).[56,86] DQB1*0602 may exert a dominant protective effect, it protects from IDDM even in the presence of high-risk alleles such as DQB1*0302 and DQB1*0201.[63] It is presently not known whether the few patients reported in the literature[80] with DQB1*0602 carry a mutated allele (which therefore may lose its protective effect) or if they have atypical forms of IDDM such as Wolfram's syndrome (diabetes mellitus, diabetes insipidus, and deafness that do not have autoimmune etiology.)[87] In fact, the only patient with IDDM and DQB1*0602 we have observed has the type I polyendocrine autoimmune syndrome, which is associated with mucocutaneous candidiasis, hypoparathyroidism, adrenal insufficiency, and other autoimmune disorders.[88] We speculate that a generalized immune deficiency in this patient may have impaired the IDDM protective mechanism associated with DQB1*0602. This suggests that protection may actually be an active response and not simply a passive mechanism usually explained by intrathymic deletion of autoreactive T cells. For instance, no evidence for thymic deletion has been found in I-E transgenic NOD mice[89] in which IDDM was prevented by inducing expression of the I-E (homologous to HLA-DR) molecule that NOD mice lack.[90–93]

We have recently reported an association between DQB1*0602 and high titers of autoantibodies against glutamic acid decarboxylase (GAD) in first-degree relatives of diabetic patients at very low risk of IDDM.[94,95] Moreover, we have found a negative association of IDDM with DQB1*0602 and sequence-related DQB1*06 alleles also in patients with stiff-man syndrome,[96] a rare neurological disorder of likely autoimmune origin associated with a strong humoral response to GAD and with diabetes in approximately 30% of cases.[97,98] In addition, a report has suggested that this strong humoral response to GAD may be inversely correlated to T cell proliferation, indicating the possibility of a Th2 response in these subjects as opposed to the usual Th1 response associated with T cell proliferation and β-cell loss.[99]

It is interesting to note that DQB1*0602 seems to be protective after the triggering of pancreatic autoimmunity as measured by ICA positivity. We have identified eight ICA-positive first-degree relatives with DQB1*0602, none of whom has developed diabetes or shown any decline in insulin secretion during the follow-up (Fig. 7.2) despite years of expression of ICA.[125]

Whether the protective mechanism of DQB1*0602 is active or passive is unknown, but protection is almost absolute. Transgenic mice[100,101] may present a useful tool to investigate the mechanism by which DQB1*0602 protects from IDDM, and indeed transgenic mice colonies expressing the DQA1*0104/DQB1*0601 heterodimer (DQw6) are already established.[102] Although this transgene has not prevented IDDM in the NOD mouse,[103] further

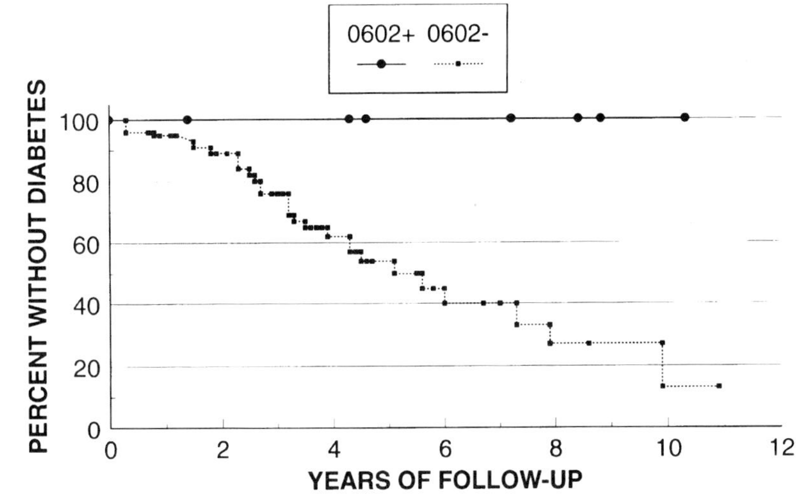

0602+: 8	7	7	4	3	1
0602-: 64	46	24	9	4	1

Figure 7.2. Lifetable analysis of 72 islet cell antibody (ICA) positive "at-risk" first-degree relatives. Despite ICA positivity, none of eight relatives with the protective allele DQB1*0602 has developed IDDM on follow-up, in contrast to 28 of 64 relatives without it.

investigation is necessary to fully assess the validity of this approach. For instance, the heterodimer chosen for these studies (DQA1*0104/DQB1*0601) protects from IDDM among Japanese but may be neutral in whites. Moreover, the human DQ transgene may not be able to generate an adequate immune response cooperating with immune accessory molecules of the murine host.

In conclusion, selected MHC genes are strongly associated with resistance to IDDM, even among first-degree relatives with ongoing pancreatic autoimmunity. The outstanding progress made in the field of gene therapy leads us to forecast that such protective genes could be delivered to individuals at high IDDM risk to prevent further progression of the disease. However, our understanding of the mechanisms by which such protective genes prevent diabetes is essential before a reasonable protocol for gene therapy can be developed.

IDDM Susceptibility and Resistance from Non-MHC Genes

Unlike animal models of diabetes, for which non-MHC susceptibility genes are currently being identified, little is known for human IDDM, mainly because different non-MHC genes may determine diabetes in different families and such genes are likely abundant in the general population. Without the possibility of analyzing several generations within a short time frame and manipulating inbreeding as we do in experimental mice, the identification of other susceptibility genes outside the MHC will require analysis of a very large number of families.

Linkage with IDDM has been suggested but not fully demonstrated for several non-MHC loci, including genes for the Kidd blood group on chromosome 18,[104–106] the immunoglobulin G heavy chain (Gm) on chromosome 14,[107,108] and the T cell receptor β gene chromosome 7.[109–111]

More recently, primarily through the analysis of sibling pairs provided by the Warren repository of the British Diabetes Association and the Human Biologic Data Interchange (HBDI), a number of additional loci have been associated with risk for type I diabetes. The technology underlying all such studies has involved typing with anonymous microsatellite DNA markers throughout the human genome and attempting to identify regions of the human genome shared by diabetes-affected sibling pairs more often than expected by chance.

The MHC region is designated IDDM1, the insulin gene IDDM2, and IDDM3 was assigned to the long arm of chromosome 15, 15q2.6 by the work of Field and coworkers.[28] Owerbach and coworkers and Copeman and coworkers have implicated a loci on the long arm of chromosome 2 (2q3.1-2q3.3, IDDM7).[25,26] Also two groups have implicated a region of the long arm of chromosome 11 in addition to the insulin gene on the short arm of 11.[27,123] The current evidence for each of the loci is somewhat tentative in that no single study in the absence of subdividing data has provided evidence for linkage or association at the level that geneticists studying monogenic disorders have generally considered definitive ($p < .001$, corrected for approximately 50 linkage groups being analyzed, giving a $p < .05$). Even the subdivision of data relative to HLA risk is somewhat controversial in that opposite subdivisions were utilized to attempt to strengthen, for example, the association of diabetes with the long arm of chromosome 11.[27,123] It is nevertheless likely that several of the above assignments will stand the test of time, with confirmation in some populations, and lack of confirmation in others. The task is to define polymorphisms or "mutations" of a gene in the identified region which relates to the association with type I diabetes. This will be attempted with linkage dysequilibrium analysis, analysis of a larger number of sibling pairs, and the study of unique families with multiple generations of type I diabetes. At present the assignments with their large degree of uncertainty provide no information to aid in the prediction even within families of risk for type I diabetes.

Several studies have indicated an association between IDDM and a 4.1 kb segment of DNA comprising the insulin gene and its 5′ and 3′ flanking regions (INS region) on chromosome 11p15.51.[112–120] As shown in Figure 7.3, several polymorphisms have been described in the INS region and they are organized in extended haplotypes because of strong linkage disequilibrium, with all polymorphism conferring similar relative risks.[118] In particular, alleles at the 1,127 PstI and 1,428 FokI sites of the 3′ flanking region of the insulin gene were reported to be strongly associated with IDDM risk and more frequently

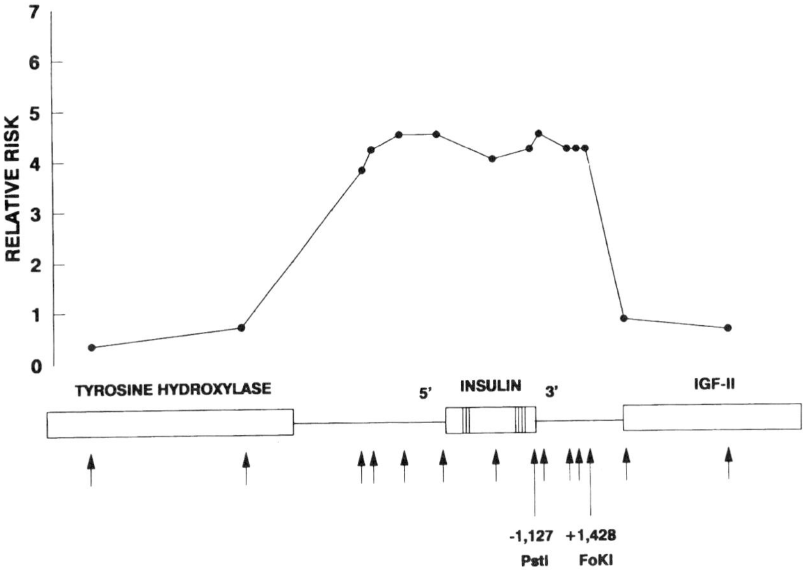

Figure 7.3. The insulin gene region (INS) on chromosome 11 and the relative risk for IDDM associated with several polymorphisms throughout the region. Arrows indicate sites of polymorphisms. The most commonly typed PstI and FokI sites are indicated (modified from Lucassen et al.[112]).

analyzed. However, a recent report suggested that susceptibility may be closer to the 5′ of the insulin gene.[119] Although there is now evidence to demonstrate genetic linkage of the INS region with IDDM, typing at the PstI or FokI loci has shown that the disease-associated "AA" INS genotype is widely represented in the general population. Approximately 85% of patients with IDDM as well as 50%–60% of the general population are AA homozygous. In contrast, the INS "AB" genotype is significantly reduced in frequency in IDDM (~15%) and the "BB" genotype is extremely rare in patients, with only one subject being BB homozygous among 244 patients with IDDM from our family study.[117] Moreover, the frequency of the B allele is lower in patients from multiplex families (12%) than in sporadic cases (24%) (Pugliese A, personal observation).

It is still controversial whether the INS contribution to IDDM susceptibility is HLA-DR4–dependent and strongest in paternal meioses, as suggested by a study in a French population.[114] Other studies have failed to show such an interaction with DR4[115,120] and found no evidence for maternal imprinting.[115,119] We have evaluated the transmission of the INS B allele to the diabetic offspring in informative families with only one AB parent. As shown in Figure 7.4, the maternal B allele segregates independently from the disease while the paternal B allele is very rarely seen in the diabetic offspring of AB fathers. The same trend has been recently reported also for another group of US families.[116] These findings are consistent with the hypothesis that some B

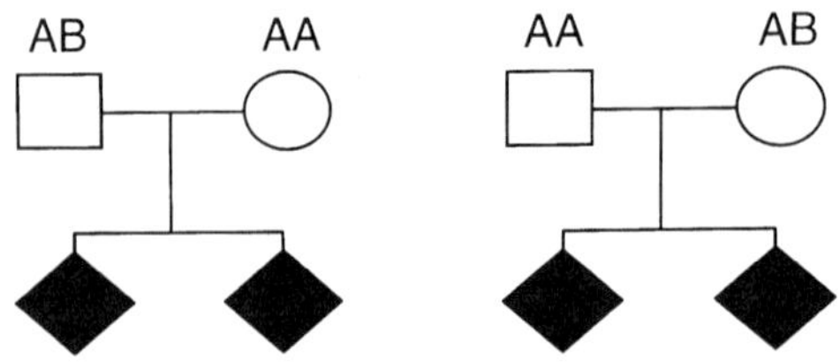

	AB	AA	AB	AA
U.S.A.	4	22	19	16
FRANCE	10	30	11	12
U.K.	8	18	6	18

Figure 7.4. Segregation analysis of the INS B allele. Informative families were collected from the United States (Pugliese et al.[111]), France (Julier et al.[108]), and the United Kingdom (Bain et al.[109]). The B allele is rarely passed to the diabetic offspring of INS AB fathers in families from U.S.A. and France, while no difference is apparent in British families.

alleles are protective, but only when paternally inherited, suggesting that maternal imprinting may inactivate the maternal allele determining loss of the protective effect. Interestingly, imprinting has been recently demonstrated for the human insulin growth factor–2 gene (IGF-2), which is the next gene telomeric to the insulin gene on the short arm of chromosome 11.[121,122] Although the protective effect of the B allele may not be absolute, depending on other genes, environmental factors, and its parental origin, in our prospective analysis of first-degree relatives at increased IDDM risk (autoantibody positive), the INS B allele has a strong negative predictive value.

Because the polymorphisms of the INS region are localized within introns and at the 5′ and 3′ untranslated regions of the insulin gene, but do not alter its coding sequence, we hypothesize that the INS alleles may determine differential regulation and expression of the insulin gene.[126,127] For example, we have evidence of expression of a human insulin message by the thymus (Pugliese A, unpublished observation). Different levels, timing, or site of expression of the insulin molecule may affect the development of the autoimmune response to insulin. However, INS alleles do not affect significantly prevalence and levels of insulin autoantibodies in first-degree relatives. Whether INS alleles are associated with qualitatively or quantitatively different T cell responses to insulin during the prediabetic period has yet to be determined.

Conclusion

Genetic factors confer susceptibility to the autoimmune process leading to the onset of IDDM. Both MHC and non-MHC genes appear to be involved in creating IDDM susceptibility, and it is likely that MHC genes may determine or limit autoimmunity targeted at specific organs while non-MHC genes determine the propensity for autoimmunity. Several research centers around the world are now concentrating their efforts to identify such genes. Many hundreds of families with at least two affected siblings (sib-pairs) have been collected and they are becoming available to researchers through two main repositories in the United States (Human Biologic Data Interchange, HBDI) and United Kingdom (British Diabetic Association, BDA). Although we already know that the average penetrance of an IDDM susceptibility gene would barely exceed 50%, genetic markers could still be very useful in combination with immunological testing in improving our ability to predict IDDM.

Moreover, a somatic mutation (perhaps in an immune cell type) could be the unknown "environmental" factor triggering pancreatic autoimmunity in genetically susceptible individuals. In this case, although such a mutation would be very difficult to identify, especially if occuring in a very limited number of cells, the genetic contribution to the pathogenesis of IDDM would extend far beyond susceptibility to a true causative role.

Finally, most recent studies have provided evidence that some alleles may provide genetic resistance to IDDM. Both the DQB1*0602 and some INS haplotypes are associated with a strong protective effect from IDDM. The DQ molecule DQA1*0102/DQB1*0602 confers dominant protection; certain INS haplotypes are protective but only when paternally inherited because of likely maternal imprinting. Our analysis of first-degree relatives with ongoing pancreatic autoimmunity suggests that those relatives carrying the above protective alleles have a very low IDDM risk and may not develop IDDM despite the presence of autoantibodies. This observation implies that such relatives should not be enrolled in preventive trials unless other immunological or metabolic parameters suggest otherwise. Further investigation on the mechanisms by which DQB1*0602 and the INS B allele confer resistance to IDDM is necessary, especially because the DR2, DQB1*0602 haplotype may confer susceptibility to multiple sclerosis. With a deeper understanding of the mechanism of disease prevention, such genes may be delivered as gene therapy or their effects mimicked for individuals at high risk for insulin-dependent diabetes.

References

1. Castano L, Eisenbarth GS. Type I diabetes: a chronic autoimmune disease of man, mouse and rat. *Annu Rev Immunol.* 1990; 8:647–679.
2. Atkinson MA, Maclaren NK. What causes diabetes? *Sci Am.* 1990; 263:62–71.
3. Todd JA. Genetic control of autoimmunity in type I diabetes. *Immun Today.* 1990; 11:122–129.
4. Rotter JI, Vadheim CM, Rimoin DL. Diabetes mellitus. In: King RA, Rotter JI, Motulsky AG, eds, New York, Oxford: *Genetic Basis of Common Diseases.* 1992; 413–481.

5. Pugliese A, Eisenbarth GS. Type I diabetes mellitus: lessons for human autoimmunity. *J Lab Clin Med.* 1992; 120:363–366.
6. Barnett AH, Eff C, Leslie RDG, Pyke DA. Diabetes in identical twins. *Diabetologia.* 1981; 20:87–93.
7. Johnston C, Pyke DA, Cudworth AG, Wolf E. HLA-DR typing in identical twins with insulin dependent diabetes, difference between concordant and discordant pairs. *Br Med J (Clin Res ED).* 1983; 286:253–255.
8. Srikanta S, Ganda OP, Eisenbarth GS, Soeldner JS. Islet cell antibodies and beta cell function in monozygotic triplets and twins initially discordant for type I diabetes mellitus. *N Engl J Med.* 1983; 308:322–325.
9. Srikanta S, Ganda OP, Jackson RA, et al. Type I diabetes mellitus in monozygotic twins: chronic progressive beta cell dysfunction. *Ann Intern Med.* 1983; 99:320–326.
10. Dib S, Vardi P. Connelly J, Eisenbarth GS, Soeldner JS. Immune changes associated with insulin dependent diabetes may remit without causing the disease: a study in identical twins. *Br Med J.* 1986; 1670:292.
11. Olmos P, Hern RA, Heaton DA, et al. The significance of the concordance rate for type I (insulin-dependent) diabetes in identical twins. *Diabetologia.* 1988; 31:747–750.
12. Leslie RDG, Millward BA, Hoskins P, et al. Prediction of diabetes in non-diabetic identical twins of insulin-dependent diabetic. *Diabetes.* 1988; 37:23A.
13. Beer SF, Heaton DA, Alberti G, Pyke DA, Leslie RDG. Impaired glucose tolerance precedes but does not predict insulin-dependent diabetes mellitus: a study of identical twins. *Diabetologia.* 1990; 33:497–502.
14. Kumar D, Gemayel NS, Deapen D, et al. Genetic, etiological, and clinical significance of disease concordance according to age, zygosity, and the interval after diagnosis in first twin. *Diabetes.* 1993; 42:1351–1363.
15. Rich SS. Mapping genes in diabetes. *Diabetes.* 1990; 39:1315–1319.
16. Rotter JI, Landaw EM. Measuring the genetic contribution of a single locus to a multilocus disease. *Clin Genet.* 1984; 26:529–542.
17. Hattori M, Buse JB, Jackson RA, et al. The NOD mouse: recessive diabetogenic gene within the major histocompatability complex. *Science.* 1986; 231:733–735.
18. Ikegami H, Makino S. Genetic susceptibility to insulin-dependent diabetes mellitus: form NOD mice to humans. In: Shafir E, ed. *Lessons from Animal Diabetes.* 4th Ed., Great Britain: Smith-Gordon; 1993: 39–50.
19. Chappel CI, Chappel WR. The discovery and development of the BB rat colony: an animal model of spontaneous diabetes mellitus. *Metabolism.* 1983; 32:8–10.
20. Colle E, Guttmann RD, Seemayer T. Spontaneous diabetes mellitus syndrome in the rat. I. Association with the major histocompatibility complex. *J Exp Med.* 1981; 154:1237–1242.
21. Colle E, Guttmann RD, Fuks A. Insulin-dependent diabetes mellitus is associated with genes that map to the right of the class I RTI: a locus of the major histocompatibilty complex of the rat. *Diabetes.* 1986; 35:454–458.
22. Colle E, Guttmann RD, Fuks A, Seemayer TA, Prud'homme GJ. Genetics of the spontaneous diabetic syndrome: interaction of the MHC and non-MHC associated factors. *Mol Biol Med.* 1986; 3:13–23.
23. Buse JB, Ben-Nun A, Klein KA, Eisenbarth GS, Seidman JG, Jackson RA. Specific class II histocompatibility gene polymorphism in BB rats. *Diabetes.* 1984; 33:700–703.
24. Buse JB, Ben-Nun A, Klien KA, Eisenbarth GS, Seidman JG, Jackson RA. Class I, II,

and III major histocompatibility complex gene polymorphisms in BB rats. *Diabetologia.* 1984; 22:77–79.

25. Owerbach D, Gabbay KH. The HOXD8 locus (2q31) is linked to type I diabetes: interaction with chromosome 6 and 11 disease susceptibility genes. *Diabetes.* 1995; 44:132–136.
26. Copeman JB, Cucca F, Hearne CM, et al. Linkage disequilibrium mapping of a type I diabetes susceptibility gene (IDDM7) to chromosome 2q31-q33. *Nature Genet.* 1995; 9:80.
27. Davies JL, KawaguchiY, Bennett ST, et al. A genome-wide search for human type I diabetes susceptibility genes. *Nature.* 1994; 371:130–136.
28. Field LL, Tobias R, Magnus T. A locus on chromosome 15q26 (IDDM3) produces susceptibility to insulin-dependent mellitus. *Nature Genet.* 1994; 8:189–194.
29. Todd JA, Aitman TJ, Cornall RJ, et al. Genetic analysis of autoimmune type I diabetes mellitus in mice *Nature.* 1991; 351:542–547.
30. Ghosh S, Palmer SM, Rodrigues NR, et al. Polygenic control of autoimmune diabetes in nonobese diabetic mice. *Nature Genetics.* 1993; 4:404–409.
31. Jacob HJ, Pettersson A, Wilson D, Mao Y, Lernmark A, Lander ES. Genetic dissection of autoimmune type I diabetes in the BB rat. *Nature Genetics.* 1992; 2:56–60.
32. Luo D-F, Bui MM, Muir A, Maclaren NK, Thomson G, She J-X. Affected sib-pair mapping of a novel susceptibility gene to insulin-dependent diabetes mellitus (IDDM8) on chromosome 6q25-q27. *Am J Hum Genet.* 1995; 57:911–919.
33. Todd JA, Bain SC. A practical approach to identification of susceptibilty genes for IDDM. *Diabetes.* 1992; 41:1029–1034.
34. Strominger JL. Biology of the human histocompatinilty leukocyte antigen (HLA) system and a hypothesis regarding the generation of autoimmune disease. *J Clin Invest.* 1986; 77:1411–1415.
35. Johnson AH, Hurley CK, Hartzman RJ, Alper CA, Yunis EJ. HLA: the major histocompatibility complex of man. In: Henry JB, ed, *Clinical Diagnosis & Management by Laboratory Methods.* 18th ed, Philadelphia: WB Saunders; 1991: 761–794.
36. Nepom GT. Immunogenetics of HLA-associated diseases. *Concepts Immunopathol.* 1988; 37:1112–1119.
37. Nepom GT, Erlich H. MHC class-II molecules and autoimmunity. *Annu Rev Immunol.* 1991; 9:493–525.
38. Singal DP, Blajchmann MA. Histocompatibility (HL-A) antigens, lymphotoxic antibodies and tissue antibodies in patients with diabetes mellitus. *Diabetes.* 1973; 22:429–432.
39. Nerup J, Platz P, Ortved-Anderson O, et al. HLA antigens and diabetes mellitus. *Lancet.* 1974; 2:864–866.
40. Cudworth AG, Woodrow JC. HLA system and diabetes mellitus. *Diabetes.* 1975; 24:345–349.
41. Platz P, Jakobsen BK, Morling N, et al. H:A-D and DR antigens in genetic analysis of insulin-dependent diabetes mellitus. *Diabetologia.* 1981; 21:108–115.
42. Wolf E, Spencer KM, Cudworth AG. The gnetic susceptibility to type I (insulin-dependent) diabetes: analysis of the HLA-DR association. *Diabetologia.* 1983; 24:224–230.
43. Bertrams J, Baur MP. Insulin-dependent diabetes mellitus. In: Albert ED, Baur MP, Mayr WR, eds, *Histocompatibility Testing 1984.* Berlin: Springer-Verlag; 1984:348–358.

44. Thomson G, Robinson WP, Kuhner MK, et al. Genetic heterogeneity, modes of inheritance, and risk estimates for a joint study of Caucasians with insulin-dependent diabetes mellitus. *Am J Hum Genet.* 1988; 43:700–816.

45. Rotter JI, Anderson CE, Rubin R, Congleton JE, Terasaki PI, Rimoin DL. HLA genotype study of insulin-dependent diabetes, the excess of DR3/DR4 heterozygotes allows rejection of the recessive hypothesis. *Diabetes.* 1983; 32:169–174.

46. Raum D, Awdeh Z, Yunis EJ, Alper CA, Gabbay KH. Extended major hitocompatibility complex haplotypes in type I diabetes mellitus. *J Clin Invest.* 1984; 74:449–454.

47. Todd JA, Bell JI, McDevitt HO. HLA-DQ beta gene contribution to susceptibility and resistance to insulin-dependent mellitus. *Nature.* 1987; 329:599–604.

48. Horn GT, Bugawan TL, Long CM, Erlich HA. Allelic sequence variation of the HLA-DQ loci: Relationship to serology and to insulin-dependent diabetes mellitus susceptibility. *Proc Natl Acad Sci U S A.* 1988; 85:6012–6016.

49. Erlich HA, Bugawan TL, Scharf S, Nepom GT, Tait B, Griffith RL. HLA-DQB sequence polymorphism and genetic susceptibility to IDDM. *Diabetes.* 1990; 39:96–103.

50. Thorsby E, Ronningen KS. Particular HLA-DQ molecules play a dominant role in determining susceptibility or resistance to type I (insulin-dependent) diabetes mellitus. *Diabetologia.* 1993; 36:371–377.

51. Begovich AB, McClure GR, Suraj VC, et al. Polymorphism, recombination, and linkage disequilibrium within the HLA class II region. *J Immunol.* 1992; 148:249–258.

52. Morel PA, Dorman JS, Todd JA, McDevitt HO, Trucco M. Aspartic acid at position 57 of the HLA-DQ beta chain protects against type I diabetes: a family study. *Proc Natl Acad Sci U S A.* 1988; 85:8111–8115.

53. Trucco M. To be or not to be ASP 57, that is the question. *Diabetes Care.* 1992; 15:705–715.

54. Todd JA, Mijovic C, Fletcher J, Jenkins D, Bradwell AR, Barnett AH. Identification of susceptibility loci for insulin-dependent diabetes mellitus by trans-racial gene mapping. *Nature.* 1989; 338:587–589.

55. Ronningen KS, Iwe T, Halstensen TS, Spurkland A, Thorsby E. The amino acid at position 57 of the HLA-DQ beta chain and susceptibility to develop insulin-dependent mellitus. *Hum Immunol.* 1989; 26:215–225.

56. Ronningen KS, Spurkland A, Tait BD, et al. HLA class II associations in insulin-dependent diabetes mellitus among Blacks, Caucasoids, and Japanese. In: Tsuji K, Aizawa M, Sasazuki T, eds, *HLA 1991,* Oxford, New York, Tokyo, Oxford University Press; 1991: 713–722.

57. Awata T, Kuzuya T, Matsuda A, et al. High frequency of aspartic acid at position 57 of the HLA-DQ β-cahin in Japanese IDDM patients and nondiabetic subjects. *Diabetes.* 1990; 37:266–269.

58. Ikegami H, Kawaguchi Y, Yamato E, et al. Analysis by polymerase chain reaction of histocompatibility leucocyte antigen-DR9-linked susceptibility to insulin-dependent diabetes mellitus. *J Clin Endocrinol Metab.* 1992; 75:1381–1385.

59. Penny MA, Jenkins D, Mijovic CH, et al. Susceptibility to IDDM in a Chinese population. *Diabetes.* 1992; 41:914–919.

60. Sanjeevi CB, Zeidler A, Shaw S, et al. Anaylsis of HLA-DQA1 and -DQB1 genes in Mexican Americans with insulin-dependent diabetes mellitus. *Tissue Antigens.* 1993; 42:72–77.

61. Mijovic CH, Jenkins D, Jacobs KH, Penny MA, Fletcher JA, Barnett AH. HLA-DQA1 and -DQB1 alleles associated with genetic susceptibility to IDDM in a black population. *Diabetes.* 1991; 40:748–753.
62. Erlich HA, Griffith RL, Bugawan TL, Ziegler R, Alper C, Eisenbarth GS. Implication of specific DQB1 alleles in genetic susceptibility and resistance by identification of IDDM siblings with novel HLA-DQB1 allele and unusual DR2 and DR1 haplotypes. *Diabetes.* 1991; 40:478–481.
63. Baisch Jm, Weeks T, Giles R, Hoover M, Stastny P, Capra JD. Analysis of HLA-DQ genotypes ans susceptibility in insulin-diabetes mellitus. *N Engl J Med.* 1990; 322:1836–1841.
64. Khalil I, D'Auroil L, Gobet M, et al. A combination of HLA-DQ beta Asp57-negative and HLA-DQ alpha Arg52 confers susceptibility to insulin-dependent diabetes mellitus. *J Clin Invest.* 1990; 85:1315–1319.
65. Ronningen KS, Gjertsen HA, Iwe T, Spurkland A, Hansen T, Thorsby E. Particular HLA-DQ alpha beta heterodimer associated with IDDM susceptibility in both DR4-Dqw4 Japanese and DR4-DQw8/DRw8-DQw4 whites. *Diabetes.* 1991; 40:759–763.
66. Nepom BS, Schwarz D, Palmer JP, Nepom GT. Transcomplementation of HLA genes in IDDM: HLA-DQ α- and β-chains produce hybrid molecules in DR3/DR4 heterozygotes. *Diabetes.* 1987; 36:114–117.
67. Khalil I, Deschamps I, Lepage V, Al-Daccak R, Degos L, Hors J. Dose effect of cis- and trans-encoded HLA-DQ alpha/beta heterodimers in IDDM susceptibility. *Diabetes.* 1992; 41:378–384.
68. Sheehy MJ, Scharf SJ, Rowe JR, et al. A diabetes susceptible HLA haplotype is best defined by a combination of HLA-DR and DQ alleles. *J Clin Invest.* 1989; 83:830–835.
69. Spies T, Bresnahan M, Bahram S, et al. A gene in the human major histocompatibility complex class II region controlling the class I antigen presenting pathway. *Nature.* 1990; 348:744–747.
70. Colonna M, Bresnahan M, Bahram S, Strominger JL, Spies T. Allelic variants of the human putative peptide teansporter involved in antigen processing. *Proc Natl Acad Sci U S A.* 1992; 89:3932–3936.
71. Caillat-Zucman S, Bertin E, Timsit J, Boitard C, Assan R, Bach JF. Protection from insulin-dependent diabetes mellitus is linked to a peptide transporter gene. *Eur J Immunol.* 1993; 23:1784–1788.
72. Ronningen KS, Undlien DE, Ploski R, et al. Linkage disequilibrium between TAP2 variants and HLA class II alleles; no primary association between TAP2 variants and insulin-dependent diabetes mellitus. *Eur J Immunol.* 1993; 23:1050–1056.
73. Van Endert PM, Liblau RS, Patel SD, et al. Major histocompatibility complex-encoded antigen processing gene polymorphism in IDDM. *Diabetes.* 1994; 43:110–117.
74. Faustman D, Li X, Lin HY, et al. Linkage of faulty major histocmpatibility complex class I to autoimmune diabetes. *Science.* 1991; 254:1756–1761.
75. Faustman D, Xiangping L, Lin H, et al. Abnormal MHC class I presentation linked to autoimmunity. *Diabetes.* 1992; 41(supp 1):99A.
76. Gaskins HR, Monaco JJ, Leiter EH. Expression of intra-MHC transporter (Ham) genes and class I antigens in diabetes-susceptible NOD mice. *Science.* 1992; 256:1826–1828.
77. Degli Esposti MA, Abraham LJ, McCann V, Spies T, Christiansen FT, Dawkins RL.

Ancestral haplotypes reveal the role of central MHC in the immunogenetics of IDDM. *Immunonogenetics.* 1992; 36:345–356.

78. Ikegawi H, Kawaguchi Y, Ueda H, et al. MHC-linked diabetogenic gene of the NOD mouse: molecular mapping of the 3′ boundary of the diabetogenic region. *Biochem Biophys Res Commun.* 1993; 192:677–682.
79. Karjalainen J, Salmela P, Ilonen J, Surcel HM, Knip M. A comparison of childhood and adult type I diabetes mellitus. *N Engl J Med.* 1989; 320:881–886.
80. Caillat-Zucman S, Garchon H-J, Timsit J, et al. Age-dependent HLA genetic heterogeneity of type I insulin-dependent diabetes mellitus. *J Clin Invest.* 1992; 90:2242–2250.
81. Gyllensten UB, Erlich HA. Ancient roots for polymorphism at the HLA-DQ alpha locus in primates. *Proc Natl Acad Sci U S A.* 1989; 86:9986–9990.
82. Erlich HA, Gyllensten UB. The evolution of allelic diversity at the primate major histocompatibility omplex class II loci. *Hum Immunol.* 1991; 30:110–118.
83. Pugliese A, Moromisato R, Gianani R, at al. Two subsets of HLA-DQA1 alleles mark phenotypic variation in levels of insulin autoantibodies in first degree relatives at risk for insulin-dependent diabetes. *J Clin Invest.* 1994; 93:2447–2452.
84. Sorrentino R, DeGrazia U, Buzzetti R, et al. An explanation for the neutral effect of DR2 on IDDM susceptibility in central Italy. *Diabetes.* 1992; 41:904–908.
85. Zelisewski D, Tiercy J, Boitard C, et al. Extensive study of DRbeta, DQalpha, and DQ beta gene polymorphism in 23 DR2-positive, insulin-dependent diabetes mellitus patients. *Hum Immunol.* 1992; 33:140–147.
86. Mijovic CH, Todd JA, Barnett AH. Trans-racial gene mapping studies. *Clin Endocrinol Metab.* 1993; 5:321–340.
87. Fishman L, Ehrlich RM. Wolfram syndrome: a report of four new cases and a review of literature. *Diabetes Care.* 1986; 9:405–408.
88. Eisenbarth GS, Jackson RA. The immunoendocrinopathy syndromes. In: Wilson JD, Foster DW, eds. 8th ed. Philadelphia: Wb Saunders; 1992: 1555–1566.
89. Bohme J, Schuhbaur B, Kanagawa O, Benoist C, Mathis D. MHC-linked protection from diabetes dissociated from clonal deletion of T cells. *Science.* 1990; 249:293–295.
90. Nishimoto H, Kikutani H, Yamamura K, Kishimoto T. Prevention of autoimmune insulitus by expression of I-E molecules in NOD mice. *Nature.* 1987; 328:432–434.
91. Lo D, Burkly LC, Widera G, et al. Diabetes and tolerance in transgenic mice expressing class II MHC molecules in pancreatic beta cells. *Cell.* 1988; 53:159–168.
92. Lund T, O'Reilly L, Hutchings P, et al. Prevention of insulin-dependent diabetes mellitus in non-obese diabetic mice by transgenes encoding modified I-A beta chain or normal I-E alpha chain. *Nature.* 1990; 345:727–729.
93. Slattery RM, Kjer-Neilsen L, Allison J, Charlton B, Mandel TE, Miller JFAP. Prevention of diabetes in non-obese diabetic I-Ak transgenic mice. *Nature.* 1990; 345:724–726.
94. Gianani R, Pugliese A, Bonner-Weir S, et al. Prognostically significant heterogeneity of cytoplasmic islet cell antibodies in relatives of patients with type I diabetes. *Diabetes.* 1992; 41:347–353.
95. Pugliese A, Gianani R, Eisenbarth GS, et al. Genetics of susceptibility and resistance to insulin-dependent diabetes in stiff-man syndrome. *Lancet.* 1994; 341:1027–1028.

96. Pugliese A, Solimena M, Awdeh ZL, et al. Association of HLA-DQB1*0201 with stiff-man syndrome. *J Clin Endocrinol Metab.* 1993; 77:1550–1553.
97. Solimena M, Folli F, Aparisi R, Pozza G, DeCamilli P. (1990).Autoantibodies to GABA-ergic neurons and pancreatic beta cells in stiff-man syndrome. *N Engl J Med.* 1990; 322:1555–1560.
98. McEvoy KM. Stiff-man syndrome. *Mayo Clin Proc.* 1991; 66:300–304.
99. Harrison LC, Honeyman MC, DeAizpurua HJ, et al. Inverse relation between humoral and cellular immunity to glutamic acid decarboxylase in subjects at risk of insulin-dependent diabetes. *Lancet.* 1993; 341:1365–1369.
100. Hanahan D. Transgenic mice as probes into complex systems. *Science.* 1990; 246:1265–1275.
101. Lipes M, Eisenbarth GS. Transgenic mouse models of type I diabetes. *Diabetes.* 1990; 39: 879–884.
102. Nishimura Y, Iwanaga T, Inamitsu T, et al. Expression of the human MHC, HLA-DQw6 genes alters the immune response in C57BL/6 mice. *J Immunol.* 1990; 145:353–360.
103. Fukui Y, Nishimura Y, Iwanga T, et al. Glycosuria and insulitis in NOD mice expressing the HLA-DQw6 molecule. *J Immunogenetics.* 1989; 16:445–453.
104. Hodge SE, Anderson CE, Neiswanger K, et al. Close linkage between IDDM and the Kidd blood group. *Lancet.* 1981; 2:893–895.
105. Barbosa J, Rich SS, Dunsworth T, Swanson J. Linkage disequilibrium between insulin-dependent diabetes and the Kidd blood group Jkb allele. *J Clin Endocrinol Metab.* 1982; 55:193–195.
106. Dunksworth TS, Tich SS, Swanson J, Barbosa J. No evidence for linkage between diabetes and the Kidd marker. *Diabetes.* 1982; 31:991–993.
107. Nakao Y, Matsumoto H, Miyazaki T, et al. IgG heavychain (Gm) allotypes and immune response to insulin in insulin-requiring diabetes mellitus. *N Engl J Med.* 1981; 304:407–409.
108. Rich SS, Weitkamp LR, Guttormsen S, Barbosa J. Gm, Km, and HLA in insulin-dependent type I diabetes mellitus. *Diabetes.* 1986; 35:927–932.
109. Hoover ML, Capra JD. HLA and T-cell receptor genes in insulin-dependent diabetes mellitus. *Diabetes Metab Rev.* 1987; 3:835–856.
110. Millward BA, Welsh KI, Leslie RDG, Pyke DA, Demaine AG. T-cell receptor beta chain polymorphisms are associated with insulin-dependent diabetes. *Clin Exp Immunol.* 1987; 70:152–157.
111. Reijonen H, Silvennoinen-Kassinen S, Ilonen J, Knip M. Lack of association of T-cell receptor beta-chain constant region polymorphism with insulin-dependent diabetes mellitus in Finland. *Clin Exp Immunol.* 1990; 81:396–399.
112. Bell GI, Horita S, Karam JH. A polymorphic locus near the human insulin gene is associated with insulin-dependent diabetes mellitus. *Diabetes.* 1984; 33:176–183.
113. Hitman GA, Tarn AC, Winter RM, et al. Type I (insulin-dependent) diabetes and a highly variable locus close to the insulin gene on chromosone 11. *Diabetologia.* 1985; 28:218–222.
114. Julier C, Hyer RN, Davies J, et al. Insulin-IGF2 region encodes a gene implicated in HLA-DR4-dependent diabetes susceptibility. *Nature.* 1991; 354:155–159.
115. Bain SC, Prins JB, Hearne CM, et al. Insulin gene region-encoded susceptibility to type I diabetes is not restricted to HLA-DR4-positive individuals. *Nature Genetics.* 1992; 2:212–215.
116. Ma Bui M, Muir A, Maclaren N, She JX. Linkage of the insulin gene (INS) with

insulin-dependent diabetes (IDD) in Caucasians suggest a maternal imprinting effect. *Diabetes.* 1993; 42(suppl. 1):63A.

117. Pugliese A, Awdeh ZL, Alper CA, Jackson RA, Eisenbarth GS. The paternally inherited insulin gene B allele (1,428 FoKI site) confers protection from insulin-dependent diabetes in families. *Autoimmunity.* 1994; 7:687–694.
118. Lucassen A, Julier C, Beressi J-P, et al. Susceptibility to insulin-dependent diabetes mellitus maps to a 4.1 kb degment of DNA spanning the insulin gene and associated VNTR. *Nature Genetics.* 1993; 4:305–310.
119. Owerbach D, Gabbay KH. Localization of a Type I diabetes susceptibility locus to the variable tandem repeat flanking the insulin gene. *Diabetes.* 1993; 42:1708–1714.
120. Van Der Auwera BJ, Heimberg H, Schrevens AF, Van Waeynberge C, Flament J, Schuit FC. 5′ insulin gene polymorphism confers risk to IDDM independently of HLA class II susceptibility. *Diabetes.* 1993; 42:851–854.
121. Giannoukakis N, Deal C. Paquette J, Goodyear CG, Polychronakos C. Parental geonomic imprinting of the human IGF2 gene. *Nature Genetics.* 1993; 4:98–101.
122. Ohlsson R, Nystrom A, Pfeifer-Ohlsson S, et al. IGF2 is parentally imprinted during the human embryogenesis and in the Beckwith-Wiedemann syndrome. *Nature Genetics.* 1993; 4:94–97.
123. Hashimoto L, Habita C, Beressi JP, et al. Genetic mapping of a susceptibility locus for insulin-dependent diabetes mellitus on chromosome 11q. *Nature.* 1994; 371:161–164.
124. Verge CF, Gianani R, Yu L, Pietropaolo M, Smith T, Jackson RA, Soeldner JS, Eisenbarth GS. Late progression to diabetes and evidence for chronic β-cell autoimmunity in identical twins of patients with type I diabetes. *Diabetes.* 1995; 44:1176–1179.
125. Pugliese A, Gianani R, Moromisato R, Awdeh ZL, Alper CA, Erlich HA, Jackson RA, Eisenbarth GS. HLA-DQB1*0602 is associated with dominant protection from diabetes even among islet cell antibody positive first degree relatives of patients with insulin-dependent diabetes. *Diabetes.* 1995; 44:608–613.
126. Bennett ST, Lucassen AM, Gough SCL, et al. Susceptibility to human type I diabetes at IDDM2 is determined by tandem repeat variation at the insulin gene minisatellite locus. *Nature Genetics.* 1995; 9:284–292.
127. Castignani A, Kennedy G, German MS, Rutter WJ. The minisatellite in the diabetes susceptibility locus IDDM2 regulates insulin transcription. *Nature Genetics.* 1995; 9:293–298.

8

Autoimmune Polyendocrine Syndromes

S. K. Garg
G. J. Klingensmith
G. S. Eisenbarth

Polyglandular autoimmune syndromes include the autoimmune polyglandular syndrome type II (APS II, Schmidt's syndrome),[1–3] autoimmune polyglandular syndrome type I[4] (APS I, APECED: autoimmune polyendocrinopathy–candidiasis–ectodermal dystrophy, MIM number 240300), non–organ-specific autoimmunity (eg, lupus erythematosus) associated with anti-insulin receptor antibodies,[5–7] thymic tumors with associated endocrinopathy,[8–10] Graves' disease associated with insulin autoimmune syndrome, and POEMS syndrome[11,12] (plasma cell dyscrasia with polyneuropathy, organomegaly, endocrinopathy, monoclonal gammopathy, and skin changes). The two major autoimmune endocrine syndromes, APS I and APS II, both have Addison's disease as a prominent component. The major autoimmune polyendocrine syndromes have a strong genetic component with the type II syndrome occurring in multiple generations and the type I syndrome primarily appearing in affected siblings. Both syndromes are associated with type I diabetes.

Table 8.1. Type I Diabetes and Polyendocrine Autoimmunity

- 50% of APS II and 5% of APS I patients become diabetic
- "Restricted" or GAD-ICA is common among APS II patients
- APS I: DQA1*0102/DQB1*0602 may not protect from diabetes
- APS II: Later mean age of diabetes onset
- APS I: Anti-GAD autoantibodies react with GAD on Western blots and inhibit enzymatic activity[13]

Table 8.2. Disease Associations*

Autoimmune Polyendocrine Syndrome Type I	*Incidence*	*Autoimmune Polyendroceine Syndrome Type II*	*Incidence*
Mucocutaneous candidiasis[4]	C		
Addison's disease[4]	C	Addison's disease[14]	C
Hypoparathyroidism	C		
Chronic active hepatitis[4]	C		
Graves' disease	C	Graves' disease	C
Hashimoto's thyroiditis	C	Hashimoto's thyroiditis[15]	C
Pernicious anemia	C	Pernicious anemia[16,17]	C
Vitiligo	C	Vitiligo[16,18–20]	C
Type I DM (5%)[4]	I	Type I DM (50%)	C
Alopecia[21,22]	I	Alopecia	I
		Myasthenia gravis[23]	C
Malabsorption syndrome[24]	I	Celiac disease, dermatitis herpetiformis[26,27]	C
IgA deficiency	I	IgA deficiency[20,28]	I
		Serositis[29]	R
Asplenism[30]	C		
Ectodermial dysplasia[4]	C		
Hypogonadism[31]	C	Hypogonadism[31–33]	I
		Stiff-man syndrome[34]	R
		Parkinson's disease[35]	I
Dental enamel and nail dystrophy[4]	C		
		Idiopathic heart block[16]	R
Pure red cell aplasia[36,37]	R		
		Idiopathic thrombocytopenia[38,39]	I
		Hypophysititis[40,41]	R

*C=common within syndrome; R=rare; I=intermediate.

Approximately 50% of APS II patients with Addison's disease are diabetic, whereas 5% of patients with APS I are diabetic (Table 8.1). The diverse names gives to the polyendocrine autoimmune syndromes reflect the large number of studies and case reports concerning these patients and heterogeneity in their clinical presentation.

The major illnesses associated with both APS I and APS II are listed in Table 8.2 and differences between the syndromes are defined in Table 8.3. Knowledge of disease associations and inheritance pattern makes early diagnosis of component illnesses of the above syndromes possible.

Patients with APS I and APS II develop additional diseases over time and approximately one out of seven relatives of such patients have an undiagnosed autoimmune disorder (most often hypothyroidism).[42,43] The individual polyendocrine autoimmune syndromes, their immunogenetics, pathogenesis, and selected aspects of therapy will be reviewed in this chapter.

Autoimmune Polyglandular Syndrome Type II (APS II, Schmidt's Syndrome)

The type II syndrome is the most common autoimmune polyendocrine syndrome. In 1926, Schmidt described two subjects with thyroiditis and Addison's disease.[1] Other diseases of the APS II include Graves' disease (thyrotoxicosis), primary hypothyroidism,[15] insulin-dependent or type I diabetes mellitus (IDDM), celiac disease,[25,26,27] vitiligo,[18–20] serositis,[20,44] IgA deficiency,[28,45] primary hypogonadism,[31] stiff-man syndrome,[34] alopecia, pernicious anemia,[17] myasthenia gravis,[23] and Parkinson's disease.[35] Organ-specific autoantibodies in the absence of overt disease is also frequently present in patients and their relatives. Genetic abnormalities underlying disease susceptibility are partially defined and include human leukocyte (HLA) haplotypes with DR3 and DR4 for the type II syndrome.[42,46–48] The only identified major environmental factor initiating a component disease is the wheat protein gliadin for celiac disease.[25]

Both autoreactive T cells and autoantibodies are pathogenic, depending on the specific disease, and most often are associated with tissue destruction. In Graves' disease, anti–thyrotropin (TSH) autoantibodies lead to thyroid hyperfunction[49] and anti–insulin receptor autoantibodies can result in either hypoglycemia or insulin resistance with hyperglycemia.[7,38]

Families with the type II polyglandular syndrome should be evaluated over time to detect the presence of organ-specific antibodies indicating the possibility of a future endocrine malfunction (Table 8.4). All such relatives should be advised of the early symptoms and signs of the principal component diseases. Even though the early signs and symptoms may be absent, patients with multiple disorders should be screened annually with measurement of

Table 8.3. Comparison of APS I and APS II

APS I	*APS II*
Onset infancy	Older onset
Siblings affected (autosomal recessive, chromosome 21)	Multiple generations
NOT HLA class II associated	DR3/DR4 associated
Immunodeficiency Asplenism Mucocutaneous candidiasis	No defined immunodeficiency
5% type I DM	50% type I DM

fasting glucose, anti-islet antibodies,[50] a sensitive thyrotropin assay, measurement of serum B12 levels, and cosyntropin-stimulated cortisol. An assay of anti–islet cell antibodies,[51,52] anti-thyroid[53–56] and anti-adrenal antibodies,[14,57–59] and anti-ovarian antibodies[33,60] may help identify subjects at increased disease risk. More than 20 years may elapse between the onset of one endocrinopathy and the diagnosis of the next. As many as 40–50% of subjects with Addison's disease will develop an associated endocrinopathy over time. A distinction must be made for subjects with isolated thyroid disease (relatively frequent in the general population) who have no family history of polyglandular syndrome type II. Such individuals have a relatively low incidence of additional autoimmune disorders in comparison with individuals with rare autoimmune disorders such as Addison's disease or myasthenia gravis.

Many of the diseases of the type II syndrome are associated with HLA antigens HLA-DR3 or HLA-DR4[2,61,62] (Table 8.4). In that the B locus allele HLA B8 is in linkage disequilibrium with HLA DR3 (associated at a population level), B8 is also associated with APS II.[42] Primary adrenal insufficiency in the type II, but not the type I syndrome, is strongly associated with both HLA-DR3 and HLA-DR4.[61] The association of HLA markers with disease can correlate with an inheritance of a common HLA-haplotype within families, but haplotypes with DR3 are often introduced into the family by more than one relative.[62] Several diseases that manifest in patients with polyendocrine autoimmune syndromes are not associated with HLA-B8 or HLA-DR3 in population studies. These disorders include vitiligo,[63] pernicious anemia,[64] and autoimmune goitrous thyroiditis.[65–66] This suggests the presence of more than one pathogenic mechanism resulting in similar manifestations of pleuriglandular autoimmune syndromes.

Rarely, hypoparathyroidism, a specific endocrine disturbance present in type I syndrome, is identified in a patient with the type II syndrome. Hypoparathyroidism in such type II polyendocrine autoimmune patients may result from a "suppressive" autoantibody[71,79] rather that parathyroid destruction as in the type I syndrome. In a patient with the type II syndrome, celiac disease is a more frequent cause of hypocalcemia than hypoparathyroidism. Other HLA-B8 and DR3 associated illnesses such as selective IgA deficiency,[45,80–82] juvenile dermatomyositis, and dermatitis herpetiformis[64] are also associated with the type II syndrome. There are case reports and clinical series linking polyendocrine autoimmunity with dermatitis herpetiformis,[26] alopecia,[22] scleroderma,[83] autoimmune thrombocytopenia purpura,[39,84] multiple endocrine neoplasia, hypophysitis,[40,42,85] metaphyseal osteopenia,[86] and serositis.[44]

Pathogenesis

Initiating factors for the type II syndrome and its component illnesses are not established except for celiac disease (wheat protein gliadin). Patients with celiac diseases, which is characterized by atrophy of intestinal villi associated

Table 8.4. Polyendocrine Type II Syndrome Diseases

Disease	*HLA Association*	*Initiator*	*Predominant Mediator*	*Autoantigen*
Graves' disease	DR3	Iodine (rare)	Antibody	TSH receptor[49]
Myasthenia gravis	DR3, DR7[68,69]	Thymoma[10] (rare) Penicillamine[69] (rare)	Antibody	Acetylcholine receptor
Hypoglycemia/ diabetes (rare cause)	?	?	Antibody[7,70]	Insulin receptor
Hypoparathyroidism "geriatric"	?	?	Antibody[71]	Cell surface inhibitor
Insulin autoimmune	DR4, DRB1*0406[72]	Methimazole	Antibody	Insulin
Celiac disease	DR3/DR7	Gluten (common)	?	"Gliadin," endomysial
Type I DM	DR3, DQA1*0502/ DQB1*0201 DR4, DQA1*0301/ DQB1*0302[73]	Rubella[74,75] (rare) ? Milk[76]	T cell	Insulin, GAD, ICA69, ICA512, GM2-1, ganglioside, etc.
Addison's disease	DR3, DR4	?	T cell	21-Hydroxylase P450-5cc
Thyroiditis	DQB1*0201, DQA1*0301[65–67]	Iodine[77]	T cell	Thyroglobulin, Thyroid peroxidase[54]
Pernicious anemia		?	T cell	Intrinsic factor H^+/K^+ ATPase
Vitiligo		?	?	Melanocyte[78]

with lymphocytic infiltration, have autoantibodies reacting with gliadin. Removal of gliadin from the diet restores intestinal villi to normal.[25] In a similar manner, recent controversial data suggest that ingestion of the milk protein bovine albumin in the first few months of life may be associated with type I diabetes.[87,88]

Several autoantibodies are both disease specific (eg, anti–acetylcholine receptor antibodies in myasthenia gravis[23,89] and anti–TSH receptor antibodies in Graves' disease[49,56]) and causal. "Causal" autoantibodies are associated with transplacental disease transmission. Other autoantibodies (eg, antithyroid autoantibodies including anti–thyroid peroxidase,[54] formerly termed anti-microsomal, and anti-thyroglobulin) are so frequent among patients and relatives as to be of little predictive value. For example, a relative with anti–thyroid peroxidase autoantibodies has a low risk of hypothyroidism unless biochemical evidence of abnormal thyroid function is also present (eg, elevated

TSH). In a similar manner, many individuals may have antibodies to parietal cells, H^+/K^+ adenosine triphosphatase of the stomach,[90] and intrinsic factor, but the autoantibodies do not correlate with abnormal gastric acid secretion and the future development of pernicious anemia.[64]

In the type II syndrome, many ICA-positive individuals appear to not progress to diabetes, and diabetes risk is much lower than for ICA-positive first-degree relatives of subjects with type I diabetes.[51,52] A major portion of ICA-positive polyendocrine patients express what has been termed "selective" or restricted ICA.[52,91] Such ICA reacts only with the β cells of rat islets and fails to react with mouse islets, and represents unusual high titer autoantibodies reacting with glutamic acid decarboxylase (GAD). This unusual form of ICA confers a lower risk of type I diabetes as compared with nonrestricted ICA for both polyendocrine patients and relatives of patients with type I diabetes.

Other autoantibodies associated with the type II syndrome include anti-melanocytic,[78] anti-adrenal[58,59] and anti-gonadal autoantibodies.[32,92] Anti-adrenal cortical antibodies have been used to predict adrenal insufficiency in the type I syndrome. The targets of anti-adrenal antibodies of the APS II syndrome are tissue-specific enzymes including 21 hydroxylase and potentially 17 alpha hydroxylase,[93] essential for steroid biosynthesis.

It is noteworthy that many of the polyendocrine autoantibodies react with intracellular enzymes, including thyroid peroxidase (Hashimoto's thyroiditis),[54] glutamic acid decarboxylase (type I diabetes[94] and stiff-man syndrome[34]), 21 hydroxylase,[59] and cytochrome P450 cholesterol side chain cleavage enzyme,[59] (Addison's disease). In addition, antibodies to hormones are often present, including anti-insulin,[72,95–97] anti-thyroxine,[98–101] and anti–intrinsic factor antibodies (pernicious anemia).

The insulin autoimmune syndrome, associated with Graves' disease and methimazole therapy, is of particular interest.[102] Such patients with elevated titers of anti-insulin autoantibodies frequently present with hypoglycemia. The disease in Japan is essentially confined to DR4-positive individuals with DRB1*0406.[72]

Finally, antibodies to specific receptors can be characteristic of given disorders (anti–acetylcholine receptor antibodies of myasthenia gravis,[23] anti–TSH receptor antibodies of Graves' disease[49] or hypothyroidism,[103] and oocyte sperm receptor autoantibodies associated with oophoritis).[92] The large variety of target molecules, at times for a single disease (eg, type I diabetes), presence of high-affinity IgG autoantibodies, and the sequential appearance over years of specific antibodies or disorders suggest that most autoantibodies are secondary to tissue destruction and are "driven" by their relevant autoantigen.

T cell autoimmunity has been much more difficult to study and correlate with disease. Recent advances in T cell immunobiology, studies of animal models, and transfer of autoreactive T lymphocytes or affected human organs into immunodeficient mice should lead to more rapid progress in understanding T cell autoimmunity.

For decades, experimental animal models of organ-specific autoimmunity have been studied. These were dependent upon the injection of putative autoantigens into animals in the presence of adjuvants that enhance inflammation.[92,104] Thus, thyroiditis can readily be induced in selective strains of mice following injection of thyroglobulin or thyroid peroxidase in Freund's adjuvant. T cell clones reacting with these molecules, or selected peptides, can be generated, and such clones when transferred into naive animals induce disease. Of note, several forms of immunization with such autoreactive clones can be used to make animals refractory to disease induction.[105] These studies provide clear evidence that autoreactive T cells are present in normal animals and can be rapidly activated, given "appropriate" antigen stimulation.

In addition, a recent study by Tung and associates suggest one mechanism whereby properties of T cell recognition may lead to multiple autoimmune disorders.[60,92] In studying experimental autoimmune oophoritis, they identified a peptide of the oocyte sperm receptor (ZP3) that upon injection in adjuvant induced disease. They then identified which of nine amino acids of this peptide was essential to activate autoimmune T cell clones or induce disease. T cells recognize only short peptides presented in the groove of class I or class II major histocompatibility complex (MHC) molecules on antigen-presenting cells. As few as three properly spaced amino acids of nine interacting with a T cell receptor can be sufficient to trigger T cell responses. Noting that a peptide of the acetylcholine receptor had the appropriate T cell binding motif associated with experimental oophoritis, they demonstrated that this peptide stimulated an oophoritis-derived T cell clone in vitro and when administered in vivo induced oophoritis. The requirement for sharing of as few as three of nine amino acids of a linear sequence for activation of autoreactive T cells provides a mechanism whereby inflammation directed at one organ may generalize to additional tissues. Such a model may also help explain specific disease associations. For example, Graves' thyroid disease is frequently complicated by autoimmunity directed at extraocular muscles leading to Graves' ophthalmopathy.[106] If such a mechanism for the "spreading" of autoimmunity is operative, it implies that mechanisms to suppress autoreactivity are particularly important. The possibilities that "molecular mimicry" may induce autoimmunity are greatly increased if short homologous sequences are sufficient to stimulate cross-reactive T cell clones.

Evidence for the importance of normal immune function for suppressing disease is derived from the induction of autoimmunity in animals by neonatal thymectomy or neonatal cyclosporine therapy. Interruption of normal T cell development can result in multiple autoimmune disorders. The BB rat develops type I diabetes and thyroiditis in association with a severe autosomally determined T cell immunodeficiency.[107–109]

Autoimmune disorders appear to share a number of "non-specific" abnormalities of T cell function or enumeration including increased numbers of cells expressing class II molecules ("Ia" positive T cells),[110–112] IL2 receptors, depressed autologous mixed lymphocyte responses,[113] and depressed class I antigen expression.[114,115] These abnormalities appear not to be disease specific and may relate to fundamental abnormalities predisposing to autoimmunity or reflect disease activity.

Autoimmune Polyendocrine Syndrome Type I (APS I)

Major components of the APS I autoimmune polyendrocrine syndrome include hypoparathyroidism, mucocutaneous candidiasis, Addison's disease, and chronic active hepatitis[4] (Table 8.2). Other diseases associated with APS I include primary hypothyroidism, a malabsorption syndrome,[24] vitiligo, pernicious anemia, type I diabetes, alopecia,[22] primary hypogonadism,[31] cutaneous abnormalities,[4] and pure red cell aplasia.[36,116] The onset of the disease is usually in infancy and there is no HLA class II Association (Table 8.2). Of note, in a study by Friedman and coworkers[30] four of nine patients with the syndrome were asplenic. Chronic mucocutaneous candidiasis is often the first disease detected, followed by the later development of adrenal insufficiency. Decades may elapse between the diagnosis of one disease and another in the same individual and the order of disease appearance is not invariant.

The syndrome is inherited in a autosomal recessive manner linked to a gene on chromosome 21 in the absence of HLA haplotype sharing among affected siblings.[136] It is likely that the immunodeficiency underlying disease susceptibility may be secondary to a simple autosomal recessive allele and application of molecular genetic typing to this syndrome is just beginning with a tentative (not definitive) assignment of the APS I locus to chromosome 22.[117] The etiology of the mucocutaneous candidiasis in the absence of systemic candidiasis in unknown but suggests an underlying immunodeficiency. The orally active antifungal drug ketoconazole has significantly improved the mucocutaneous candidiasis associated with this disorder.

Particular patterns of anti-adrenal autoantibodies are associated with this syndrome (eg, anti–P450 cholesterol side chain cleavage enzyme[59] rather than anti–21 hydroxylase antibodies). The presence of anti-adrenal autoantibodies is strongly associated with subsequent development of Addison's disease. In addition, anti-GAD autoantibodies of patients with the APS I syndrome differ from anti-GAD autoantibodies in terms of being able to detect GAD on Western blots and inhibit enzymatic activity.[13] A small minority of patients with APS I develop type I diabetes and their ICA and anti-GAD autoantibodies appear similar to "restricted" ICA, which is infrequently associated with progression to diabetes both in relatives of patients with type I diabetes and in APS II patients.

POEMS Syndrome

These patients usually present with a sensory motor polyneuropathy, diabetes mellitus (50%), primary gonadal failure (70%), and a plasma cell dyscrasia with sclerotic bony lesions.[11,12,118] Temporary remission in bone disease may result following radiotherapy. The syndrome is assumed to be secondary to circulating immunoglobulins.

Anti-Insulin Receptor Antibodies

The presence of anti-insulin receptor autoantibodies is characterized by marked insulin resistance, but paradoxically, patients can also have severe hypoglycemia.[6,7] Approximately one third of the subjects have other autoimmune disorders. Characteristically, associated autoimmune diseases are non–organ specific.

Thymic Tumors

Thymomas and thymic hyperplasias are associated with series of autoimmune diseases.[8,9,119] The most common autoimmune diseases are myasthenia gravis and red cell aplasia. Graves' disease, type I diabetes, and Addison's disease may also be associated with thymic tumors. Unique anti–acetylcholine receptor autoantibodies may be present with thymoma[89] and disease may be initiated by transcription of molecules within the tumor related to acetylcholine receptors.[120]

Other Disorders

Other diseases with polyglandular autoimmunity are Kearns-Sayre syndrome,[121] diabetes and thyroiditis associated with trisomy 21,[122] DIDMOAD syndrome (diabetes insipidus, diabetes mellitus, optic atrophy, and nerve deafness), and congenital rubella[75,123–125] associated with thyroiditis and/or diabetes. Karounos and coworkers have described a rubella protein with homology to an islet protein, suggesting that molecular mimicry may initiate disease.[75] An alternative hypothesis has been proposed by Rabinowe and coworkers.[124] They described long-term T cell subset abnormalities in patients following congenital rubella.

Trials of "Isohormonal" Therapy of Endocrine Autoimmunity

A general property of endocrine glands is feedback inhibition of hormonal secretion. Such feedback control relates not only to the specific hormone (eg, thyroxine, insulin, or glucocorticoids) but in a general manner to metabolism of the relevant endocrine cell. Thus, exogeneous insulin suppresses beta cell synthesis of a large number of molecules and beta cell volume shrinks dramatically. Autoantigens such as GAD disappear from rat islets with maximal insulin feedback inhibition. In a similar manner, thyroxine, by inhibiting TSH secretion, and glucocorticoids, by inhibiting corticotropin (ACTH) secretion from the pituitary, lead to thyroid and adrenal cortical cell atrophy. Such suppression of glandular function may have a profound effect on endocrine autoimmunity, and pilot trials of such therapy for the prevention of type I diabetes, Addison's disease, and Graves' disease have been reported.[137]

Chapter 12 provides more detail concerning trials of insulin therapy in prediabetics. In animal models (BB rat and NOD mouse) subcutaneous insulin suppresses the development of both the diabetes and insulitis.[126,127] It is not known whether the effect of insulin is secondary to its metabolic action in "resting" beta cells, or related to modifying the immune system. Suppression of disease is specific to islets; for example, thyroiditis of the BB rat is not affected. Evidence supports an important role of beta cell suppression and there is suggestive evidence of an immune effect in the BB rat model, high doses of insulin are required[128]; in the NOD mouse model, immunization with the B chain of insulin can decrease the development of diabetes.[129] In addition, oral insulin to induce "oral tolerance" may be important for disease suppression. The findings of Dale Wegmann and coworkers that insulin-reactive T cell clones are present in NOD islets and that such clones can transfer diabetes (see Chapter 4) strongly suggest that an immune response to insulin may be an important regulatory component of the pathogenesis of diabetes. In man a small pilot trial has been completed,[130] and a larger randomized trial of parenteral insulin therapy initiated.

Hashizume and coworkers have reported that thyroxine therapy of individuals at risk for recurrence of Graves' disease markedly decreases disease relapse.[131–133] These studies also suggest that such therapy decreases anti–TSH receptor autoantibodies. Studies in animal models suggest that thyroxine therapy, for example of the BB rat, decreases thyroiditis. It is possible that a portion of the self-immunization that leads to persistence of autoimmunity occurs within the thyroid gland, and thus decreasing thyroid cell activity would limit autoimmunity.

Recently, DeBellis and coworkers described the development of Addison's disease in a series of patients with anti-adrenal autoantibodies.[14] Three of the patients were treated with 6 months of glucocorticoids for Graves' ophthalmopathy. Remarkably, anti-adrenal autoantibodies disappeared in all three of these individuals and, in contrast to other patients with high titers of anti-adrenal autoantibodies, development of Addison's disease appears to have been prevented. The patients remained with normal adrenal function after the discontinuation of glucocorticoid therapy.

Conclusions

Polyendrocrine autoimmune syndromes have historically played an important role in understanding several autoimmune disorders and in particular for type I diabetes. The initial evidence that type I diabetes was an autoimmune disorder came from its association with spontaneous Addison's disease, and lack of association with tuberculous Addison's disease.[134] The first demonstration of cytoplasmic islet cell autoantibodies occurred in patients with polyendocrine autoimmunity.[135] It is now recognized that a major subset of such ICA in polyendocrine patients is unusual anti-GAD autoantibodies.[52,91]

The existence of families of related autoimmune disorders not only is clinically important but suggests that the pathogenesis of these diseases are related. This relationship probably is a result of two distinct pathogenic phenomena. The first is inherited abnormalities of immune function, predisposing to the loss of tolerance to a series of self antigens. Given such a predisposition, alleles within the major histocompatibility complex may then target specific organs. Differences between characteristic diseases of the syndromes may also be related to immunogenetic differences. For example, the only patient with type I diabetes we have observed with the protective allele DQB1*0602 (among 250 typed) is a patient with polyendocrine autoimmune syndrome type I. In this syndrome, Addison's disease is also not HLA associated, in contrast to Addison's disease of the type II polyendocrine autoimmune syndrome. The second phenomenon that may link these disorders, especially for tightly linked diseases such as Graves' ophthalmopathy and Graves' thyroid disease, is creation of pathogenic T cells reacting with components of more than one tissue. In that T cell clones can respond to peptides that share only three of nine identical amino acids, depending upon the linear sequence, the potential for such cross-reactivity must be enormous.

Finally, the relationships between these diverse disorders suggest that as disease pathogenesis is elucidated and antigen-specific therapies are developed, they will find wide applicability for many autoimmune diseases.

References

1. Schmidt MB. Eine biglandulare Erkrankung (Nebennieren und Schilddruse) bei Morbus Addisonii. *Verh Dtsch Ges Pathol.* 1926; 21:212–221.
2. Eisenbarth GS, Jackson RA. The immunoendocrinopathy syndromes. In: Wilson JD, Foster DW, eds. *Williams Textbook of Endocrinology.* 8th ed. Philadelphia: W. B. Saunders Company; 1992; 1555–1566.
3. Neufeld M, Maclaren NK, Blizzard BM. Two types of autoimmune Addison's disease associated with different polyglandular autoimmune (PGA) syndromes. *Medicine.* 1981; 60:355–362.
4. Ahonen P, Myllarniemi S, Śipila J. Clinical variation of autoimmune polyendocrinopathy–candidiasis–ectodermal dystrophy (APECED) in a series of 68 patients. *N Engl J Med.* 1990; 322:1830–1836.
5. Flier JS, Kahn CR, Roth J, Bar RS. Antibodies that impair insulin receptor binding in an unusual diabetic syndrome with severe insulin resistance. *Science.* 1975; 190:63–65.
6. Flier JS, Bar RS, Muggeo M, Kahn CR, Roth J, Gorden P. The evolving clinical course of patients with insulin receptor autoantibodies: spontaneous remission or receptor proliferation with hypoglycemia. *J Clin Endocrinol Metab.* 1978; 47:985–995.
7. Taylor SI, Grunberger G, Marcus-Samuels B, et al. Hypoglycemia associated with antibodies to the insulin receptor. *N Engl J Med.* 1982; 307:1422–1426.

8. Souadjian JV, Enriquez P, Silverstein MN, Pepin J-M. The spectrum of diseases associated with thymoma. *Arch Intern Med.* 1974; 134:374–379.
9. Combs RM. Malignant thymoma, hyperthyroidism and immune disorder. *South Med J.* 1968; 61:337–341.
10. Maggi G, Casadio C, Cavallo A, Cianci R, Molinatti M, Ruffini E. Thymoma: results of 241 operated cases. *Ann Thorac Surg.* 1991; 51:152–156.
11. Imawari M, Akatsuka N, Ishibashi M, Beppu H, Suzuki H, Yoshitoshi Y. Syndrome of plasma cell dyscrasia, polyneuropathy, and endocrine disturbances. *Ann Intern Med.* 1974; 81:490–493.
12. Miralles GD, O'Fallon JR, Talley NJ. Plasma-cell dyscrasia with polyneuropathy: the spectrum of POEMS syndrome. *N Engl J Med.* 1992; 327:1919–1923.
13. Bjork E, Velloso LA, Kampe O, Karlsson FA. GAD autoantibodies in IDDM, stiff-man syndrome, and autoimmune polyendocrine syndrome type I recognize different epitopes. *Diabetes.* 1994; 43:161–165.
14. De Bellis A, Bizzarro A, Rossi R, et al. Remission of subclinical adrenocortical failure in subjects with adrenal autoantibodies. *J Clin Endocrinol Metab.* 1993; 76:1002–1007.
15. Landin-Olsson M, Karlsson FA, Lernmark A, Sundkvist G, and the Diabetes Incidence Study in Sweden Group. Islet cell and thyrogastric antibodies in 633 consecutive 15- to 34-yr-old patients in the diabetes incidence study in Sweden. *Diabetes.* 1992; 41:1022–1027.
16. Fairfax AJ, Leatham A. Idiopathic heart block: association with vitiligo, thyroid disease, pernicious anemia, and diabetes mellitus. *Br Med J.* 1975; 4:322–324.
17. Campbell IL, Harrison LC. Molecular pathology of type I diabetes. *Mol Biol Med.* 1989; 6:1–11.
18. Peserico A, Rigon F, Semsenzato G, Caretto A, Pasini CV, Betterle C. Vitiligo and polyglandular autoimmune disease with autoantibodies to melanin-producing cells. *arch Dermatol.* 1981; 117:751–752.
19. Peserico A, Rigon F, Semenzato G, Caretto A, Pasini CV, Betterle C. Vitiligo and polyglandular autoimmune disease with autoantibodies to melanin-producing cells. A new syndrome? *Arch Dermatol.* 1981; 117:751–752.
20. Torrelo A, Espana A, Balsa L, Ledo A. Vitiligo and polyglandular autoimmune syndrome with selective IgA deficiency. *Int J Dermatol.* 1992; 31:343–344.
21. Stankler L, Bewsher PD. Chronic mucocutaneous candidiasis endocrine deficiency and alopecia areata. *Br J Dermatol.* 1972; 86:238–245.
22. Garty BZ, Kauli R. Alopecia universalis in autoimmune polyglandular syndrome type I [letter; comment]. *West J Med.* 1990; 152:76–77.
23. Protti MP, Manfredi AA, Horton RM, Bellone M, Conti-Tronconi B. Myasthenia gravis: recognition of a human autoantigen at the molecular level. *Immunol Today.* 1993.
24. Scire G, Magliocca FM, Cianfarani S, Scalamandre A, Petrozza V, Bonamico M. Autoimmune polyendocrine candidiasis syndrome with associated chronic diarrhea caused by intestinal infection and pancreas insufficiency. *J Pediatr Gastroenterol Nutr.* 1991; 13:224–227.
25. Savilahti E, Simell O, Koskimies S, Rilva A, Akerblom AK. Celiac disease in insulin dependent diabetes mellitus. *J Pediatr.* 1986; 108(1):690–693.
26. Teunala T, Salmi J, Karvonen J. Dermatitis herpetiformis and celiac disease associated with Addison's disease. *Arch Dermatol.* 1987; 123:930–932.
27. Papadopoulos KI, Hallengren B. Polyglandular autoimmune syndrome type III associated with coeliac disease and sarcoidosis. *Postgrad Med J.* 1993; 69:72–75.

28. Volanakis JE, Zhu Z, Schaffer FM, et al. Major histocompatibility complex class III genes and susceptibility to immunoglobulin A deficiency and common variable immunodeficiency. *J Clin Invest.* 1992; 89:1914–1922.
29. Tucker WS, Niblack GD, McLean RH, et al. Serositis with autoimmune endocrinopathy; clinical and immunogenetic features. *Medicine.* 1987; 64:?.
30. friedman TC, Thomas PM, Fleisher TA, et al. Frequent occurrence of asplenism and cholelithiasis in patients with autoimmune polyglandular disease type I. *Am J Med.* 1991; 91:625–630.
31. Ahonen P, Miettinen A, Perheentupa J. Adrenal and steroidal cell antibodies in patients with autoimmune polyglandular disease type I and risk of adrenocortical and ovarian failure. *J Clin Endocrinol Metab.* 1987; 64:494–500.
32. Irvine WJ, Chand MMM, Scarth L, et al. Immunological aspects of premature ovarian failure associated with idiopathic Addison's disease. *Lancet.* 1968; 2:883–887.
33. Turkington RW, Lebovitz HE. Extra-adrenal endocrine deficiencies in Addison's disease. *Am J Med.* 1967; 43:499–507.
34. Solimena M, Folli F, Aparisi R, Pozza G, DeCamilli P. Autoantibodies to GABA-ergic neurons and pancreatic beta cells in stiff-man syndrome. *N Engl J Med.* 1990; 322:1555–1560.
35. Brown FM, Freeman R, Tyler HR, Watts M, Rabinowe SL. Polyglandular autoimmunity and Parkinson's disease. *Clin Res.* 1989; in press.
36. Mandel M, Etzoni A, Theodor R, Passwell JH. Pure red cell hypoplasia associated with polyglandular autoimmune syndrome type I. *Isr J Med Sci.* 1989; 25:138–141.
37. Lucas-Martin A, Foz-Sala M, Todd I, Bottazzo GF, Pujol-Borrell R. Occurrence of thyrocyte HLA class II expression in a wide variety of thyroid diseases: relationship with lymphocytic infiltration and thyroid autoantibodies. *J Clin Endocrinol Metab.* 1988; 66:367–375.
38. Selinger S, tsai J, Pulini M, Saperstein A, Taylor S. Autoimmune thrombocytopenia and primary bilary cirrhosis with hypoglycemia and insulin receptor autoantibodies. *Ann Intern Med.* 1987; 107:686–688.
39. Candrina R, Giustina A. Development of type II autoimmune polyglandular syndrome in a patient with idiopathic thrombocytopenic purpura. *Isr J Med Sci.* 1988; 24:57–58.
40. Muir A, Maclaren NK. Autoimmune diseases of the adrenal glands, parathyroid glands, gonads, and hypothalamic-pituitary axis. *Endocrinol Metab Clin North Am.* 1991; 20:619–644.
41. Barkan AL, Kelch RP, Marshall JC. Isolated gonadotrope failure in the polyglandular autoimmune syndrome. *N Engl J Med.* 1985; 312:1535–1540.
42. Eisenbarth GS, Wilson P, Ward F, Lebovitz HE. HLA type and disease occurrence in familial polyglandular failure. *N Engl J Med.* 1978; 298:92–94.
43. Eisenbarth GS, Wilson P, Ward F, Buckley C, Lebovitz HE. The polyglandular failure syndrome: disease inheritance, HLA-type and immune functions. *Ann Intern Med.* 1979; 91:528–533.
44. Tucker WS, Niblack GD, McLean RH, et al. Serositis with autoimmune endocrinopathy: clinical and immunogenetic features. *D.* 1992; 66:138–147.
45. Liblau R, Fischer AM, Shapiro DE, Morel E, Bach JF. The frequency of selective IgA deficiency in myasthenia gravis. *Neurology.* 1992; 42:516–518.
46. Maclaren NK, Riley WJ. Inherited susceptibility to autoimmune Addison's disease is linked to human leukocyte antigens-DR3 and/or DR4 except when associated

with type I autoimmune polyglandular syndrome. *J Clin Endocrinol Metab.* 1986; 62:455–459.

47. Butler MG, Hodes ME, Conneally PM, Biegel AA, Wright JC. Linkage analysis in a large kindred with autosomal dominant transmission of polyglandular autoimmune disease type II (Schmidt syndrome). *Am J Med Genet.* 1984; 18:61–65.
48. Farid NR, Larsen B, Payne R, Noel EP, Sampson L. Polyglandular autoimmune disease and HLA. *Tissue Antigens.* 1980; 16:23–29.
49. Costagliola S, Swillens S, Niccoli P, Dumont JE, Vassart G, Ludgate M. Binding assay for thyrotropin receptor autoantibodies using the recombinant receptor protein. *J Clin Endocrinol Metab.* 1992; 75:1540–1544.
50. Betterle C, Presotto F, Pedini B, et al. Islet cell and insulin autoantibodies in organ-specific autoimmune patients: their behavior and predictive value for the development of Type I (insulin-dependent) diabetes mellitus: a 10 year follow up study. *Diabetologia.* 1987; 30:292–297.
51. Bosi E, Becker F, Bonifacio E, et al. Progression to Type I (insulin-dependent) diabetes in autoimmune endocrine patients with islet cell antibodies. *Diabetes.* 1991; 40:977–984.
52. Genovese S, Bonifacio E, McNally JM, et al. Distinct cytoplasmic islet cell antibodies with different risks for type I (insulin-dependent) diabetes mellitus. *Diabetologia.* 1992; 35:385–388.
53. Kohno Y, Yamaguchi F, Saito K, Miimi H, Nishikawa T, Hosoya T. Anti-thyroid peroxidase antibodies in sera from healthy subjects and from patients with chronic thyroiditis: differences in the ability to inhibit thyroid peroxidase activities. *Clin Exp Immunol.* 1991; 85:459–463.
54. Maastricht J, Koenig RJ, Kaplan MM, Arscott P, Thompson N, Baker JR. Identification of localized autoantibody epitopes in thyroid peroxidase. *J Clin Endocrinol Metab.* 1992; 75:121–126.
55. Chase HP, Garg SK, Cockerhams RS, Wilcox WD, Walravens PA. Thyroid hormone replacement and growth of children with subclinical hypothyroidism and diabetes. *Diabetic Med.* 1990; 7:299–303.
56. Nagayama Y, Rapoport B. Thyroid stimulatory autoantibodies in different patients with autoimmune thyroid disease do not all recognize the same components of the human thyrotropin receptor: selective role of receptor amino acids Ser25-Glu30. *J Clin Invest.* 1992; 75:1425–1430.
57. Blizzard RM, Kyle M. Studies of the adrenal antigens and antibodies in Addison's disease. *J Clin Invest.* 1963; 42:1653–1660.
58. Wardle CA, Weetman AP, Mitchell R, Peers N, Robertson WR. Adrenocorticotropic hormone receptor-blocking immunoglobulins in serum from patients with Addison's disease: a reexamination. *J Clin Endocrinol Metab.* 1993; 77:750–753.
59. Winqvist O, Gustafsson J, Rorsman F, Karlsson FA, Kampe O. Two different cytochrome P450 enzymes are the adrenal antigens in autoimmune polyendrocrine syndrome type I and Addison's disease. *J Clin Invest.* 1993; 92:2377–2385.
60. Luo A-M, Garza KM, Hunt D, Tung KSK. Antigen mimicry in autoimmune disease sharing of amino acid residues critical for pathogenic T cell activation. *J Clin Invest.* 1993; 92:2117–2123.
61. Maclaren NK, Riley WJ. Inherited susceptibility to autoimmune Addison's disease is linked to human leukocyte antigens DR3 and/or DR4, except when associated

with type 1 autoimmune polyglandular syndrome. *J Clin Endocrinol Metab.* 1986; 62(3):455–459.

62. Valenta LJ, Bull RW, Hackel E, Bottazzo GF. Correlation of the HLA-A1, B8 haplotypes with circulating autoantibodies in a family with increased incidence of autoimmune disease. *Acta Endocrinol.* 1982; 100:143–149.
63. Bloch MH, Sowers JR. Vitiligo and polyglandular autoimmune endocrinopathy. *Cutis.* 1985; 36:417–419.
64. Petite J, Rosset N, Chapuis B, Jeannet M. Genetic factors predisposing to autoimmune diseases: study of HLA antigens in a family with pernicious anemia and thyroid diseases. *Schweiz Med Wochenschr.* 1987; 117:2032–2037.
65. Inoue D, Sato K, Sugawa H, et al. Apparent genetic difference between hypothyroid patients with blocking-type thyrotropin receptor antibody and those without, as shown by restriction fragment length polymorphism analyses of HLA-DP loci. *J Clin Endocrinol Metab.* 1993; 77:606–610.
66. Farid NR. Understanding the genetics of autoimmune thyroid disease–still an elusive goal! [editorial]. *J Clin Endocrinol Metab.* 1992; 74:485A–495B.
67. Shi Y, Zou M, Robb D, Farid NR. Typing for major histocompatibility complex class II antigens in thyroid tissue blocks: association of Hashimoto's thyroiditis with HLA-DQA0301 and DQB0201 alleles. *J Clin Endocrinol Metab.* 1992; 75:943–946.
68. Matsuki K, Juji T, Tokunaga K, et al. HLA antigens in Japanese patients with myasthenia gravis. *J Clin Invest.* 1990: 392:399.
69. Garlepp MJ, Dawkins RL, Christiansen FT. HLA antigens and acetylcholine receptor antibodies in penicillamine induced myasthenia gravis. *Br Med J.* 1983; 286:338–340.
70. Dons RF, Havlik R, Taylor SI, Baird KL, Chernick SS, Gorden P. Clinical disorders associated with autoantibodies to the insulin receptor. *J Clin Invest.* 1992; ?.
71. Posillico JT, Wortsman J, Srikanta S, Eisenbarth GS, Malette L, Brown EM. Parathyroid cell surface autoantibodies that inhibit parathyroid hormone secretion from dispersed human parathyroid cells. *Bone Miner Res.* 1986; 5:475–485.
72. Uchigata Y, Kuwata S, Tsushima T, et al. Patients with Graves' disease who developed insulin autoimmune syndrome (Hirata disease) possess HLA-Bw62/Cw4?DR4 carrying DRB1*0406. *J Clin Endocrinol Metab.* 1993; 77:249–254.
73. Nepom GT. Immunogenetics and IDDM. *Diabetes Rev.* 1993; 1:93–103.
74. Rubenstein P. The HLA system in congenital rubella patients with and without diabetes. *Diabetes.* 1982; 31:1088–1091.
75. Karounos DG, Wolinsky JS, Thomas JW. Monoclonal antibody to rubella virus capsid protein recognizes a B-cell antigen. *J Immunol.* 1993; 150:3080–3085.
76. Virtanen S, Rasanen L, Aro A, et al. Infant feeding in Finnish children <7 yr. of age with newly diagnosed IDDM. *Diabetes Care.* 1991; 14(5):415–417.
77. Rabinowe SL, Larsen PR, Antman EM, et al. Amiodarone therapy and autoimmune thyroid disease: elevation of a new monoclonal antibody defined T cell subset. *Am J Med.* 1986; 81:53–57.
78. Naughton GK, Eisenger M, Bystryn J-C. Detection of antibodies to melanocytes in vitiligo by specific immunoprecipitation. *J Invest Dermatol.* 1983; 81:540–542.
79. Posillico JT, Srikanta S, Eisenbarth GS, Quaranta V, Kajiji S, Brown EM. Binding of monoclonal antibody (4F2) to its cell surface antigen on dispersed adenomatous parathyroid cells raises cytosolic calcium and inhibits parathyroid secretion. *J Clin Endocrinol Metab.* 1987; 64:43–50.

80. French MAH, Dawkins RL. Central MHC genes, IgA deficiency and autoimmune disease. *Immunology Today.* 1990; 11(8):?.
81. Deschamps I, Goderel I, Lestradet H, et al. Segregation of HLA-DR2 among affected and non-affected offspring of 66 families with Type I (insulin-dependent) diabetes. *Diabetologia.* 1984; 27:80–82.
82. Liblau RS, Caillat-Zucman S, Fischer AM, Bach JF, Boitard C. The prevalence of selective IgA deficiency in type 1 diabetes mellitus. *APMIS.* 1992; 100:709–712.
83. Valenta LJ, Elias AN. Familial scleroderma in a kindred with high incidence of autoimmune disease: correlation with HLA-A1/B8 haplotype. *Arch Dermatol.* 1987; 123:1438–1440.
84. Dobersen MJ, Scharff JE. Preferential lysis of pancreatic B cells by islet cell surface antibodies. *Diabetes.* 1982; 31:459–462.
85. Bottazzo GF, Vandelli G, Mirakian R. The detection of autoantibodies to discrete endocrine cells in complex endocrine organs. In: Pinchera A, Doniach D, Fenzi GF, Baschieri, eds. *Autoimmune Aspects of Endocrine Disorders.* London: Academic Press; 1980:366–377.
86. Vela BS, Dorin RI, Hartshorne MF. Case report 631: neo-osseous porosis (metaphyseal osteopenia) in polyglandular autoimmune (Schmidt) syndrome. *Skeletal Radiol.* 1990; 19:468–471.
87. Karjalainen J, Martin JM, Knip M, et al. A bovine albumin peptide as a possible trigger of insulin-dependent diabetes mellitus. *N Engl J Med.* 1992; 327:302–307.
88. Atkinson MA, Bowman MA, Kuo-Jang K, et al. Lack of immune responsiveness to bovine serum albumin in insulin-dependent diabetes. *N Engl J Med.* 1993; 329;1853–1858.
89. Mygland A, Tysnes O-B, Aarli JA, Matre R, Gilhus NE. IgG subclass distribution of ryanodine receptor autoantibodies in patients with myasthenia gravis and thymoma. *J Autoimm.* 1993; 6:507–515.
90. Karlsson FA, Burman P, Loof L, Mardh S. Major parietal cell antigen in autoimmune gastritis and pernicious anemia is the acid producing H^+, K adenosine triphosphatase of the stomach. *J Clin Invest.* 1988; 81:475–479.
91. Gianani R, Pugliese A, Bonner-Weir S, et al. Prognostically significant heterogeneity of cytoplasmic islet cell antibodies in relatives of patients with type I diabetes. *Diabetes.* 1992; 41:347–353.
92. Rhim SH, Millar SE, Robey F, et al. Autoimmune disease of the ovary induced by a ZP3 peptide from the mouse zona pellucida. *J Clin Invest.* 1992; 89:28–35.
93. Krohn K, Uibo R, Aavik E, Peterson P, Savilahit K. Identification by molecular cloning of an autoantigen associated with Addison's disease as steroid 17alpha-hydroxylase. *Lancet.* 1992; 339:770–773.
94. Baekkeskov S, Aanstoot H, Christgau S, et al. Identification of the 64K autoantigen in insulin dependent diabetes as the GABA-synthesizing enzyme glutamic acid decarboxylase. *Nature.* 1990; 347:151–156.
95. Palmer JP, Asplin CM, Clemons P, et al. Insulin antibodies in insulin-dependent diabetics before insulin treatment. *Science.* 1983; 222:1337–1339.
96. Greenbaum C, Palmer JP, Kuglin B, Kolb H, and Participating Laboratories. Insulin autoantibodies measured by radioimmunoassay methodology are more related to insulin-dependent diabetes mellitus than those measured by enzyme-linked immunosorbent assay: results of the Fourth International Workshop on the Standardization of Insulin Autoantibody Measurement. *J Clin Endocrinol Metab.* 1992; 74:1040–1044.
97. Vardi P, Ziegler AG, Matthews JH, et al. Concentration of insulin autoantibodies at

onset of type I diabetes: inverse log-linear correlation with age. *Diabetes Care.* 1988; 11:736–739.

98. Robbins J, Rall je, Rawson RW. An unusual instance of thyroxine-binding by human serum gamma globulins. *J Clin Endocrinol Metab.* 1956; 16:573–579.
99. Staeheli V, Vallotton MB, Burger A. Detection of human anti-thyroxine and anti-triiodothyronine antibodies in different thyroid conditions. *J Clin Endocrinol Metab.* 1975; 41:669–675.
100. Inada M, Nishikawa M, Naito K, Oishi M, Kurata S, Imura H. Triiodothyronine-binding immunoglobulin in a patient with Graves' disease and its effect on metabolism and radioimmunoassay of triiodothyronine. *Am J Med.* 1980; 68:787–792.
101. Papo T, Oksenhendler E, Izembart M, Leger A, Clauvel J-P. Antithyroid hormone antibodies induced by interferon-a. *J Clin Endocrinol Metab.* 1992; 75:1484–1486.
102. Hirata Y. Methimazole and insulin autoimmune syndrome with hypoglycemia. *Lancet.* 1983; 99:182–184.
103. Takasu N, Yamada T, Takasu M, et al. Disappearance of thyrotropin-blocking antibodies and spontaneous recovery from hypothyroidism in autoimmune thyroiditis. *N Engl J Med.* 1992; 326:513–518.
104. McKeever U, Mordes JP, Greiner DL, et al. Adoptive transfer of autoimmune diabetes and thyroiditis to athymic rats. *Proc Natl Acad Sci U S A.* 1990; 87:7618–7622.
105. Cohen IR, Young DB. Autoimmunity, microbial immunity and the immunological homunculus. *Immunol Today.* 1991; 105:105–110.
106. Heufelder AE, Wenzel BE, Bahn RS. Cell surface localization of a 72 kilodalton heat shock protein in retroocular fibroblasts from patients with Graves' ophthalmopathy. *J Clin Endocrinol Metab.* 1992; 74:732–736.
107. Rossini AA, Greiner DL, Friedman HP, Mordes JP. Immunopathogenesis of diabetes mellitus. *Diabetes Rev.* 1993; 1:43–75.
108. Jackson R, RASSI N, Crump A, Haynes BF, Eisenbarth GS. The BB diabetic rat: profound T cell lymphocytopenia. *Diabetes.* 1981; 30:887–889.
109. Jacob HJ, Pettersson A, Wilson D, Mao Y, Lernmark A, Lander ES. Genetic dissection of autoimmune type I diabetes in the BB rat. *Nature Genetics.* 1992; 2:56–60.
110. Jackson RA, Haynes BF, Burch WM, Shimizu K, Bowring MA, Eisenbarth GS. Ia^+ T cells in new onset Graves' disease. *J Clin Endocrinol Metab.* 1984; 114:1–6.
111. Jackson Ra, Morris MA, Haynes BF, Eisenbarth GS. Increased circulating Ia-antigen-bearing T cells in type I diabetes mellitus. *N Engl J Med.* 1982; 306:785–788.
112. Alviggi L, Hoskins PJ, Pyke DA, et al. Pathogenesis of insulin-dependent diabetes: a role for activated T lymphocytes. *Lancet.* 1984; 1:4–6.
113. Kaye WA, Adri MNS, Soeldner JS, et al. Acquired interleukin-2 production defect in patients with type I diabetes mellitus. *N Engl J Med.* 1986; 315:920–924.
114. Faustman D, Li X, Lin HY, et al. Linkage of faulty major histocompatibility complex class I to autoimmune diabetes. *Science.* 1991; 254:1756–1761.
115. LI X, Golden J, Faustman DL. Faulty major histocompatibility complex class II I-E expression is associated with autoimmunity in diverse strains of mice. *Diabetes.* 1993; 42:1166–1172.
116. Hara T, Mizuno Y, Nagata M, et al. Human gamma delta T-cell receptor-positive cell-mediated inhibition of erythropoiesis in vitro in a patient with type I

autoimmune polyglandular syndrome and pure red blood cell aplasia. *Blood.* 1990; 75:941–950.

117. Aaltonen J, Komulainen J, Vikman A, et al. Autoimmune polyglandular disease type I. *Eur J Hum Genet.* 1993; 1:164–171.
118. Amiel LL, Machover D, Droz JP. Dyscrasie plasmocytaire avec arteriopathie, polyneuropathie, syndrome endocrinien. *Ann Med Interne.* 1975; 745:749.
119. Piccolo G, Martino G, Moglia A, Arrigo A, Cosi V. Autoimmune myasthenia gravis with thymoma following the spontaneous remission of stiff-man syndrome. *Ital J Neurol Sci.* 1990; 11(2):177–180.
120. Elliot RB, Martin JM. Dietary protein: a trigger of insulin-dependent diabetes in the BB rats? *Diabetologia.* 1984; 26:297–299.
121. Scully RE, Mark EJ, McNeely WF, McNeely BU. Case records of the Massachusetts General Hospital: Case 34-1987. *N Engl J Med.* 1987; 317:493–501.
122. Rabinowe SL, Rubin L, George KL, Adri MNS, Eisenbarth GS. Trisomy 21 (Down's syndrome): autoimmunity, aging and monoclonal antibody defined T cell abnormalities. *J Autoimmun.* 1989; 2:25–30.
123. Clarke W, Shaver K, Bright GA, Rogal AD, Nance WE. Autoimmunity in congenital rubella syndrome. *J Pediatr.* 1984; 104:370–373.
124. Rabinowe SL, George KL, Laughlin R, Soeldner JS, Eisenbarth GS. Congenital rubella: monoclonal antibody defined T cell abnormalities in young children. *Am J Med.* 1986; 81:779–782.
125. Rubinstein P, Walker ME, Fedun B, Witt ME, Cooper LZ, Ginsberg-Fellner F. The HLA system in congenital rubella patients with and without diabetes. *Diabetes.* 1982; 31:1088–1091.
126. Gottsfredsen Cf, Buschard K, Frandsen EK. Reduction of diabetes incidence of BB Wistar rats by early prophylactic insulin treatment of diabetes-prone animals. *Diabetologia.* 1985; 28:933–935.
127. Atkinson M, Maclaren N, Luchetta R, Burr I. Insulitis and diabetes in NOD mice reduced by prophylactic insulin therapy. *Diabetes.* 1990; 39:933–937.
128. Like AA. Insulin injections prevent diabetes in BB/Wor rats. *Diabetes.* 1986; 35(Suppl 1):75a. Abstract.
129. Muir A, Luchetta R, Song H-Y, Peck A, Krischer J, Maclaren N. Insulin immunization protects NOD mice from disease. *Autoimmunity.* 1993; 15:58. Abstract.
130. Keller RJ, Eisenbarth GS, Jackson RA. Insulin prophylaxis in individuals at high risk of type I diabetes. *Lancet.* 1993; 341:927–928.
131. Hashizume K, Ichikawa K, Sakurai A, et al. Administration of thyroxine in treated Graves' disease: effects on the level of antibodies to thyroid-stimulatory hormone receptors and on the risk of recurrence of hyperthyroidism. *N Engl J Med.* 1991; 324:947–953.
132. Hashizume K, Ichikawa K, Nishi Y, et al. Effect of administration of thyroxine on the risk of postpartum recurrence of hyperthyroid Graves' disease. *J Clin Endocrinol Metab.* 1992; 75:6–10.
133. Singer PA. Editorial: Will postpartum recurrence of Graves' hyperthyroidism become a thing of the past? *J Clin Endocrinol Metab.* 1992; ?.
134. Nerup J. Addison's disease—clinical studies: a report of 108 cases. *Acta Endocrinol.* 1974; 76:127–141.
135. Olmos P, A'Hearn R, Heaton DA, Risley D, Pyke DA, Leslie RDG. The significance of concordance rate of type I (insulin dependent) diabetes mellitus in identical twins. *Diabetologia.* 1988; 31:747–750.

136. Aaltonen J, Bjorses P, Sandkijl L, Peerheentupa J, Peltonen L. An autosomal locus causing autoimmune disease: autoimmune polyglandular disease type I assigned to chromosome 21. *Nature Genet.* 1994; 8:83–87.
137. Schloot N, Eisenbarth GS. Isohormonal therapy of endocrine autoimmunity. *Immunol Today.* 1995; 16:289–294.

9

Epidemiology of Type I Diabetes

M. Rewers
J. M. Norris

Type I diabetes (insulin-dependent diabetes mellitus, IDDM) is one of the most common of chronic childhood illnesses, affecting in the United States over 11,000 new cases annually and 2–3/1000 children by the age of 20 years.[1] It is the leading cause of end-stage renal disease, blindness, and amputation and a major cause of cardiovascular disease and premature death in the general population.[2] This disease results in over $5 billion in medical care expenditures per year, with costs for patients over 10 times that for nondiabetics.[3] Both the U.S. Public Health Service[4] and the American Diabetes Assocation[5] have recently identified needs in the area of prevention of type I diabetes. The information gained from laboratory, family, and population screening studies has made it possible today to plan secondary prevention of diabetes in persons with ongoing β-cell autoimmunity, but this information remains insufficient to plan primary prevention of β-cell autoimmunity. This chapter considers the whole spectrum of type I diabetes—from genetic susceptibility, through β-cell autoimmunity without diabetes, to clinical IDDM. Special emphasis is given to epidemiological data relevant to the primary and secondary prevention of IDDM.

Descriptive Epidemiology of IDDM

For the purposes of epidemiological research, a standard definition of IDDM has been developed and widely used. The definition consists of the following criteria: 1) diagnosis of diabetes by a physician, 2) daily insulin injections instituted at the time of diagnosis, 3) residence by the patient in the area of registration at the time of the first insulin administration, and 4) diagnosis prior to an age specified by the study (ie, <15 years or <20 years, etc.). The risk of IDDM varies considerably based on family history of IDDM, geographic location, race, age, gender, and time period. There are a number of exciting features about IDDM epidemiology that, if elucidated, could lead to a better understanding of the etiology of the disease.

Prevalence

Initial examination of a disease generally begins with cross-sectional data on its prevalence (ie, the number of people in the population who have the disease). Selected estimates of IDDM prevalence in different populations with at least 90% ascertainment are compared in Table 9.1. Comparisons based upon prevalence data may be subject to considerable bias, since prevalence is determined not only by disease incidence (ie, the rate at which disease appears in the population), but also by case survival, which may vary markedly in populations. Prevalence data are useful in determining the public health impact of IDDM. For example, it is estimated that there are approximately 123,000 individuals aged 0–19 years in the United States who currently have IDDM.[6]

Incidence

Family History of IDDM. The risk of IDDM by the age of 15 years is approximately 1/400 for children in the general (Colorado) population.[17] The risk is increased to about 1/40 in offspring of IDDM fathers and to 1/66 in offspring of IDDM mothers (J. S. Dorman and B. McCarthy, unpublished

Table 9.1. Prevalence of Insulin-Dependent Diabetes Mellitus (IDDM), from Selected Studies

Location	*Year of Study*	*Age (y)*	*Prevalence Rate (per 100,000)*
United States			
Rochester, MN[7]	1970	0–14	57
Kentucky[8]	1978–79	0–17	208
Erie County, PA[9]	1961	0–15	61
Europe			
Denmark[10]	1973	0–14	83
Finland[11]	1979	0–14	191
Sweden[12]	1977	0–14	300
Leicester[13]	1984–85	0–14	99
Estonia[14]	1988	0–14	60
Oceania			
Canterbury, NZ[15]	1986	0–19	105
Tasmania, Australia[16]	1984	0–14	57

observation). The risk to siblings of IDDM probands, reported from several U.S. populations, ranges from 1/12 to 1/35[18–22] and it is 1/4 for human leukocyte antigen (HLA) identical siblings. Family history of IDDM serves as a surrogate measure for genes associated with IDDM and, probably, for some of the shared environmental exposure(s). For comparison, the estimated risk to HLA-DR3/4 heterozygous children in the general population ranges from 1/35 to 1/90, by age 15 years.[23] The genetic susceptibility for IDDM is discussed in a separate chapter of this volume.

"Familial" and "sporadic" cases of IDDM do not appear to be etiologically different subtypes. In fact, the body of published evidence, reviewed by O'Leary and coworkers,[24] indicates that there is no difference between these subgroups in terms of the HLA phenotype distribution, seasonality of onset, prevalence of islet cell antibodies (ICAs), insulin autoantibodies, or IgM against Coxsackie virus B. Familial cases tend to have lower hemoglobin A_1 and higher C peptide levels than sporadic cases, because relatives recognize diabetes symptoms earlier; however, these differences disappear within 1 year of diagnosis. If IDDM is heterogeneous, age at onset[25] or HLA phenotypes[26] are likely to be better discriminators than family history.

Geographic Location. Approximately 3 out of 1000 children will develop IDDM by the age of 20 years.[27] In the United States, the incidence of IDDM is approximately 15 per 100,000 persons per year.[17,28] One of the most striking characteristics of IDDM is the large geographic variability in the incidence, which has been summarized in several reports[27,29,30] (Fig. 9.1). Scandinavia has the highest incidence of IDDM in the world. Interestingly, the island of Sardinia has rates of IDDM that equal those of Scandinavian countries. Asian countries, such as Japan and China, have the lowest IDDM incidence. Overall, a child in Finland is 35 times more likely to develop diabetes than a child in Japan. While clearcut differences in the occurrence of diabetes exist across geographic boundaries, the severity of the disease remains constant,[31] making it unlikely that the observed difference in incidence throughout the world is confounded by misclassification of different types of diabetes. The situation remains complex because a multitude of factors may contribute to the geographic variability of IDDM. Therefore, identification of the reasons for the geographic variability will be valuable for the understanding and, it is hoped, prevention of IDDM.

The farther an individual is from the equator, the greater the risk of developing IDDM.[27] Populations located around the equator have a risk of disease that is at least one-tenth that of populations bordering the Arctic and Antarctic circles.[32] The increased incidence in cooler climates argues for an environmental factor, such as virus, although people living in cooler climates differ genetically from those in the equatorial zone, as well. Geographic analyses of multiple sclerosis have revealed that, similarly to IDDM,[29] the risk of multiple sclerosis tends to increase with latitude in all three racial groups in the United States.[33] This may suggest that environmental rather than genetic

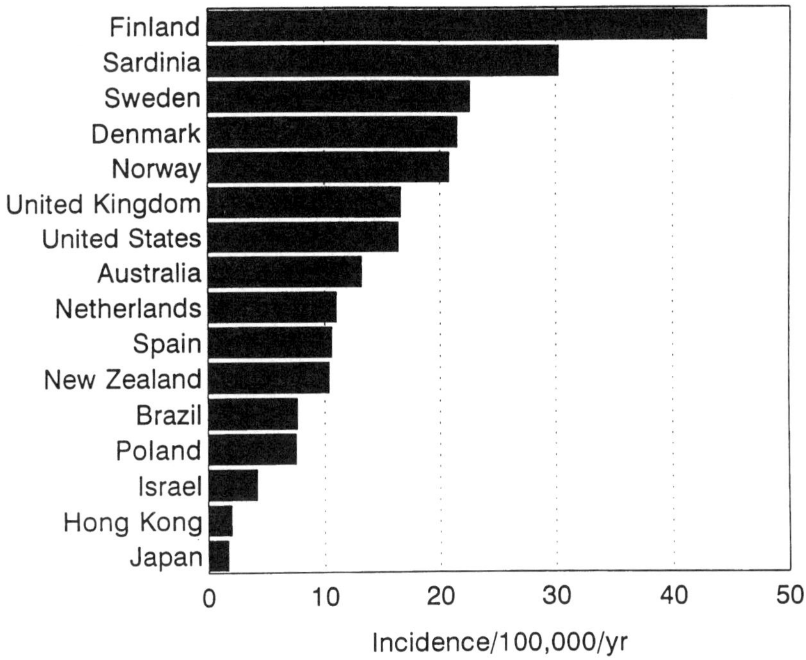

Figure 9.1. Incidence of IDDM in selected countries. Data were obtained from three reviews.[27,29,30]

factors underlie the north to south gradients in the incidence of autoimmune diseases.

Race and Ethnicity. Racial differences in IDDM risk within the same population are striking, although they are not of the same magnitude as the geographic differences (Table 9.2).[34] American whites are about one and a half times as likely to develop IDDM as American blacks or Hispanics. This is similar to the differences reported from Montreal, where children of British descent had about one and a half the risk of IDDM as children of French descent.

Age. The age at onset of diabetes provides important clues as to the etiology of the disease. Across all geographic areas there is an increasing risk of developing IDDM until puberty, followed by an apparent decline in risk, as demonstrated by data from Colorado (Fig. 9.2). Some studies have reported an early peak in incidence around age 5 years,[9,35,36] which is possibly caused by an increased exposure to certain diabetogenic factors related to school entry. At puberty the risk for developing IDDM is over two times that of both younger and older ages at onset. The incidence peak at puberty may be related to the physiological changes occurring at this time, such as increases in levels of sex hormones and associated increase in insulin resistance or alterations in lifestyle and associated change in the pattern of infections. There

Table 2. Age-Adjusted Incidence of IDDM per 100,000 Person-Years (ages 0–14 years) and the 95% Confidence Intervals by Racial and Ethnic Groups

Location	*Incidence*	*95% Confidence Interval*
Allegheny County, PA[29]		
White	16.2	14.1–18.4
Black	11.8	7.9–17.2
Colorado[29]		
Non-Hispanic	16.4	15.0–17.8
Hispanic	9.7	7.4–12.4
Montreal, Canada[34]		
French	8.2	7.5– 8.9
British	15.3	12.8–17.8
Italian	10.7	7.5–13.9
Jewish	17.2	10.4–24.0
Other	13.1	10.9–15.3

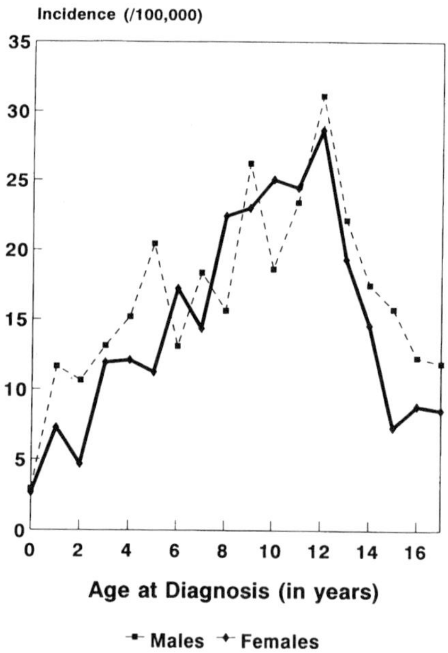

Figure 9.2. Age at diagnosis of IDDM for males and females. Data from the Colorado iddm Registry, 1978–1988.[17]

have been only a few studies that have examined the incidence of IDDM in older groups (ie, over 20 years of age), mainly because of the difficulty of distinguishing IDDM from insulin-requiring type II diabetes in older individuals. In Sardinia the incidence of IDDM is decreased from 30/100,000 in the 0–14-year-olds to 19/100,000 in the 15–29-year-olds.[37] In Turin, Italy,[38]

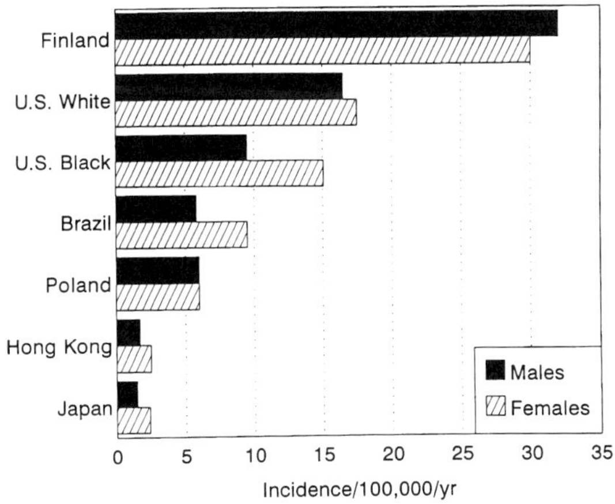

Figure 9.3. Differences in the incidence of IDDM (0–14 year olds) by sex. Data from Finland,[27] the United States,[27] Brazil,[45] Poland,[27] Hong Kong[44] and Japan.[27]

incidence was 7.4 and 5.8/100,000 for the age groups 0–14 and 15–29 years, respectively, and in Norway[39] the incidence was 20 and 17/100,000 in these two age groups, respectively. It has been speculated that the incidence of IDDM is again increased in the fifth decade of life[40] or after the age of 60.[41] However, there is no hard evidence that such an increase really exists and that all the insulin-dependent cases diagnosed at these ages are etiologically similar to those diagnosed in childhood.

Gender. In general, males and females have similar risk of IDDM. However, in low-risk countries, such as Japan, there is a female preponderance, whereas in very high-risk areas, there is a slight male excess (Fig. 9.3, refs.[11,36,42–45]).

Time. There is evidence for marked variation in the incidence in IDDM over time. This variation occurs both seasonally and yearly. In the northern hemisphere, there is a decline in the incidence of IDDM during the warm summer months. Conversely, in the southern hemisphere, the seasonal pattern exhibits a decline during the warm months of December, January, and February, implicating a climatic factor. A number of studies have reported this seasonal pattern to be present specifically in children diagnosed after the age of 4 years.[42,43,46–51] The seasonal pattern, which appears to occur only in school-age children, suggests that factors related to attending school (eg, infections, stress) may be related to diabetes etiology or clinical diagnosis. Because the pathological process leading to IDDM may start years before the diagnosis or the appearance of symptoms, the seasonal variation probably reflects the operation of triggering rather than initiating factors, at least in a majority of cases. Because the timing of the clinical diagnosis of diabetes may

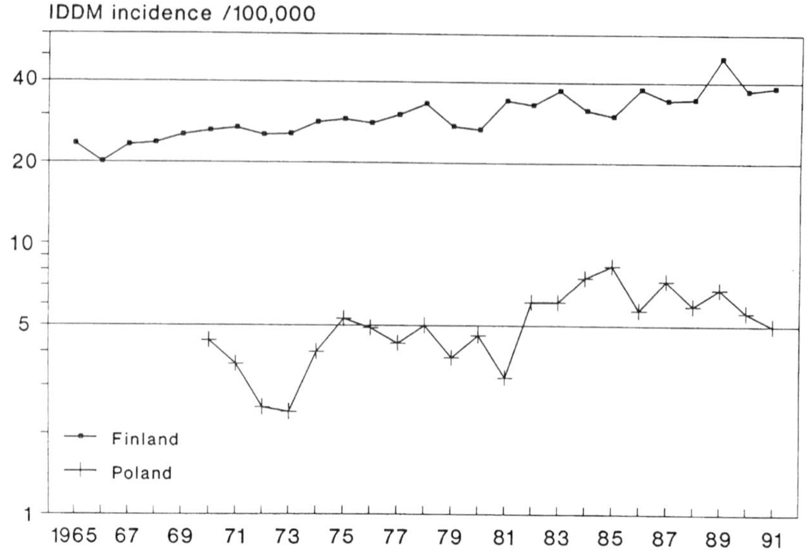

Figure 9.4. Contrasting forms of temporal changes in the incidence of IDDM: a secular trend with superimposed outbreaks (Finland[55]) and outbreaks with no clear secular increase (Poland).

depend on factors such as health care access, investigators have examined the appearance of diabetes symptoms as a more accurate marker of onset of the disease. Evidence for appearance of symptoms with peaks predominantly in the autumn and winter months,[11,36,52–54] which may be weaker in preschool children,[52] indicates that the observed seasonality is not an artifact of health care seeking or access.

A number of studies using population-based registries have shown an increasing incidence of insulin-dependent diabetes mellitus over time,[25,36,47,50,51,55,56] while others have shown no trend.[42,49,57,58] Some of the inconsistencies may be attributed to differences in ascertainment over time. Cases need to be collected over a sufficient number of years to detect a temporal change in the incidence. For example, initial studies from Sweden and Norway showed no temporal trend in the incidence of insulin-dependent diabetes mellitus with 3 years and 5 years of data, respectively.[48,59] Analysis of the patterns of diabetes incidence over 10 years, however, showed an increase in both countries.[50,56] Figure 9.4 displays examples of the two types of changes in the incidence of IDDM that have been observed—periodic outbreaks superimposed on a steady secular increase (Finland) or outbreaks with little secular increase (Poland).

Remission of IDDM

After clinical onset, the natural course of IDDM is characterized by a transient fall in insulin requirement associated with improved beta cell function, which is called remission. Partial remission is defined as a decrease in the insulin requirement, whereas total remission is defined as the lack of an insulin requirement to maintain appropriate glycemia. One study showed that during the first 18 months of the disease, 12% of the patients entered total remission and 18% entered partial remission.[60] It has been suggested that remission is more common in adolescents than in preschoolers and that males may be more likely to experience a remission than females.[61] Recent reports of spontaneous remission in young adults with IDDM have come from the observation of the placebo groups of randomized controlled clinical trials studying the effects of immunosuppression on diabetes remission. Total remission 3 months after diagnosis of IDDM was observed in 22–27% of the placebo group of randomized trials of cyclosporin A[62,63] and at 1 year, 10% still did not need insulin.[62] Unfortunately, the observed remission is almost always temporary and is marked by an abrupt or gradual decline in insulin secretory capacity, so that 1–2 years after diagnosis, most patients have lost this residual beta cell function.

Analytic Epidemiology of IDDM

Environmental Candidate Factors

The aforementioned geographic and ethnic variation in IDDM risk may reflect either different population pools of susceptibility genes or different prevalence of causative environmental factors or a combination of both. Increasing rates of IDDM in some countries and "epidemics" of IDDM have been attributed to environmental factors such as viruses and diet.

Viruses. IDDM incidence data from Colorado[17] show periodic increases in incidence rather than a secular trend, which is consistent with findings in other U.S. locations[64,65] and suggests than an infectious factor may play a role. In 1984, we reported an epidemic of childhood IDDM in Poland, associated with a concurrent epidemic of piconaviruses in the area.[36] The incidence of IDDM almost doubled, from 3.5/100,000 during 1970–81 to 6.6/100,000 in 1982–84. This ecologic observation was later confirmed by a case-control study in the epidemic area conducted in cooperation with the Enteroviral Branch of the Centers for Disease Control in Atlanta.[66] Using a novel monotypic detector system,[67] 98 cases of IDDM and 66 control children were examined for the presence of IgM and IgA antiviral antibodies against Coxsackie viruses B1, 2, 3, 4, 5, 6 A9, echo viruses 4, 6, 9, 11, 30, 34, and enterovirus 71. These serotypes included all picornaviruses found to be prevalent in the epidemic area by culture and traditional neutralizing assay.[36] During the peak epidemic years of 1983–84, presence of IgM against Coxsackie virus B5 was higher in cases than controls, odds ratio (OR) = 3.2 (95% CI 1.1–8.8). Strikingly similar observations have recently been reported from Birmingham, Alabama, where an epidemic of IDDM was observed in

1983–84 as well,[65] corresponding temporally to an epidemic of Coxsackie virus B5 that occurred in 1983. The overall incidence in the year beginning July 1983, the month of the first isolation of Coxsackie virus B5, was 18.5/100,000, an excess of 6.7/100,000 over the average annual incidence for the previous 4 years. These data, although suggestive of a role for Coxsackie virus B5 as a cause of epidemic outbreaks of IDDM, indicate that a recent picornavirus infection can be responsible only for about 20% of the cases.

Multiple cross-sectional studies of the association between Coxsackie virus antibodies and IDDM were reviewed in 1985 by Barrett-Connor[68] with the conclusion that odds ratios, ranging in those studies from 0.7 to 20, were inconclusive but weighed more for an association than against it. Case reports linked picornavirus infection to β-cell necrosis on autopsy[69] and isolates of Coxsackie virus B from a newly diabetic patient induced diabetes in mice.[70,71] Susceptibility to "diabetogenic" picornavirus in humans appears to be genetically restricted,[72] similar to the animal model of IDDM caused by the encephalomyocarditis (EMC) virus. In addition, compelling evidence has accumulated that picornaviruses trigger other chronic autoimmune diseases in humans, such as myocarditis,[73] hepatitis,[74] and myositis.[75] Theiler's virus causes persistent infection of the central nervous system and demyelinating lesions similar to those seen in sclerosis multiplex.[73] In addition to picornaviruses, herpesviruses,[76,77] mumps,[78] rubella,[79] and retroviruses[80,219] are candidate viruses to cause IDDM.

An increased incidence of IDDM has been found in patients with congenital rubella syndrome (CRS).[79,81–83] CRS does not appear to be associated with particular HLA-DR alleles; however, the distribution of DR alleles in CRS patients with diabetes resembles that in non-CRS IDDM patients,[81] ie, the diabetogenic DR (and likely DQ) alleles are required for the development of IDDM. In the CRS, the incubation period of IDDM is 5–20 years.[82] Persistent infection of the pancreas with rubella virus has been demonstrated in some cases on autopsy.[84] Recently, molecular mimicry has been suggested to exist between an antigenic determinant on a rubella virus protein and a 52-kd β-cell autoantigen.[85] In any case, CRS is responsible for only a minute proportion of IDDM cases and there is little evidence that postnatal rubella infection either with the wild strain[86–87] or after the measles-mumps-rubella (MMR) vaccination[89] is associated with IDDM.

Evidence also exists that viral infection may protect the host from developing IDDM. Persistent infection with exogenous viruses prevents IDDM in mice[90,91] and rats.[92] However, evidence for a similar protective effect in humans is not available. Immunization with live measles virus appears to decrease risk of IDDM,[89] but the effect of current mass immunization programs against potentially diabetogenic viruses, eg, mumps or rubella, is virtually unknown.

Infant and Childhood Diet. In 1984, scientists in Scandinavia reported a nationwide decrease in breast-feeding and a corresponding increase in the incidence of IDDM between 1940 and 1980.[93] Subsequent case-control studies have shown that: (1) diabetic children were significantly *less* likely to have been breast-fed than nondiabetic children,[94–97] (2) there was no significant difference in the frequency of breast-feeding between diabetic and nondiabetic children,[93,98–104] or (3) diabetic children were significantly *more* likely to have been breast-fed than nondiabetic children.[105] Certain studies suggested that the longer children had been breast-fed, the lower was their risk for developing diabetes[93,95,96,106–108]; other studies did not show increased protection with longer duration of breast-feeding.[102–105]

These inconsistent results suggest that breast-feeding initiation and duration may be inadequate measures of the diabetogenic exposure. For example, rather than simply regarding breast milk as protective, the breast-feeding variable could be viewed as a surrogate for the avoidance of perinatal food diabetogens either in breast-milk substitutes or in the weaning foods. Indeed, several studies have reported that children with diabetes were more likely to have received breast-milk substitutes prior to 3 or 4 months of age than children without diabetes.[97,106–108] This was also true for cow's milk–based breast-milk substitutes.[97,106–108] However, most odds ratios were relatively weak; and these associations were not seen in all populations.[97,100,103] Two meta-analyses have been performed on these data and have found a 50% increase in IDDM risk associated with a breast-feeding duration of less than 3 months, and exposure to breast-milk substitutes (any or cow's milk based) prior to 3 months of age.[109,110]

Kostraba and coworkers[100] examined exposure to whole cow's milk in children at high and low risk for IDDM, as defined by a genetic susceptibility marker in the HLA region. Exposure to whole cow's milk by 3 months of age was associated with an odds ratio of 3.7 in high-risk children, which was not statistically significant and was not markedly higher than the odds ratio associated with exposure in nonsusceptible children (OR=2.9). However, the authors did demonstrate a gene-environment interaction, where having only one of the risk factors (eg, exposure to whole cow's milk prior to 3 months of age or having the high-risk gene) resulted in a moderately increased risk of IDDM, while having both risk factors resulted in an 11-fold increased risk of IDDM compared with those without any risk factors (Fig. 9.5).

Other exposures in the infant diet have not been evaluated as extensively as whole cow's milk and cow's milk–based formulas. Exposure to solid foods by 3 months of age was associated with a 2.5-fold increased risk of IDDM. These findings warrant further study given that wheat- and soy-based diets have been found to be diabetogenic in the Bio Breeding (BB) rat and nonobese diabetic (NOD) mouse.[111–113] The interrelationship of the timing of the introduction of formulas, cow's milk, and solid foods into the infant's diet makes it difficult to disentangle, both conceptually and statistically, the independent effects of these dietary exposures.

It may be that diabetes risk is related to exposures in the childhood diet, rather than the infant diet. Two ecologic analyses showed that national consumption of milk proteins was directly related to the national IDDM incidence,[114,115] which could reflect either childhood or infant diet. Additional

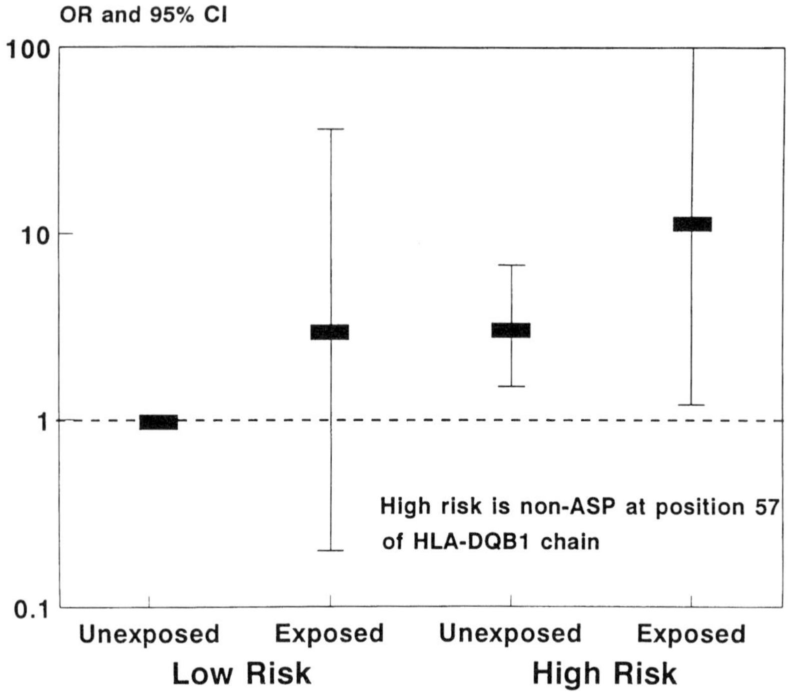

Figure 9.5. Odds ratios for IDDM by exposure to whole cow's milk prior to 3 months of age in low- and high-risk individuals, as determined by a genetic marker on the HLA-DQB1 chain.[101]

evidence of an association between cow's milk and IDDM risk was provided by several studies that showed that children with newly diagnosed IDDM had higher levels of serum IgA against cow's milk, IgA and IgG against beta-lactoglobulin,[116] and IgG against bovine serum albumin (BSA)[117] than age-matched controls. It has been difficult to reproduce a report that 100% of IDDM children studies within 4 months of diagnosis had elevated serum levels of anti-BSA antibodies, compared to less than 4% of controls.[117] These findings may indicate differences between cases and controls in either current consumption or past consumption. Ecologic studies have been used to generate hypotheses concerning other components in the diet and IDDM incidence. Average coffee[118] and sugar consumption[119] is positively correlated with IDDM incidence, whereby countries with the highest consumption rates also have the highest rates of IDDM and vice versa. Investigators from Sweden found that children with diabetes were consuming larger quantities of protein prior to diagnosis than age-matched controls.[120]

Circumstantial evidence first suggested a connection between IDDM in males and consumption of nitrosamine-rich smoked mutton by their parents at the time of conception.[121] A study from Sweden showed that diabetic children consumed a greater amount of foods containing nitrates, nitrites, or nitrosamines prior to diagnosis than nondiabetic children.[120] An ecologic study from the Colorado IDDM Registry suggested that higher insulin-dependent diabetes mellitus (IDDM) incidence rates occurred in areas with high nitrate levels in their potable water supplies.[122] Adverse health effects of nitrates, which are found in vegetables, processed meats, and water, are related to the reduction of nitrate to nitrite and, in the presence of secondary amines or amides, to *N*-nitroso compounds in the body. Anecdotal reports have shown that toxic doses of nitrosamine-containing compounds can cause diabetes. The well-documented diabetogenic properties of toxins containing *N*-nitroso compounds, such as the rodenticide Vacor,[123] are associated with the generation of free radicals. The beta cell toxins streptozocin and alloxan have been used extensively to induce diabetes mellitus in animals for experimental research.[124,125]

Spectrum of IDDM, from Genetic Susceptibility through β-Cell Autoimmunity to Overt Diabetes

Autoimmunity Against β-Cells

IDDM results from a chronic autoimmune destruction of the pancreatic β-cells, probably initiated by exposure of a genetically susceptible host to an environmental agent. There is a long preclinical phase of the disease, called here β-cell autoimmunity, lasting up to 9–13 years.[126–128] The pathological process is mediated by T lymphocytes, with CD4 cells playing a central role.[129] Several mechanisms have been proposed for the induction and failure of self-tolerance.[130] When this tolerance fails, β-cells are selectively destroyed, likely by a cellular mechanism.[131] Concurrently, circulating antibodies to various β-cell antigens, called jointly islet cell antibodies (ICAs), can be detected.[2,132–137] Because ICAs seldom have cytotoxic properties, they are regarded as a marker of β-cell autoimmunity but not a direct cause of β-cell damage.[132] Studies of β-cell autoimmunity, to date, have used almost exclusively humoral markers of autoimmunity, because their measurement requires less cost and smaller blood volume and its partially standardized across laboratories, in contrast to the cellular markers. In this chapter, the epidemiology of β-cell autoimmunity is described in terms of humoral autoimmunity; however, it is recognized that the epidemiology of cellular autoimmunity may differ from that defined by humoral markers.

Genetic Markers for β-Cell Autoimmunity and for IDDM

No particular HLA type seems to predict β-cell autoimmunity or its absence in relatives of IDDM subjects. For instance, the HLA-DR2 associated alleles DQA1*0102, DQB1*0602, which almost completely protect from IDDM, are found in a significant proportion of ICA-positive relatives. In a combined

Barbara Davis Center (BDC) and Joslin Clinic study (unpublished data), the frequency of DQB1*0602 was similar in ICA positive relatives—13% (10/75)—and in all HLA-typed relatives—12% (39/125). However, HLA phenotype frequencies in relatives who remain persistently ICA positive appear to be similar to those in IDDM patients, ie, 94% of the subjects are HLA-DR3 or DR4.[138] Similarly, children identified with β-cell autoimmunity on screening of the general population show a large number of different HLA phenotypes,[139] but among those who remain persistently ICA positive, 91% are DQB1$_{57nAsp/nAsp}$ or $_{57nAsp/Asp}$.[140] The high prevalence of glutamic acid decarboxylase (GAD) autoantibodies in offspring and siblings of IDDM probands (L. Yu and G. S. Eisenbarth, unpublished data) led to speculation that β-cell autoimmunity may develop as a joint effect of a widespread environmental exposure and a dominant autosomal gene. More subjects with β-cell autoimmunity need to be genotyped in order to show convincingly that a non-HLA gene determines who develops β-cell autoimmunity, but that it is the HLA genotype that determines progression to persistent autoimmunity and overt IDDM.

The primary loci of genetic susceptibility to IDDM have been mapped to the HLA-DR and DQ regions[141,142] and new gene candidates outside the HLA region are being identified.[143] We have previously reviewed the genetic markers that could be used to identify children at increased risk of IDDM in the general population.[23] Family history of IDDM and the HLA-DR3/4 phenotype are approximately equally related to the risk of IDDM and can identify, respectively, 12% and 30% of IDDM cases, yet they are present in only 2–5% of persons in the general population. Since only a fraction of susceptible subjects actually develop IDDM, in those who do not, either the penetrance or number of susceptibility gene(s) may be insufficient or the environmental exposure is too low to trigger autoimmunity.

Natural History of β-Cell Autoimmunity

Similar to most infectious and chronic diseases, there appears to be a broad spectrum of the disease process leading to IDDM. Many genetically susceptible persons are exposed to the etiologic agent; in fewer persons, it leads to β-cell autoimmunity, to end up in clinical diabetes in just a few (Fig. 9.6). β-cell autoimmunity does not end with the clinical onset of diabetes and is probably lifelong; however, in this review, β-cell autoimmunity denotes the subclinical, ie, normoglycemic period in the natural history of the disease. Four specific questions, listed below and identified by corresponding numbers in Figure 9.6, appear to be particularly relevant to the epidemiology of β-cell autoimmunity and are now being answered by the Diabetes Autoimmunity Study in the Young (DAISY) in Colorado.

1. What is the incidence of β-cell autoimmunity, by family history of IDDM, geographic location, race and ethnicity, age, and other characteristics?

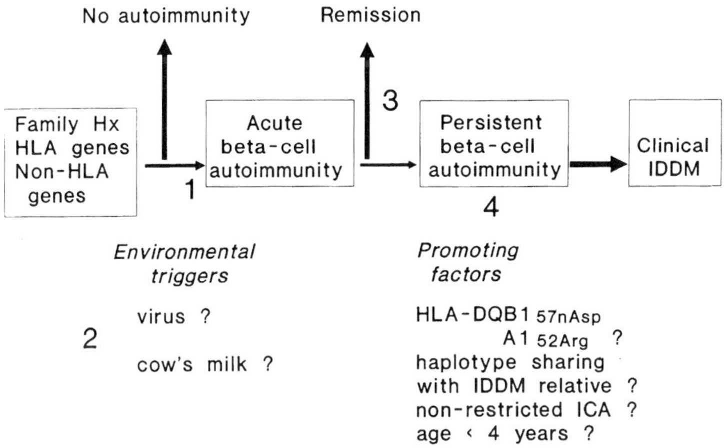

Figure 9.6. Proposed model of the natural history of pre-IDDM. The outstanding research questions are denoted by numbers 1 through 4 and listed in the text.

2. Is the onset of β-cell autoimmunity associated with the exposure of a genetically susceptible child, in a susceptible age range, to a virus or to a nutritional factor?
3. Does β-cell autoimmunity remit and if so, how often?
4. What are the risk factors for persistence of β-cell autoimmunity and progression to clinical IDDM?

Does autoimmunity to different β-cell antigens develop simultaneously or sequentially? This question will be best addressed in very young children, of the age when conversion to antibody positivity primarily occurs. We hypothesize that the appearance is sequential and the order is relatively "fixed," The first autoantibody to appear may aid in determining which if any autoantigen is most important for the development of IDDM. Also, the autoantibody that appears earliest would be preferred as a screening test because a positive result would allow the most time for an intervention.

Descriptive Epidemiology of β-Cell Autoimmunity

Prevalence and Incidence of β-Cell Autoimmunity

Family History of IDDM. The prevalence of β-cell autoimmunity among the first degree relatives of persons with IDDM varies from 1.9% to 7.2% (Table 9.3). Unexpectedly, the prevalence of β-cell autoimmunity in schoolchildren with no family history of IDDM is as high as 0.2–4.4% (Table 9.3), although only one in 3–10 of these children will develop IDDM by the age of 20 years.

Table 9.3. Geographic Dierences in the Prevalence of β-Cell Autoimmunity, Defined as ICA Positivity, in the General Population and in the First Degree Relatives of IDDM Persons

	Prevalence of β-cell Autoimmunity				
	General population		*First-degree relatives*		*IDDM incidence/ 100,000*
Country	*Percent*	*Age (y)*	*Percent*	*Relation*	
Italy					
Sardinia[148]	4.4	6–14			30[30]
Finland[149]	4.1	3–18	7.2*[150]	Siblings	30[29]
Sweden[151]	3.3	1–15	6.5[152]	Siblings	22[29]
United Kingdom	2.8	9–13	6.6[153]	Siblings	16[30]
			2.7[126]	Parents	
New Zealand[154]	1.2	5–7	4.9†[155]	Siblings and offspring (ages 0–14)	12[65]
France[156]	1.8	6–17	2.9[157]	Siblings	8[30]
			1.9[157]	Parents	
United States					9–21[29]
Washington[158]	1.7	12–18			
Florida[138]	0.6	6–17	4.2[147]	Siblings	
			2.5[147]	Parents	
Estonia[159]	1.6	3–18			10[159]
Germany[139]	1.2	7–15	5.5[160]	Siblings	7[29]
			3.8[160]	Parents	
Australia[161]	1.1	4–18			14[162]
Spain[163]	0.4	14–17			11[164]
Japan[165]	0.4	7–18			2[29]
Netherlands[166]	0.2	5–19			11[30]

*An additional 3.4% of the siblings developed ICA within 17–49 months after the initial testing.
†An additional 2.5% of the relatives developed ICA within 7–26 months after the initial testing.

Race and Ethnicity. Some incompletely validated studies have reported very low prevalence of ICA at onset of IDDM in African Americans[144,145] and Nigerians.[146] First-degree relatives of African American IDDM probands in Florida had somewhat higher prevalence of ICA positives (9/199; 4.5%) than the relatives of white probands (116/3, 816; 3%).[148] Ethnic differences in the specificity of ICA cannot be ruled out and the appropriateness of using Caucasian pancreata to assess ICA positivity in other racial groups has been questioned. Little data concerning β-cell autoimmunity is available for other nonwhite populations (Table 9.3).

Geographic Location. Table 9.3 summarizes available data concerning the prevalence of β-cell autoimmunity by geographic location. The prevalence in schoolchildren, defined by ICA positivity, varies from 0.2% in Dutch (sera stored for 10 years) to 4.4% in Sardinians. The prevalence of β-cell autoimmunity appears to be roughly proportional to IDDM incidence in the population; however, the rates are not strictly comparable, because of differences in age structure of the populations screened and different cut-off values for ICA positivity. Most of the studies defined ICA positivity as greater than 4–5 Juvenile Diabetes Foundation (JDF) units; however, it could be as low as 0.6 JDF units in the Dutch study and as high as 20 JDF units in Florida. In contrast to that in the general population, prevalence of β-cell autoimmunity in relatives does not appear to differ dramatically between high and low IDDM risk countries (eg, Sweden or Finland vs France of Germany).

The incidence of β-cell autoimmunity in the background population has not been studied systematically. The family studies only very recently have begun to recognize "incident" cases of β-cell autoimmunity. The Barts-Windsor study[126] and the Gainesville study[147] reported, respectively, 14 and 21 ICA-negative relatives who apparently developed ICA during follow-up. In Finland, 732/1036 siblings of IDDM children diagnosed in 1986–89 and enrolled in the DIME study have been followed prospectively. At baseline, 2.7% of the siblings were already diabetic and 7.2% were ICA positive.[150] During the initial 17–49 months of follow-up, an additional 3.4% of the siblings developed ICA positivity and 2.3% developed IDDM (0.4% were ICA negative at baseline). No loss of ICA positivity has been reported. Thus, the prevalence of combined β-cell autoimmunity plus IDDM was 9.9% at baseline and 14.7% at the end of this initial follow-up, with an incidence of about 1.4% per year.

Pilcher and coworkers[155] retested 1007 initially ICA negative first-degree relatives and found that 17/460 (3.7%) of those younger than 5 years seroconverted over a period of 1 year, 3/191 (1.6%) of those 5–9 years old converted over a period of 3 years, while none of the 356 relatives older than 10 converted over a period of 5 years.

Age. Since the incubation period of IDDM may be as long as 9–13 years,[126,128] if not longer, it is very likely that the process begins in early childhood in the majority of cases. Between 20–25% of IDDM cases have already been diagnosed by the age of 5 years[29] and seroconversion to β-cell autoimmunity appears to be infrequent after that age.

The prevalence of β-cell autoimmunity in children aged 0–6 years was estimated in a series of 127 high-risk siblings and offspring screened at the Barbara Davis Center (BDC) in Denver (P. Chase, unpublished data) and in 868 relatives tested at the Joslin Clinic (G. S. Eisenbarth and R. Jackson, unpublished data). These studies are summarized in Table 9.4.

Children tested before the first year of life were excluded because they were too few to produce reliable estimates. In addition, passive transplacental transfer of autoantibodies, observed in 34% and 97% of newborns, for ICA and IAA, respectively (A.-G. Ziegler, personal communication), could not be

Table 9.4. Studies of β-Cell Autoimmunity in Early Childhood

Study	*Barbara Davis Center*	*Joslin Clinic*
Subjects	Siblings/offspring	Siblings/offspring
Age	1–4	1–6
Autoimmunity definition	ICA+	ICA+ or IAA+
Number tested	117	868
Number prevalent, positive	11	103
Number reverting to negative	3/7 (43%)	25/55 (45%)
Number converting to positive	0	10
Person-years of follow-up	13	180

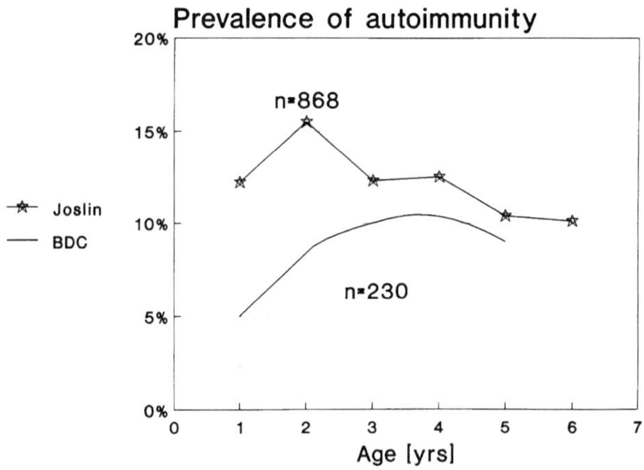

Figure 9.7. Age-specific prevalence of β-cell autoimmunity in first-degree relatives aged 1–6 years of IDDM probands seen in the Joslin Clinic (*———*) and in the Barbara Davis Center (———).

excluded on the basis of the data available. For the whole age range 1–6 years, the prevalence of autoimmunity was higher in the Joslin Clinic than in the BDC series, due to the higher sensitivity of the combination of two tests (ICA and IAA) used in the former series (Fig. 9.7). The difference was profound at the ages of 1–2 years, for which there were very few observations in the BDC series.

In these two studies, approximately 13% of first-degree relatives had β-cell autoimmunity at the age of 4 years but the prevalence decreased to 6–7% in the relatives aged 5–9 years[167,168] and to 4–5% at ages 10–19 years.[147,168] Such a rapid decrease in the prevalence cannot be explained solely by development of IDDM in some of the relatives, because the cumulative incidence of IDDM in the relatives is only 2–3% by the age of 10 years. This supports the hypothesis that few children develop β-cell autoimmunity after the age of 5[168] and that some may recover from autoimmunity.[169] We estimated (Fig. 9.8) the

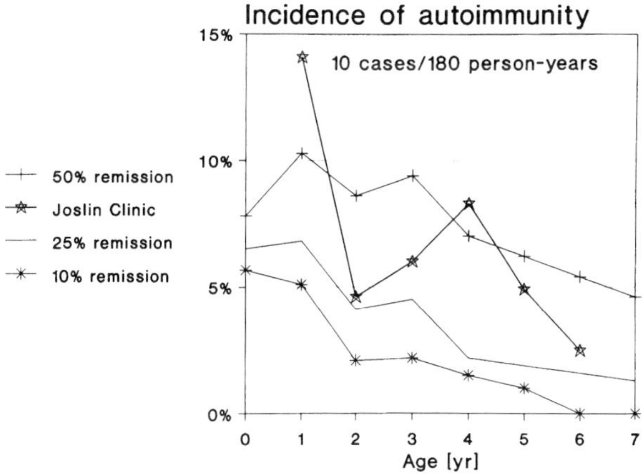

Figure 9.8. Incidence of β-cell autoimmunity in early childhood predicted from the prevalence data (in Fig. 9.7) and three hypothesized rates of remission: 50% (+——+), 25% (———), and 10% (*———*). The fourth line, denoted by stars, shows incidence of β-cell autoimmunity observed in the Joslin Clinic series of first-degree relatives of IDDM persons.

age-specific incidence of β-cell autoimmunity in first-degree relatives aged 0–6 years, based on the Joslin Clinic data and those from other selected studies.[126,168,170] The Joslin Clinic data were based on only 180 person-years of follow-up and the other curves are "guesstimates" based on an assumption of variable rate of remission of β-cell autoimmunity. This will be discussed in more detail in the section concerned with remission of β-cell autoimmunity.

Although the first 5 years of life are most likely critical for the initiation of autoimmunity, there are only a few case reports[70,171] concerning this age group. Existing prospective family studies typically exclude young children and the baseline measurement is rarely taken before the age of 5–6 years. To determine possible triggers of autoimmunity and ultimately to identify ways to prevent diabetes, it is necessary to study this age group.

Gender. No significant gender difference has been reported in the prevalence of β-cell autoimmunity, either in first-degree relatives or in general population screening.

Time. Population-based studies of β-cell autoimmunity has been initiated only a few years ago and no information is available concerning potential seasonal or annual variation in the incidence od β-cell autoimmunity. However, given other similarities between descriptive epidemiology of β-cell autoimmunity and IDDM, temporal changes in the incidence of the former are likely to occur and may reflect acute changes in the causal environmental exposures.

Remission of β-Cell Autoimmunity

First-Degree Relatives. Evidence has accumulated that β-cell autoimmunity may remit without causing diabetes.[128,169,170] The early reports from family studies, concerning fluctuation or disappearance of ICA during follow-up,[172] had unproven value because of the problems with standardization of ICA assays, especially in the low titer range. More recently, several studies that use reliable ICA assays have reported cases of first-degree relatives with ICA levels greater than 20 JDF units who become ICA negative at follow-up.[169,170,173] With the current progress in standardization[135,174] and development of quantitative ICA assays, these doubts will be resolved in the near future.

In Figure 9.8, the *observed* incidence of β-cell autoimmunity in the Joslin Clinic series lays between *predicted* incidence assuming a 25% remission rate and a 50% remission rate. This is consistent with the observed remission rates (43% in the BDC series and 45% in the Joslin Clinic series). Interestingly, a Swiss study[170] reported the remission rate to be as high as 80%. The most conservative estimates of the incidence of β-cell autoimmunity come from the study of Elliott and coworkers[168] that suggests no conversion after the age of 5 and slowly declining prevalence, consistent with a remission rate of about 10%.

If only a subset of relatives positive for autoantibodies by age 5 develop IDDM, in the great majority of relatives autoimmunity is suppressed (remits). In animal models, a number of environmental factors (eg, Freund's adjuvant, see Chapter 3) prevent diabetes.

General Population. Population studies of the natural history of ICA in schoolchildren in Florida,[138] Sweden,[175] and Finland[149] have reported ICA remission rates between 10–78%. Moreover, the prevalence of ICA positivity in schoolchildren is 3–10 times higher than the cumulative incidence of IDDM by the age of 20, suggesting that autoimmunity will remit in most of these ICA-positive children.[156] If the HLA genes associated with IDDM promote persistence of autoimmunity, it would be natural that children who lack this susceptibility (most schoolchildren) "fight back" β-cell autoimmunity and lose detectable ICA.

Although it is still possible that some of these "remissions" were artifacts due to imprecise assays, it is biologically plausible that β-cell autoimmunity remits spontaneously or after the offending factor is removed. This plausibility is based on the follow-up of high-risk relatives or patients with celiac disease,[176] chronic autoimmune hepatitis,[74] and autoimmune thyroiditis.[177] The phenomenon of transient metabolic remission in the first year of IDDM is also well recognized.[178] It would be premature to speculate whether specific protective factor(s) operate in children who experience remission of β-cell autoimmunity. It may be due simply to the lack of factors promoting ICA persistence, discussed below. It is possible that β-cell autoimmunity may remit and reappear in the course of subsequent viral infections and the cumulative insult may eventually cause diabetes at any age. This "multiple hits" theory[179] could include factors that increase insulin resistance (obesity, physical inactivity) and, thus, provide a link between early life events and development of "NIDDM" at later ages. It has been reported that 14–33% of NIDDM patients[180,181] may be positive for GAD autoantibodies and that this is associated with early failure of oral hypoglycemic drug therapy and insulin dependence in these patients.

Analytical Epidemiology of β-Cell Autoimmunity

Environmental Candidate Factors Triggering β-Cell Autoimmunity

Geographic and ethnic variation in the prevalence of β-cell autoimmunity in the general population[138,139,148,149,151,168] may reflect either different population pools of susceptibility genes or different prevalence of causative environmental factors or a combination of both. There is a paucity of analytic epidemiological data concerning the determinants of β-cell autoimmunity; however, a number of anecdotal reports suggest that an infectious or dietary factor(s) plays a role.

Viruses. It can be hypothesized that viral infection initiates β-cell autoimmunity rather than merely precipitates diabetes symptoms in subjects with ongoing β-cell autoimmunity. Such a relationship has been demonstrated to exist between picornaviral infection and chronic autoimmune hepatitis type 1 in a prospective study of high-risk relatives.[76] Transgenic mice expressing a viral protein in the β-cells do not develop anti-islet autoimmunity unless the host is exposed to the same virus later in life,[182] even if cytotoxic T cells specific to this viral antigen are present.[183] This may indicate that two episodes of viral infection are needed to cause β-cell autoimmunity—the first resulting in persistent expression of a viral antigen in β-cells and the second, with an antigenetically similar agent, initiating autoimmunity. Alternative scenarios are plausible[184,185] but lie beyond the scope of this review.

Picornaviruses,[186] herpesviruses,[76,77] mumps,[78] rubella,[79] and retroviruses[80,219] are candidates as the cause of β-cell autoimmunity. Currently, the body of evidence for a role in the etiology of human IDDM is the strongest for picornaviruses, small RNA viruses that include human (enteroviruses and rhinoviruses) and animal pathogens (eg, mouse EMC virus and Theiler's virus). It has been suggested that molecular mimicry due to homology between the P2-C protein of Coxsackie virus and the GAD protein[137,187] is responsible for β-cell autoimmunity. A case-control study of anti-GAD antibodies in newly diagnosed IDDM patients and friend controls found 54% of subjects with high titers of IgM against Coxsackie virus B (cases and controls combined) to be positive for GAD autoantibodies, compared to 35% GAD positive among those with low anti–Coxsackie virus B IgM levels.[188] This moderate difference in GAD autoantibody positivity appeared to be stronger in controls than in IDDM cases.

At least two case reports have linked acute Coxsackie virus infection with development of ICA. In one, seroconversion to ICA and Coxsackie virus antibodies coincided with the onset of IDDM[189]; in the other, the infection and ICA positivity preceded IDDM by 3 years.[171] In the latter study, concurrent ICA and Coxsackie virus antibodies seroconversion was not actually observed—titers of both were already high in the first sample available. A report from Cuba[190] suggested that ICA may develop following echovirus 4 infection. Several years later, 17 patients were studied during an echovirus 4 outbreak in Glasgow.[191] The group mean insulin levels were found to transiently increase following the infection and one subject showed ICA positivity just after the infection, with the ICA titer declining in follow-up. A pre-infection ICA measurement was, however, not available in this subject.

A French study of first-degree relatives[192] found a positive anti-Coxsackie virus IgG in seven of eight (88%) and IgM in one of eight (13%) of ICA-positive relatives, proportions that were not very different from those in ICA-negative relatives (84% and 39%), nonrelated controls (60% and 28%), and recent-onset IDDM cases (100% and 67%, respectively). All the groups studied included, however, young adults, rather than children. A German study of schoolchildren aged 7–19 and screened for ICA[86] found anti-Coxsackie virus IgM in 14 of 44 ICA-positive children and in 7 of 44 age-sex–matched ICA-negative controls. This difference was statistically not significant. No important differences were found for IgM antibodies against mumps, rubella, or cytomegalovirus (CMV) as well.

ICA positivity after mumps infection in children from the general population has been reported to be as high as 78%[193] and 62%[194] and as low as 0%.[87] One study[87] reported ICA positivity, though not a true conversion, after rubella and measles, as well as elevated insulin autoantibodies, especially following chickenpox. Among patients with congenital rubella syndrome, 70% have been found to be ICA positive.[79] An Italian study of first-degree relatives[195] found a high prevalence of anti-CMV IgG (but not IgM) antibodies in ICA-positive relatives (75%), compared with ICA-negative relatives (20%) or age-sex–matched controls (25%).

The degree of tolerance to a viral antigen may depend on the host's age at the time of antigen presentation. Newborns and infants are particularly likely to develop a chronic infection, due to their immature immunological systems. Such an "age-window" model has been suggested for poliomyelitis and multiple sclerosis[196] and it could be tested for candidate viruses and β-cell autoimmunity. Picornavirus (PV) has been shown to persist in hypo- or agammaglobulinemic patients[197] and in subjects with post-polio syndrome,[198] as well as in cultured cell lines.[199] The tropism of picornaviruses to β-cells has been demonstrated in multiple studies reviewed by Foulis and coworkers[200]; however, convincing evidence for a persistent PV infection of β-cells is missing. It is possible that persistent infection with a defective noncytopathic picornavirus causes a significant proportion of β-cell autoimmunity cases.

Case-control or cross-sectional comparisons conducted at the time of clinical IDDM onset are of little value in assessing the cause of β-cell autoimmunity that might have begun several years earlier. Since IDDM onset is preceded by a long period of subclinical β-cell autoimmunity, it is necessary to measure anti-viral IgM close to the onset of *autoimmunity* rather than overt diabetes, to fully assess the role of candidate viruses. Sensitive monoclonal antibodies are now available to a nonspecific picornavirus epitope that allows screening for "footprints" of almost any picornavirus as late as 4–9 months after infection. Picornavirus nucleic acids can now be reliably detected[201] in various body fluids to evaluate whether persistent infection is present. In summary, investigation of the viral etiology of IDDM will likely shift from cross-sectional and retrospective studies of IDDM patients to prospective studies with β-cell autoimmunity as the endpoint.

Nutritional Factors. Early childhood diet may also be important for the development of β-cell autoimmunity. Exposure to wheat and cow's milk protein at weaning triggers insulitis and diabetes in BB rats[202]; however, there are virtually no data to support an association between diet and development of β-cell autoimmunity in humans.

A molecular homology between bovine serum albumin (BSA) and a rat β-cell surface protein p69 inducible by interferon gamma led to speculation[203] that β-cell autoimmunity may result from a molecular mimicry between BSA and p69. A human homologue of p69 (called ICA69) has been recently identified, sequenced, its transcribing locus mapped, and its tissue expression defined.[204] The locus transcribing ICA69 shows no nucleotide or amino acid sequence relation to any known sequence in GenBank, except for two short regions of homology with bovine serum albumin, but not with human albumin. Reactivity with ICA69 has been detected in 6 of 10 ICA-positive sera and 0 of 12 control sera. An ELISA assay for ICA69 is currently being developed and shows promise as a tool for studying the molecular mimicry between ICA69 and BSA in β-cell autoimmunity.

Sensitization to a cow's milk protein may be the initial step in the etiology of β-cell autoimmunity. It may occur as a result of a very early exposure to cow's milk prior to gut cellular tight junction closure or during an infective gastroenteritis when the intestinal barrier is compromised. A prospective collection of infant diet data is necessary to overcome the limitations of the retrospective design[205,206] in the assessment of the effect of early childhood nutrition on the development of β-cell autoimmunity.

Risk Factors for Persistence of Autoimmunity and Progression to Diabetes

The factors that determine progression of β-cell autoimmunity to overt diabetes are poorly understood. This is a major unresolved problem hampering advances in secondary prevention of β-cell autoimmunity where side effects of immunosuppression question its use in children who may recover spontaneously.

High titers of standard cytoplasmic ICA confer increased risk for IDDM.[126,147] However, the risk of progression to IDDM for a given ICA titer varies from study to study, which may reflect different subject selection criteria or the need for further standardization of the assays. Persistent β-cell autoimmunity may be defined as at least two cytoplasmic ICA titers greater than or equal to 20 JDF units measured over a period of 1 year.

Antibodies to the 64-kd islet antigen[207,208] or to its purified forms GAD_{65} and GAD_{67} have been reported to be more predictive for IDDM than the cytoplasmic ICA.[209] However, antibodies to intact GAD are less predictive than so-called nonrestricted ICA.[135] Nonrestricted ICAs react with all pancreatic islet cells (not only the β-cells) and are not absorbed with affinity purified GAD. Their predictive value for persistence of autoimmunity should be further evaluated. In addition, preliminary data (L. Yu, G. S. Eisenbarth, unpublished observations) indicate that the positive predictive value of GAD autoantibodies may be very low in the first 10 years of life.

ICA-positive relatives who were younger than 10 years at the time of the initial positive test had a three-fold increased risk of progressing to IDDM, compared with older relatives.[147] This may be similar to infections with, for example, polio, rubella, and Epstein-Barr viruses (EBV), where age at infection has been shown to determine clinical outcome.[210] Very young age at ICA conversion, eg, prior to the fourth birthday, may be more strongly associated with persistent autoimmunity.

In tuberculosis or poliomyelitis,[210] genetic background appears to determine whether infection progresses to clinical illness. A study of first-degree relatives suggested that ICA-positive individuals progress to IDDM if they possess certain HLA-DQA1, DQB1 phenotype.[211] The DRB1 alleles appear also to be important determinants of IDDM risk.[212] Sharing of one or two HLA haplotypes with a diabetic relative has been reported to predict persistence of ICA among nondiabetic ICA+ relatives.[132] It is likely that although autoimmunity may be triggered in anyone, the HLA genes may be crucial for progression of β-cell autoimmunity to IDDM. An alternative hypothesis is that the HLA phenotype determines whether or not β-cell autoimmunity occurs in the first place.

Conclusions

The determinants of progression from genetic susceptibility, through β-cell autoimmunity, to clinical IDDM are hardly testable in a cross-sectional or retrospective design. Due to the long preclinical period, footprints of exposure cannot be expected to persist until the time of clinical diagnosis. Moreover, diabetes itself modifies both the immune response to viruses and dietary patterns to such an extent that observations taken after diagnosis are likely to be invalid. Therefore, high-risk subjects must be followed prospectively to describe the temporal sequence between the candidate exposures and the onset of autoimmunity.

IDDM is likely caused by an interactive effect of genetic and environmental "exposures" within a limited age-window. Although both the susceptibility genes and the candidate environmental exposures appear to be quite common, the likelihood of these causal components meeting within the susceptibility age-window is fairly low.[213] To investigate the environmental causes of IDDM, the study subjects have to be prescreened for known susceptibility gene markers so that only the susceptible are included. In the susceptible population, the incidence of autoimmunity is likely to be high (3–14% per year) and multiple outcomes can be studied. The environmental exposures have to be measured as they occur, using sensitive and specific instruments, rather than long-term recall, to minimize misclassification and loss of power. These objectives can be achieved with the prospective design.

In spite of our imperfect understanding of IDDM etiology, several preventive trials are under way. A pilot trial of preventive insulin therapy in relatives with β-cell autoimmunity is an encouraging example that secondary prevention of IDDM may be possible.[214] However, some of the interventions proposed for the secondary prevention are associated with significant adverse effects.[215–218] More information is urgently needed to understand who would benefit from such interventions.

Despite enormous progresss, the current knowledge of IDDM etiology is insufficient to design a primary prevention program—one that would *prevent* β-cell autoimmunity, rather than merely *suppress* it. Reasonable evidence exists that early childhood viral or nutritional exposures initiate prediabetic autoimmunity. A safer and more efficient primary prevention may be possible if factors triggering autoimmunity could be identified.

Acknowledgments

This work was supported in part by NIH grant DK32493.

References

1. Patrick SL, Moy CS, LaPorte RE. The world of insulin-dependent diabetes mellitus: what international epidemiologic studies reveal about the etiology and natural history of IDDM. *Diabetes Metab Rev.* 1989; 5:571–578.
2. WHO Study Group. *Diabetics Mellitus - Technical Report Series 727.* Geneva: World Health Organization, 1985.
3. Songer TJ. Health services and costing in diabetes. *Med J Aust.* 1990; 152:115–117.
4. *Healthy people 2000.* National health promotion and disease prevention objectives. Washington, D.C.: U.S. Department of Health and Human Services, Public Health Service, 1991.

5. Skyler JS, Crofford OB, Dupre J, Eisenbarth GS, Fathman GC, Gale EAM, Goldstein D, Haymond MW, Jackson RA, Kahn R, Krischer J, MacLaren NK, Palmer JP, Silverman R, Simon R.Prevention of type 1 diabetes mellitus. *Diabetes.* 1990; 39:1151–1152.
6. Libman I, Songer T, LaPorte R. How many people in the U.S. have IDDM? (Commentary) *Diabetes Care.* 1993; 16:841–842.
7. Palumbo PH, Elevback LR, Chu CP, et al. Diabetes mellitus: Incidence, prevalence, surviorship, and causes of death in Rochester, Minnesota, 1945–1970. *Diabetes.* 1976; 25:566–573.
8. Leichter SB, et al. Diabetes in Kentucky. *Diabetes Care.* 1982; 5:126–134..
9. Sultz HA, Schlesinger ER, Mosher WE, Feldman JG. *Long-term Childhood Illness.* Pittsburg PA: University of Pittsburg Press, 1972.
10. Green A, et al. Epidemiological studies of diabetes mellitus in Denmark - II. A prevalence study based on insulin prescriptions. *Diabetologia.* 1981; 20:468–470.
11. Reunanen A, Akerblom HK, Kaar M. Prevalence and ten-year (1970–1979) incidence of insulin-dependent diabetes mellitus in children and adolescents in Finland. *Acta Paediatr Scand.* 1982; 71:893–899.
12. Hagglof b, et al. Incidence of insulin-dependent diabetes mellitus among children in North-Swedish population 1938–1977. *Hum Hered.* 1982; 32:408–417.
13. Samanta A, et al. Prevalence of insulin-dependent diabetes mellitus in Asian children. *Diabetic Med.* 1986; 4:65–67.
14. Kalits I, Podar T. Incidence and prevalence of type 1 (insulin-dependent) diabetes in Estonia in 1988. *Diabetologia.* 1990; 33:346–349.
15. Mason DR, Scott RS, Darlow BA. Epidemiology of insulin-dependent diabetes mellitus in Canterbury, New Zealand. *Diabetes Res Clin Pract.* 1987; 3:21–29.
16. King H, et al. Type 1 (insulin-dependent) diabetes in Tasmania: prevalence and apparent regional differences. *Diabetologia. 1988; 31:93–97.*
17. Kostraba JN, Gay EC, Cai Y, Cruickshanks KJ, Rewers MJ, Klingensmith GJ, Chase HP, Hamman RF. Incidence of insulin-dependent diabetes mellitus in Colorado. *Epidemiology.* 1992; 3:232–238.
18. Allen C, Palta M, D'Alessio DJ. Risk of diabetes in siblings and other relatives of IDDM subjects. *Diabetes.* 1991; 40:831–836.
19. Warram JH, Martin BC, Krolewski AS. Risk of IDDM in children of diabetic mothers decreases with increasing maternal age at pregnancy. *Diabetes.* 1991; 40:1679–1684.
20. Green A. Empirical risk estimation for relatives of insulin-dependent diabetics: theoretical considerations and practical applications. Kobberling J, Tattersall R, (eds). London: Academic Press; 1982; 21–26.
21. Wagener DK, Sacks JM, LaPorte RE, MacGregor JM. The Pittsburg study of insulin-dependent diabetes mellitus: risk for diabetes among relatives of IDDM. *Diabetes.* 1982; 31:136–144.
22. Tillil H, Kobberling J. Age-corrected empirical genetic risk estimates for first-degree relatives of IDDM patients. *Diabetes.* 1987; 36:93–99.
23. Rewers M. The changing face of the epidemiology of insulin-dependent diabetes mellitus (IDDM): research designs and models of disease causation. *Ann Med.* 1991; 23:419–426.
24. O'Leary LA, Dorman JS, LaPorte RE, Orchard TJ, Becker DJ, Kuller LH, Eberhardt MS, Cavender DE, Rabin BS, Drash AL. Familial and sporadic insulin-dependent diabetes: evidence for heterogeneous etiologies? *Diabetes Res Clin Pract.* 1991; 14:183–190.

25. Ciampi A, Schiffrin A, Thiffault J, Quintal H, Weitzner G, Poussier P, Lalla D. Cluster analysis of an insulin-dependent diabetic cohort towards the definition of clinical subtypes. *Clin Epidemiol.* 1990; 43:701–715.
26. Eberhardt MS, Wagener DK, Orchard TJ, LaPorte RE, Cavender DE, Rabin BS, Atchison RW, Kuller LH, Drash AL, Becker DJ. HLA heterogeneity of insulin-dependent diabetes mellitus at diagnosis: The Pittsburgh IDDM Study. *Diabetes.* 1985; 34:1247–1252.
27. Rewers M, LaPorte RE, King H, Tuomilehto J. Trends in the prevalence and incidence of diabetes: insulin-dependent diabetes mellitus in childhood. *World Health Stat Q.* 1988; 41:179–189.
28. LaPorte RE, Fishbein HA, Drash AL, Kuller LH, Schneider BB, Orchard TJ, Wagener DK. The Pittsburgh Insulin-Dependent Diabetes Mellitus (IDDM) Registry: The incidence of insulin-dependent diabetes mellitus in Allegheny, County, Pennsylvania (1965–1976). 1981; 30:279–284.
29. Diabetes Epidemiology Research International Group. Geographic patterns of childhood insulin-dependent diabetes mellitus. *Diabetes.* 1988; 37:1113–1119.
30. Green A, Gale EAM, Patterson CC. Incidence of childhood-onset insulin-dependent diabetes mellitus: the EURODIAB ACE study. *Lancet.* 1992; 339:905–909.
31. Kitawaga T, Fujita H, Hibi I, et al. A comparative study on the epidemiology of IDDM between Japan, Norway, Israel and the United States. *Acta Paediatr Jpn.* 1984; 26:275–281.
32. Norris JM, Dorman JS, Rewers M, LaPorte RE. The epidemiology and genetics of insulin-dependent diabetes mellitus. *Arch Pathol Lab Med.* 1987; 111:905–909.
33. Lowis GW. Ethnic factors in multiple sclerosis: a review and critque of the epidemiological literature. *Int J Epidemiol.* 1988; 17:14–20.
34. Siemiatycki J, Colle E, Campbell S, Dewar R, Aubert D, Belmonte MM. Incidence of IDDM in Montreal by ethnic group and by social class and comparisons with ethnic groups living elsewhere. *Diabetes.* 1988; 37:1096–1102.
35. Gamble DR. The epidemiology of insulin-dependent diabetes with particular reference to the relationship of virus infection to its etiology. *Epidemiol Rev. 1980; 2;49–70.*
36. Rewers M, LaPorte RE, Wlaczak M, Dmochowski K, Bogaczynska E. Apparent epidemic of insulin-dependent diabetes mellitus in midwestern Poland. *Diabetes.* 1987; 36:106–113.
37. Muntoni S, Songini M, Sardinian Collaborative Group for Epidemiology of IDDM. High incidence rate of IDDM in Sardinia. *Diabetes Care.* 1992; 15:1317–1322.
38. Bruno G, Merletti F, Vuolo A, Pisu E, Gioro M, Pagano G. Sex difference in incidence of IDDM in age-group 15–29 yr. *Diabetes Care.* 1993; 16:133-136.
39. Joner G, Sovik O. The incidence of type 1 (insulin-dependent) diabetes mellitus 15–29 years in Norway 1978–1982. *Diabetologia.* 1991; 34:271–274.
40. Melton JL, et al. Incidence of diabetes mellitus by clinical type. *Diabetes Care.* 1983; 6:75–86.
41. Christau B, Molbak AG. Further epidemiological evidence of a higher incidence level for the insulin-dependent diabetes mellitus in the older age groups. In: Advance abstracts of papers of the 19th Annual Meeting of the Scandinavian Society for the Study of Diabetes, Trondheim, 14–16 June 1984. *Acta Endocrinol.* 1984; 95(suppl 263):18.
42. LaPorte RE, Tajima N, Dorman JS, Cruickshanks KJ, Eberhardt MS, Rabin BS, Atchison RW, Wagener DK, Becker DJ, Orchard TJ, Songer TJ, Slemenda CW,

Kuller LH, Drash AL. Differences between blacks and whites in the epidemiology of insulin-dependent diabetes mellitus in Allegheny County, Pennsylvania. *Am J Epidemiol.* 1986; 123:592–603.

43. Tajima N, LaPorte RE, Hibi I, Kitagawa T, Fujita H, Drash AL. A comparison of the epidemiology of youth-onset insulin-dependent diabetes mellitus between Japan and the United States (Allegheny County, Pennsylvania). *Diabetes Care.* 1985; 8(suppl 1):17–23.
44. Wong GWK, Leung SSF, Oppenheimer SJ. Epidemiology of IDDM in Southern Chinese children in Hong Kong. *Diabetes Care.* 1993; 16:926–928.
45. Ferreira SRG, Franco LJ, Vivolo MA, Negrato CA, Simoes ACP, Venturelli CR. Population-based incidence of IDDM in the state of Sao Paulo, Brazil. *Diabetes Care.* 1993; 16:701–704.
46. Bingley PH, Gale EAM. Incidence of insulin dependent diabetes in England: a study in the Oxford region, 1985–6. *Br Med J.* 1989; 298:558–560.
47. Soltesz G, Madacsy L, Bekefi D, Danko I, and the Hungarian Childhood Diabetes Epidemiology Group. Rising incidence of type 1 diabetes in Hungarian children (1978–1987). *Diabetic Med.* 1990; 7:111–114.
48. Dahlquist G, Gustavsson KH, Holmgren G, Hagglof B, Larsson Y, Nilsson KO, Samuelsson G, Sterky G, Thalme B, Wall S. The incidence of diabetes mellitus in Swedish children 0–14 years of age. *Acta Pediatr Scand.* 1982; 71:7–14.
49. Serrano Rios M, Moy CS, Martin Serrano R, Minuesa Asenio A, de Tomas Labat ME, Zarandieta Romero G, Herrera J. Incidence of type 1 (insulin-dependent) diabetes mellitus in subjects 0–14 years of age in the Comunidad of Madrid, Spain. *Diabetologia.* 1990; 33:422–424.
50. Joner G, Sovik O. Increasing incidence of diabetes mellitus in Norwegian children 0–14 years of age 1973–1982. *Diabetologia.* 1989; 32:79–83.
51. Patterson CC, Thorogood M, Smith PG, Heasman MA, Clarke JA, Mann JI. Epidemiology of type 1 (insulin-dependent) diabetes in Scotland 1968–1976: evidence of an increasing incidence. *Diabetologia.* 1983; 24:238–243.
52. Siemiatycki J, Colle E, Aubert D, Campbell S, Belmonte MM. The distribution of type 1 (insulin-dependent) diabetes mellitus by age, sex, secular trend, seasonality, time clusters, and space-time clusters: evidence from Montreal, 1971–1983. *Am J Epidemiol.* 1986; 124:545–560.
53. Ludvigsson J, Afoke AO. Seasonality of type 1 (insulin-dependent) diabetes mellitus: values of C-peptide, insulin antibodies and haemoglobin A_{1c} show evidence of a more rapid loss of insulin secretion in epidemic patients. *Diabetologia.* 1989; 32:84–91.
54. Pagano G, Cavallo-Perin P, Cavalot F, Dall'omo AM, Masciola P, Suriani R, Amoroso A, Curtoni SE, Borelli I, Lenti G. Genetic, immunologic, and environmental heterogeneity of IDDM: incidence and 12-mo follow-up of an Italian population. *Diabetes.* 1987; 36:859–863.
55. Tuomilehto J, Rewers M, Reunanen A, Lounamaa P, Lounamaa R, Tuomilehto-Wolf E, Akerblom HK. Increasing trend in type 1 (insulin-dependent) diabetes mellitus in childhood in Finland. *Diabetologia.* 1991; 34:282–287.
56. Nystrom L, Dahlquist G, Rewers M, Wall S. The Swedish Childhood Diabetes Study: an analysis of the temporal variation in diabetes incidence 1978–1987. *Int J Epidemiol.* 1990; 19:141–146.
57. Hamman RF, Gay EC, Cruickshanks KJ, Cook M, Lezotte DC, Klingensmith GJ, Chase HP. Colorado IDDM Registry: incidence and validation of IDDM in children aged 0–17 yr. *Diabetes Care.* 1990; 13:499–506.

58. De Beaufort CE, Michel G, Glaesener G. The incidence of type 1 (insulin-dependent) diabetes mellitus in subjects aged 0–19 years in Luxembourg: a retrospective study from 1977 to 1986. *Diabetologia.* 1988; 31:758–761.
59. Joner G, Sovik O. Incidence, age at onset and seasonal variation of diabetes mellitus in Norwegian children, 1973–1977. *Acta Paediatr Scand.* 1980; 70:329–335.
60. Agner T, Damm P, Binder C. Remission in IDDM: prospective study of basal C-peptide and insulin dose in 268 consecutive patients. *Diabetes Care.* 1987; 10:164–169.
61. Drash AL. The epidemiology of insulin-dependent diabetes mellitus. *Clin Invest Med.* 1987; 10:432–436.
62. Martin S, Pawlowski B, Greulich B, Ziegler AG, Mandrup-Poulsen T, Mahon J. Natural course of remission in IDDM during 1st yr after diagnosis. *Diabetes Care.* 1992; 15:66–74.
63. Assan R, Feutren G, Sirmai J, Laborie C, Boitard C, Vexiau P, Du Rostu H, Rodier M, Figoni M, Vague P, Hors J, Bach J-F. Plasma C-peptide levels and clinical remissions in recent-onset Type 1 diabetic patients treated with cyclosporin A and insulin. *Diabetes.* 1990; 39:768–774.
64. Diabetes Epidemiology Research International Group. Secular trends in incidence of childhood IDDM in 10 countries. *Diabetes.* 1990; 39:358–864.
65. Wagenknecht LE, Roseman JM, Herman WH. Increased incidence of insulin-dependent diabetes mellitus following an epidemic of coxsackievirus B5. *Am J Epidemiol.* 1991; 133:1024–1031.
66. Rewers M, Pallansch MA, Bogaczynska E, Patrick SL, Anderson LA, Walczak M, LaPorte RE. Conflicting evidence for enterovirus as the cause of childhood diabetes epidemic in Poland. *Diabetologia.* 1990; 33(suppl 1):A198.
67. Hayward JC, Gillespie SM, Kaplan KM, Packer R, Pallansch M, Plotkin S, Schonberger LB. Outbreak of poliomyelitis-like paralysis associated with enterovirus 71. *Pediatr Infect Dis J.* 1989; 8:611–616.
68. Barrett-Connor E. Is insulin-dependent diabetes mellitus caused by Coxsackie virus B infection? A review of the epidemiologic evidence. *Rev Infect Dis.* 1985; 7:207–215.
69. Jenson AB, Rosenberg HS, Notkins AL. Pancreatic islet-cell damage in children with fatal viral infections. *Lancet.* 1980; 2:354–358.
70. Champsaur HF, Bottazzo GF, Bertrams J, Assan R, Bach C. Virologic, immunologic, and genetic factors in insulin-dependent diabetes mellitus. *J Pediatr.* 1982; 100:15–20.
71. Yoon AW, Austin M, Onodera T, Notkins AL. Virus-induced diabetes mellitus: isolation of a virus from the pancreas of a child with diabetic ketoacidosis. *N Engl J Med.* 1979; 300:1173–1179.
72. D'Alessio DJ. A case-control study of group B Coxsackievirus immunoglobulin M antibody prevalence and HLA-DR antigens in newly diagnosed cases of insulin-dependent diabetes mellitus. *Am J Epidemiol.* 1992; 135:1331–1338.
73. Rose NR, Griffin DE. Virus-induced autoimmunity. In: Talal N, ed. *Molecular Autoimmunity.* London: Academic Press Ltd; 1991; 247–272.
74. Vento S, Garofano T, DiPerri G, Dolci L, Concia E, Bassetti D. Identification of hepatitis A virus as a trigger for autoimmune chronic hepatitis type 1 in susceptible individuals. *Lancet.* 1991; 337:1181–1187.
75. Bowles NE, Dubowitz V, Sewry CA, Archard LC. Dermatomyositis, polymyositis, and Coxsackie-B-virus infection. *Lancet.* 1987; 2:1004–1007.

76. Pak CY, Hyone-Myong E, McArthur RG, Yoon JW. Association of cytomegalovirus infection with autoimmune type 1 diabetes. *Lancet.* 1988; 2:1–3.

77. Sairenji T, Daibata M, Sorli CH, et al. Relating homology between the Epstein-Barr virus BOLF1 and HLA-DQw8 beta chain to recent onset type 1 (insulin-dependent) diabetes mellitus. *Diabetologia.* 1991; 34:33–39.

78. Helmke K. In: Becker Y, ed. *Virus Infections and Diabetes Mellitus.* Boston: Martinus Nijhoff Publishing; 1987; 127–142.

79. Ginsberg-Fellner F, Witt ME, Yagihashi S, Dobersen MJ, Taub F, Fedun B, McEvoy RC, Roman SH, Davies RG, Cooper LZ, et al. Congenital rubella syndrome as a model for type 1 (insulin-dependent) diabetes mellitus: increased prevalence of islet cell surface antibodies. *Diabetologia.* 1984; 27(suppl 1):87–89.

80. Suenaga K, Yoon JW. Association of beta-cell-specific expression of endogenous retrovirus with development of insulitis and diabetes in NOD mouse. *Diabetes.* 1988; 37:1722–1726.

81. Rubinstein P, Walker ME, Fedun B, Witt ME, Cooper LZ, Ginsburg-Fellner F. The HLA system in congenital rubella patients with and without diabetes. *Diabetes.* 1982; 31:1088–1091.

82. Menser MA, Forrest JM, Bransby RD. Rubella infection and diabetes mellitus. *Lancet.* 1978; 1:57–50.

83. Forrest JM, Menser MA, Burgess JA. High frequency of diabetes mellitus in young adults with congenital rubella. *Lancet.* 1971; 2:332–334.

84. Monif GRG, Avery GB, Korones SB, Sever JL. Post-mortem isolation of rubella virus from three children with rubella-syndrome defects. *Lancet.* 1965; 1:723–724.

85. Karounos DG, Wolinsky JS, Thomas JW. Monoclonal antibody to rubella virus capsid protein recognizes a beta-cell antigen. *J Immunol.* 1993; 150:3080–3085.

86. Scherbaum WA, Hampl W, Muir P, Glück M, Seissler J, Egle H, Hauner H, Boehm BO, Heinze E, Banatvala JE, Pfeiffer EF. No association between islet cell antibodies and Coxsackie B, mumps, rubella and cytomegalovirus antibodies in non-diabetic individuals aged 7–19 years. *Diabetologia.* 1991; 34:835–838.

87. Bodansky HJ, Grant PJ, Dean BM, McNally J, Bottazzo GF, Hambling MH, Wales JK. Islet-cell antibodies and insulin autoantibodies in association with common viral infections. *Lancet.* 1986; 2:1351–1353.

88. Banatvala JE, Bryant J, Schernthaner G, Borkenstein M, Schober E, Brown D, De Silva LM, Menser MA, Silink M. Coxsackie B, mumps, rubella, and cytomegalovirus specific IgM responses in patients with juvenile-onset insulin-dependent diabetes mellitus in Britain, Austria, and Australia. *Lancet.* 1985; 1:1409–1412.

89. Blom L, Nystrom L, Dahlquist G. The Swedish Childhood Diabetes Study: vaccinations and infections as risk determinants for diabetes in childhood. *Diabetologia.* 1991; 34:176–181.

90. Oldstone MBA. Viruses as therapeutic agents. I. Treatment of nonobese insulin-dependent diabetes mice with virus prevents insulin-dependent diabetes mellitus while maintaining general immune competence. *J Exp Med.* 1990; 171:2077–2089.

91. Wilberz S, Partke HJ, Dagnaes-Hansen F, Herberg L. Persistent MHV (mouse hepatitis virus) infection reduces the incidence of diabetes mellitus in non-obese diabetic mice. *Diabetologia.* 1991; 34:2–5.

92. Like AA, Guberski DL, Butler L. Influence of environmental viral agents on frequency and tempo of diabetes mellitus in BB/Wor rats. *Diabetes.* 1991; 40:259–262.
93. Borch-Johnsen K, Joner G, Mandrup-Poulsen T, et al. Relation between breast-feeding and incidence of insulin-dependent diabetes mellitus. *Lancet.* 1984; 2:1083–1086.
94. Glatthaar C, Whittall DE, Welborn TA, et al. Diabetes in Western Australian children: descriptive epidemiology. *Med J Austral.* 1988; 148:117–123.
95. Metcalfe MA, Baum JD. Family characteristics and insulin dependent diabetes. *Arch Dis Child.* 1992; 67:731–736.
96. Mayer EJ, Hamman RF, Gay EC, Lezotte DC, Savitz DA, Klingensmith GJ. Reduced risk of IDDM among breast-fed children. *Diabetes.* 1988; 37:1625–1632.
97. Kostraba JN, Dorman JS, LaPorte RE, et al. Early infant diet and risk of IDDM in blacks and whites: a matched case-control study. *Diabetes Care.* 1992; 15:626–631.
98. Blom L, Dahlquist G, Nystrom L, Sandstrom A, Wall S. The Swedish Childhood Diabetes Study: social and perinatal determinants for diabetes in childhood. *Diabetologia.* 1989; 32:7–13.
99. Fort P, Lanes R, Dahlem S, et al. Breast feeding and insulin-dependent diabetes mellitus in children. *J Am Coll Nutr* 1986; 5:439–441.
100. Kostraba JN, Cruickshanks KJ, LAwler-Heavner J, et al. Early exposure to cow's milk and solid foods in infancy, genetic predisposition, and risk of IDDM. *Diabetes.* 1993; 42:288–295.
101. Siemiatycki J, Colle E, Campbell S, DeWar RAD, Belmonte MM. Case-control study of IDDM> *Diabetes Care.* 1989; 12:209–216.
102. Kyvik KO, Green A, Svendsen A, Mortensen K. Breast-feeding and the development of type 1 diabetes mellitus. *Diabetic Med.* 1992; 9:233–235.
103. Samuelsson U, Johansson C, Ludvigsson J. Breast-feeding seems to play a marginal role in the prevention of insulin-dependent diabetes mellitus. *Diabetes Res Clin Pract.* 1993; 19:203–210.
104. Bodington M, Burden AC. Early exposure to cow's milk or cow's milk formula does not appear to increase the risk of childhood onset of IDDM in Leicestershire. *Diabetic Med.* 1993; 10(suppl 1):S41.
105. Nigro G, Campea L, DeNovellis A, Orsini M. Breast-feeding and insulin-dependent diabetes mellitus [letter]. *Lancet.* 1985; 1:467.
106. Virtanen SM, Rasanen L, Aro A, et al. Infant feeding in Finnish children <7 yr of age with newly diagnosed IDDM. *Diabetes Care.* 1991; 14:415–417.
107. Virtanen SN, Rasanen L, Aro A, et al. Feeding in infancy and the risk of type 1 diabetes mellitus in Finnish children. *Diabetic Med.* 1992; 9:815–819.
108. Verge CF, Howard NJ, Irwig L, Simpson JM, Silink M. Childhood diabetes and infant feeding: a population based case-control study. *Diabetologia.* 1992; 35(suppl 1):25A.
109. Gerstein HC. Cow's milk exposure and type 1 diabetes mellitus—a critical overview of the clinical literature. *Diabetes Care.* 1993; 17:13–19.
110. Norris JM, Scott FW. Difficulties in examining infant diet and insulin-dependent diabetes mellitus (IDDM) risk. *Diabetes.* 1994; 43(suppl 1):213A.
111. Elliot RB, Martin JM. Dietary protein: a trigger of insulin-dependent diabetes in the BB rat? *Diabetologia.* 1984; 26:297–299.
112. Coleman DL, Kuzava JE, Leiter EH. Effect of diet on incidence of diabetes in nonobese diabetic mice. *Diabetes.* 1990; 39:432–436.

113. Scott FW, Marliss EB. Conference summary: diet as an environmental factor in development of IDDM. *Can J Physiol Pharmacol.* 1991; 69:311–319.

114. Scott FW. Cow's milk and insulin-dependent diabetes mellitus: Is there a relationship? *Am J Clin Nutr.* 1990; 51:489–491.

115. Dahl-Jorgensen K, Joner G, Hanssen KF. Relationship between cow's milk consumption and incidence of IDDM in childhood. *Diabetes Care.* 1991; 14:1081–1083.

116. Savilahti E, Akerblom HK, Tainio VM, Koskimies S. Children with newly diagnosed insulin dependent diabetes mellitus have increased levels of cow's milk antibodies. *Diabetes Res.* 1988; 7:137–140.

117. Karjalainen J, Martin JM, Knip M, et al. A bovine serum albumin peptide as a possible trigger of insulin dependent diabetes mellitus. *N Engl J Med.* 1992; 327:302–307.

118. Tuomilehto J, Tuomilehto-Wolf E, Virtala E, LaPorte R. Coffee consumption as trigger for insulin-dependent diabetes mellitus in childhood. *Br Med J.* 1990; 300:642–643.

119. Pozzilli P, Bottazzo GF. Coffee or sugar—which is to blame in IDDM? [Commentary]. *Diabetes Care.* 1991; 14:144–145.

120. Dahlquist GG, Blom LG, Persson LA, Sandstrom AIM, Wall SGI. Dietary factors and the risk of developing insulin-dependent diabetes in childhood. *Br Med J.* 1990; 300:1302–1306.

121. Helgason T, Jonasson MR. Evidence for a food additive as cause of ketosis-prone diabetes. *Lancet.* 1981; 2:716–720.

122. Kostraba JN, Gay EC, Rewers M, Hamman RF. Nitrate levels in community drinking waters and risk of IDDM. *Diabetes Care.* 1991; 15:1505–1508.

123. Pont A, Rubino JM, Bishop D. Diabetes mellitus and neuropathy following Vacor ingestion in man. *Arch Intern Med.* 1979; 139:185–187.

124. Schein PS, Alberti KGMM, Williamson DH. Effects of streptozotocin on carbohydrate and lipid metabolism in the rat. *Endocrinology.* 1971; 89:827–834.

125. LeDoux SP, Hall CR, Forbes PM, Patton NJ, Wilson GL. Mechanisms of nicotinamide and thymidine protection from Alloxan and streptozocin toxicity. *Diabetes.* 1988; 37:1015–1019.

126. Bonifacio E, Bingley PJ, Shattock M, Dean BM, Dunger D, Gale EAM, Bottazzo GF. Quantification of islet-cell antibodies and prediction of insulin-dependent diabetes. *Lancet.* 1990; 335:147–149.

127. Rosenbloom AL, Hunt SS, Rosenbloom EK, macLaren NK. Ten-year prognosis of impaired glucose tolerance in siblings of patients with insulin-dependent diabetes. *Diabetes.* 1982; 31:385–387.

128. Johnston C, Millward Ba, Hoskins P, Leslie RD, Bottazzo GF, Pyke DA. Islet-cell antibodies as predictors of the later development of type 1 (insulin-dependent) diabetes: a study in identical twins. *Diabetologia.* 1989; 32:382–386.

129. Haskins K, McDuffie M. Acceleration of diabetes in young NOD mice with a CD4+ islet-specific T cell clone. *Science.* 1990; 249:1433–1436.

130. Cooke A. An overview on possible mechanisms of destruction of the insulin-producing beta cell. *Curr Top Microbiol Immunol.* 1990; 164:125–141.

131. Santamaria P, Nakhleh RE, Sutherland DE, Barbosa JJ. Characterization of T lymphocytes infiltrating human pancreas allograft affected by isletitis and recurrent diabetes. *Diabetes.* 1992; 41:53–61.

132. Lipton R, LaPorte RE. Epidemiology of islet cell antibodies. *Epidemiol Rev.* 1989; 11:182–203.

133. Riley WH, MacLaren NK. Islet cell autoantibodies. In: Samois E, ed. *The Endocrine Pancreas.* New York: Raven Press, Ltd; 1991:409–422.
134. Lernmark A, Molenaar JL, van Beers WAM, Yamaguchi Y, Nagataki S, Ludvigsson J, MacLaren NK. The fourth international serum exchange workshop to standardize cytoplasmic islet cell antibodies. *Diabetologia.* 1991; 34:534–535.
135. Gianani R, Pugliese A, Bonner-Weir S, Shiffrin AJ, Soeldner JS, Erlich H, Awdeh Z, Alper CA, Jackson RA, Eisenbarth GS. Prognostically significant heterogeneity of cytoplasmic islet cell antibodies in relatives of patients with type 1 diabetes. *Diabetes.* 1992; 41:347–353.
136. Baekkeskov S, Aanstoot H, Christgau S, Reetz A, Solimena M, Cascaiho M, Folli F, Richter-Olesen H, DeCamilli P. Identification of the 64k autoantigen in insulin-dependent diabetes as the GABA-synthesizing enzyme glutamic acid decarboxylase. *Nature.* 1990; 347:151–156.
137. Clare-Salzler MJ, Tobin AJ, Kaufman DL. Glutamate decarboxylase: an autoantigen in IDDM. *Diabetes Care.* 1992; 15:132–135.
138. Maclaren N, Horne G, Spillar R, Brown L, Silverstein J, Shah S, Malone J, Riley W. The feasibility of using ICA to predict IDDM in U.S. school children. *Diabetes.* 1990; 39(suppl 1):122A.
139. Boehm BO, Manfras B, Seissler J, Schoffling K, Gluck M, Holzberger G, Seidl S, Kuhnl P, Trucco M, Scherbaum WA. Epidemiology and immunogenetic background of islet cell antibody–positive nondiabetic schoolchildren: Ulm-Frankfurt population study. *Diabetes.* 1991; 40:1435–1439.
140. Levy-Marchal C, Tichet J, Fajardy I, Dubois F, Czernichow P. Follow-up of children from a background population with high ICA titres. *Diabetologia.* 1992; 35(suppl 1):A32.
141. Bertrams J, Baur MP. Insulin-dependent diabetes mellitus. In: Albert ED, ed. *Histocompatibility Testing 1984.* Berlin: Springer-Verlag; 1984:348–358.
142. Todd JA. The role of MHC class II genes in susceptibility to insulin-dependent diabetes mellitus. *Curr Top Microbiol Immunol.* 1990; 164:17–40.
143. Garchon H-J, Bedossa P, Eloy L, Bach J-F. Identification and mapping to chromosome 1 of a susceptibility locus for periinsulitis in non-obese diabetic mice. *Nature.* 1991; 353:260–262.
144. Neufeld M, Maclaren NK, Riley WJ, Lezotte D, McLaughlin JV, Silverstein J, Rosenbloom AL. Islet cell and other organ-specific antibodies in U.S. Caucasians and blacks with insulin-dependent diabetes mellitus. *Diabetes.* 1980; 29:589–592.
145. St A Morrison EY, Rosenbloom AL, McLaren NK, Riley WJ, Kooperman S. Absence of islet cell autoantibodies in Jamaican blacks with diabetes mellitus. *West Indian Med J.* 1986; 35:35–37.
146. Oli JM, Bottazzo GF, Doniach D. Islet cell antibodies and diabetes in Nigerians. *Trop Geogr Med.* 1981; 33:161–164.
147. Riley WJ, MacLaren NK, Krischer J, Spillar RP, Silverstein JH, Schatz DA, Schwartz S, Malone J, Shah S, Vadheim C, Rotter JI. A prospective study of the development of diabetes in relatives of patients with insulin-dependent diabetes. *N Engl J Med.* 1990; 323:1167–1172.
148. Muntoni S, Loviselli A, Martino E, Velluzzi F, Shattock M, Balestrieri A, Songini M, Muntoni S, Bottazzo GF. High prevalence of islet cell antibodies (ICA) in healthy schoolchildren in Sardinia. *Diabetologia.* 1992; 35(suppl 1):A32.

149. Karjalainen JK. Islet cell antibodies as predictive markers for IDDM in children with high background incidence of disease. *Diabetes.* 1990; 39:1144–1150.

150. Knip M. How well do risk markers reflect future IDDM? Presented at the Annual Meeting of the Finnish Medical Association, Helsinki, January 7, 1991.

151. Landin-Olsson M, Palmer JP, Lernmark A, Blom L, Sundkvist G, Nyström L, Dahlquist G. Predictive value of islet cell and insulin autoantibodies for type 1 (insulin-dependent) diabetes mellitus in a population-based study of newly-diagnosed diabetic and matched control children. *Diabetologia.* 1992; 35:1068–1073.

152. Hägglöf B, Rabinovitch A, Mackay P, Huen A, Rubenstein AH, Marner B, Nerup J, Lernmark A. Islet cell and other organ-specific autoantibodies in healthy first-degree relatives to insulin-dependent. *Acta Paediatr Scand.* 1986; 75:611–618.

153. Bingley PJ, Dunger DB, Bonifacio E, Scott RDM, Shattock M, Bottazzo GF, Gillmor HA, Gale EAM, Sawtell PA. Can islet cell antibodies predict IDDM in the general population? *Diabetes Care.* 1993; 16:45–50.

154. Elliott RB, Pilcher CC, McGregor MA. Protection from diabetes in normal school children using nicotinamide. Presented at the 12th International Immunology and Diabetes Workshop, Orlando, Florida, April 1993.

155. Pilcher CC, Elliott RB. Ontogeny of islet cell and insulin autoantibodies in first degree relatives of IDDM. Presented at the American Diabetes Association 12th International Immunology and Diabetes Workshop, Orlando, Florida, April 1993.

156. Levy-Marchal C, Tichet J, Fajardy I, Gu XF, Dubois F, Czernichow P. Islet cell antibodies in normal French schoolchildren. *Diabetologia.* 1992; 35:577–582.

157. Thivolet C, Beaufrere B, Geburher L, Chatelain P, Orgiazzi J, François R. Autoantibodies and genetic factors associated with the development of type 1 (insulin-dependent) diabetes mellitus in first degree relatives of diabetic patients. *Diabetologia.* 1991; 34:186–191.

158. Rowe RE, Leech NJ, McCullouch DK. Persistence of ICA in a healthy teenage population. Presented at the 12th Annual Immunology and Diabetes Workshop, Orlando, Florida, April 1993.

159. Adojaan B, Knip M, Karjalainen J, Kalits I, Åkerblom HK. Relation between frequency of ICA-positivity in healthy children and incidence of type 1 diabetes: an Estonian-Finnish comparison. *Diabetologia.* 1992; 35(suppl 1):A218.

160. Becker F, Lenders W, Sauer H, Petzold R, Federlin K. Low rate of conversion to diabetes mellitus in healthy first degree relatives of German type 1 diabetic patients. Presented at the 12th International Immunology and Diabetes Workshop, Orlando, Florida, April 1993.

161. Colman PG, McNair PD, Caudwell JP, Howard N, Colaguri S, Harrison LC. Screening of an apparent 'hot spot' of IDDM for markers of preclinical IDDM. Presented at the 12th International Immunology and Diabetes Workshop, Orlando, Florida, April 1993.

162. Kelly HA, Byrne GC. Incidence of IDDM in Western Australia in children aged 0–14 yr from 1985 to 1989. *Diabetes Care.* 1992; 15:515–517.

163. Bergua M, Solé J, Marion G, Perez MC, Recasens A, Fernández J, Casamitjana R, Gomis R. Prevalence of islet cell antibodies, insulin antibodies and hyperglycaemia in 2291 schoolchildren. *Diabetologia.* 1987; 30:724–726.

164. Goday A, Castell C, Tresserras R, Canela J, Taberner JL, Lloveras G. Incidence of type 1 (insulin-dependent) diabetes mellitus in Catalonia, Spain. *Diabetologia.* 1992; 35:267–271.

165. Notsu K, Oka N, Note S, Nabeya N, Kuno S, Sakurami T. Islet cell antibodies in the Japanese population and subjects with type 1 (insulin-dependent) diabetes. *Diabetologia.* 1985; 28:660–662.
166. Bruining GJ, Molenaar JL, Grobbee DE, Hofman A, Scheffer GJ, Bruining HA, deBruyn AM, Valkenburg HA. Ten-year follow-up study of islet-cell antibodies and childhood diabetes mellitus. *Lancet.* 1989; 1:1100–1103.
167. Chase HP, Voss MA, Butler-Simon N, Hoops S, O'Brien D, Doberson MJ. Diagnosis of pre-type 1 diabetes. *J Pediatr.* 1987; 111:807–812.
168. Pilcher CC, Dickens K, Elliott RB. ICA only develop in early childhood. *Diabetes Res Clin Pract.* 1991; 14(suppl 1):s82.
169. Palmer JP, McCulloch DK. Prediction and prevention of IDDM—1991. *Diabetes.* 1991; 40:943–947.
170. Spinas GA, Matter L, Wilkin T, Staffelbach O, Berger W. Islet-cell and insulin autoantibodies in first-degree relatives of type I diabetics: a 5-year follow-up study in a Swiss population. *Adv Exp Med Biol.* 1988; 246:209–214.
171. Asplin CM, Cooney MK, Crossley JR, Dornan TL, Raghu P, Palmer JP. Coxsackie B4 infection and islet cell antibodies three years before overt diabetes. *J Pediatr.* 1982; 101:398–400.
172. Spencer KM, Dean BM, Tarn A, Lister J, Bottazzo GF. Fluctuating islet-cell autoimmunity in unaffected relatives of patients with insulin-dependent diabetes. *Lancet.* 1984; 1:764–766.
173. Thivolet C, Beaufrere B, Betuel H, Gebuhrer L, Chatelain P, Durand A, Tourniaire J, Francois R. Islet cell and insulin autoantibodies in subjects at high risk for development of type 1 (insulin-dependent) diabetes mellitus: the Lyon family study. *Diabetologia.* 1988; 31:741–746.
174. Kuglin B, Kolb H, Greenbaum C, MacLaren NK, Lernmark A, Palmer JP. The fourth international workshop on the standardisation of insulin autoantibody measurement. *Diabetologia.* 1990; 33:638–639.
175. Landin-Olsson M, Karlsson A, Dahlquist G, Blom L, Lernmark A, Sundkvist G. Islet cell and other organ specific autoantibodies in all children developing Type 1 (insulin-dependent) diabetes mellitus in Sweden during one year and in matched control children. *Diabetologia.* 1989; 32:387–395.
176. Maki M, Holm K, Lipsanen V, Hallstrom O, Viander M, Collin P, Savilahti E, Koskimies S. Serological markers and HLA genes among healthy first-degree relatives of patients with coeliac disease. *Lancet.* 1991; 338:1350–1353.
177. Takasu N, Yamada T, Takasu M, Komiys I, Nagasawa Y, Asawa T, Shinoda T, Aizawa T, Koizumi Y. Disappearance of thyrotropin-blocking antibodies and spontaneous recovery from hypothyroidism in autoimmune thyroiditis. *N Engl J Med.* 1992; 326:513–518.
178. Kobayashi T, Itoh T, Kosaka K, Sato K, Tsuji K. Time course of islet cell antibodies and β-cell function in non-insulin-dependent stage of type I diabetes. *Diabetes.* 1987; 36:510–517.
179. Rossini AA, Mordes JP, Handler ES. Speculations on etiology of diabetes mellitus: Tumbler hypothesis. *Diabetes.* 1988; 37:257–261.
180. Groop LC, Bottazzo FB, Doniach D. Islet cell antibodies identify latent type I diabetes in patients aged 35–75 at diagnosis. *Diabetes.* 1986; 35:237–241.
181. Tuomi T, Groop LC, Zimmet PZ, Rowley MJ, Knowles W, Mackay IR. Antibodies to glutamic acid decarboxylase reveal latent autoimmune diabetes mellitus in adults with a non-insulin-dependent onset of disease. *Diabetes.* 1993; 42:359–362.
182. Oldstone MB, Nerenberg M, Southern P, Price J, Lewicki H. Virus infection

triggers insulin-dependent diabetes mellitus in a transgenic model: role of anti-self (virus) immune response. *Cell.* 1991; 65:319–331.

183. Ohashi PS, Oehen S, Buerki K, Pircher H, Ohashi CT, Odermatt B, Malissen B, Zinkernagel RM, Hengartner H. Ablation of "tolerance" and induction of diabetes by virus infection in viral antigen transgenic mice. *Cell.* 1991; 65:305–317.
184. Yoon JW. The role of viruses and environmental factors in the induction of diabetes. *Curr Top Microbiol Immunol.* 1990; 164:95–123.
185. Lemon SM, Murphy PC, Shields PA, Ping L, Feinstone SM, Cromeans T, Jansen RW. Antigenic and genetic variation in cytopathic hepatitis A virus variants arising during persistent infection: evidence for genetic recombination. *J Virol.* 1991; 65:2056–2065.
186. Craighead JE, Huber SA, Sriram S. Animal models of picornavirus-induced autoimmune disease: their possible relevance to human disease. *Lab Invest.* 1990; 63:432–446.
187. Gerling I, Nejman C, Chatterjee NK. Effect of Coxsackievirus B4 infection in mice on expression of 64,000-Mr autoantigen and glucose sensitivity of islets before development of hyperglycemia. *Diabetes.* 1988; 37:1419–1425.
188. Hagopian WA, McGrew S, Kaliappan SB, Karlsen AE, D'Allessio DJ. Recent Coxsackie B virus infection associates with glutamic acid decarboxylase autoantibodies (GAD65 Ab) regardless of insulin-dependent diabetes (IDDM) status. Presented at the American Diabetes Association 12th International Immunology and Diabetes Workshop, Orlando, Florida, April 1993.
189. Orchard TJ, Becker DJ, Atchison RW, LaPorte RE, Wagener DK, Rabin BS, Kuller Lh, Drash AL. The development of type 1 (insulin-dependent) diabetes mellitus: two contrasting presentations. *Diabetologia.* 1983; 25:89–92.
190. Uriarte A, Cabrera E, Ventura R, Vargas J. Islet cell antibodies and ECHO-4 virus infection. *Diabetologia.* 1987; 30(suppl 1):590A.
191. Dronfield DM. Changes in serum insulin and islet cell antibodies following an outbreak of Echovirus 4 in Glasgow. *Diabetic Med.* 1993; 10(suppl 1):S41.
192. Vialettes B, Demicco P, Badier C, Niccoline J, Lassmann-Vague V. Anti-Coxsackie B IgG and IgM antibodies in first degree relatives of type 1 (insulin-dependent) diabetic patients: lack of association with islet cell antibodies. *Diabetologia.* 1987; 30(suppl 1):594A.
193. Ratzmann KP, Strese J, Witt S, Berling H, Keilacker H, Michaelis D. Mumps infection and insulin-dependent diabetes mellitus (IDDM). *Diabetes Care.* 1984; 7:170–173.
194. Helmke K, Otten A, Willems Wr, Brockhaus R, Mueller-Eckhardt G, Stief T, Bertrams J, Wolf H, Federlin K. Islet cell antibodies and the development of diabetes mellitus in relation to mumps infection and mumps vaccination. *Diabetologia.* 1986; 29:30–33.
195. Nicoletti F, Scalia G, Lunetta M, Concorelli F, Di Mauro M, Barcellini W, Stracuzzi S, Pagano M, Meroni PL. Correlation between islet cell antibodies and anti-cytomegalovirus IgM and IgG antibodies in healthy first-degree relatives of type 1 (insulin-dependent) diabetic patients. *Clin Immunol Immunopathol.* 1990; 55:139–147.
196. Martyn CN. In: *The Childhood Environment and Adult Disease. Ciba Foundation Symposium 156.* Chichester: Wiley; 1991:93–108.
197. McKinney RE, Katz SL, Wilfert CM. Chronic enteroviral meningoencephalitis in agammaglobulinemic patients. *Rev Infect Dis.* 1987; 9:334–356.

198. Sharief MK, Hentges R, Ciardi M. Intrathecal immune response in patients with the post-polio syndrome. *N Engl J Med.* 1991; 325:749–755.
199. Montgomery L, Lordon D, George K, Maratos-Flier E. Coxsackie infection of insulinoma cells leads to viral latency and altered insulin and class i MHC expression. *Diabetes.* 1991; 40(suppl 1):150A.
200. Foulis AK, Farquharson MA, Cameron SO, McGill M, Schönke, Kandolf R. A search for the presence of the enteroviral capsid protein VP1 in panceases of patients with type 1 (insulin-dependent) diabetes of coxsackieviral myocarditis. *Diabetologia.* 1990; 33:290–298.
201. Rotbart HA. Nucleic acid detection systems for enteroviruses. *Clin Microbiol Rev.* 1991; 4:156–168.
202. Atkinson MA, Winter WE, Skordis N, Beppu H, Riley WM, MacLaren NK. Dietary protein restriction reduces the frequency and delays the onset of insulin dependent diabetes in bb rats. *Autoimmunity.* 1988; 2:11–20.
203. Martin JM, Trink B, Daneman D, Dosch H-M, Robinson B. Milk proteins in the etiology of insulin-dependent diabetes mellitus (IDDM). *Ann Med.* 1991; 23:447–452.
204. Pietropaolo M, Castaño L, Babu S, Martin S, Martin A, Powers AC, Prochazka M, Naggert J, Leiter EH, Eisenbarth GS. Islet cell autoantigen 69 kDa (ICA69): molecular cloning and characterization of a novel diabetes associated autoantigen. *J Clin Invest.* 1993; 92:359–371.
205. Chandra RK. Long-term health effects of infant feeding. *Nutr Res.* 1989; 9:1–4.
206. Vobecky JS, Vobecky J, Froda S. The reliability of the maternal memory in a retrospective assessment of nutritional status. *J Clin Epidemiol.* 1988; 41:261–265.
207. Atkinson MA, MacLaren NK, Scharp DW, Lacy DW, Lacy PE, Riley WJ. 64,000 Mr autoantibodies as predictors of insulin-dependent diabetes. *Lancet.* 1990; 335:1357–1360.
208. Baekkeskov S, Landin M, Kristensen JK, Srikanta S, Bruining GJ, Mandrup-Poulsen T, De Beaufort C, Soeldner JS, Eisenbath G, Lindgren F, et al. Antibodies to a 64,000 Mr human islet cell antigen precede the clinical onset of insulin-dependent diabetes. *J Clin Invest.* 1987; 79:926–934.
209. Barmeier H, McCulloch DK, Neifing JL, Warnock G, Rajotte RV, Palmer JP, Lernmark A. Risk for developing type 1 (insulin-dependent) diabetes mellitus and the presence of islet 64k antibodies. *Diabetologia.* 1991; 34:727–733.
210. Evans AS. Subclinical epidemiology. *Am J Epidemiol.* 1987; 125:545–555.
211. Lipton RB, LaPorte RE, Dorman JS, Riley WJ, Trucco M, Becker DJ. A combination of HLA-DQ-beta non-Asp-57 homozygosity and positive islet cell antibody (ICA) assay predicts insulin-dependent diabetes in relatives of children with IDDM. *Diabetes.* 1991; 40(suppl 1):151A.
212. Khalil I, Deschamps I, Lepage V, al-Daccak R, Degos L, Hors J. Dose effect of cis- and trans-encoded HLA-DQ alpha beta heterodimers in IDDM susceptibility. *Diabetes.* 1992; 41:378–384.
213. Khoury MJ, Flanders WD, Greenland S, Adams MJ. On the measurement of susceptibility in epidemiologic studies. *Am J Epidemiol.* 1989; 129:183–190.
214. Keller RJ, Eisenbarth GS, Jackson RA. Insulin prophylaxis in individuals at high risk of type 1 diabetes. *Lancet.* 1993; 341:927–928.
215. Mahon JL, Dupre J, Stiller CR, Donner AP. Immunosuppression in IDDM: rationale, risks, benefits, and strategies. *Diabetes Care.* 1990; 13:806–808.
216. Marks JB, Skyler JS. Clinical review 17 immunotherapy of type 1 diabetes mellitus. *J Clin Endocrinol Metab.* 1991; 72:3–9.

217. Lipton R, LaPorte RE, Becker DJ, Dorman JS, Orchard TJ, Atchison J, Drash AL. Cyclosporin therapy for prevention and cure of IDDM: epidemiological perspective of benefits and risks. *Diabetes Care.* 1990; 13:776–784.
218. Silverstein J, Maclaren N, Riley W, Spillar R, Radjenovic D, Johnson S. Immunosuppression with azathioprine and prednisone in recent-onset insulin-dependent diabetes mellitus. *N Engl J Med.* 1988; 319:599–604.
219. Conrad B, Weidmann E, Trucco G, Rudert WA, Behbo R, Ricordi C, Rodriquez-Rilo H, Finegold D, and Trucco M. Evidence for superantigen involvement in insulin-dependent diabetes mellitus aetiology. *Nature.* 1994; 371:351–355.

10

Humoral Autoimmunity

R. Gianani
G. S. Eisenbarth

During the past 5 years there has been a remarkable increase in the number of biochemically defined autoantigens found to be targets of the autoimmune process that precedes type I diabetes. A decade ago, screening for autoantibodies associated with type I diabetes was limited to measuring cytoplasmic islet cell autoantibodies (ICAs) and insulin antibodies. Currently, sequenced autoantigens include insulin,[1] glutamic acid decarboxylase (GAD),[2] ICA512/IA-2,[72] carboxypeptidase H,[3] ICA69,[4] GT3,[5] and a GM2-1[6] islet ganglioside. In addition, there are many other autoantigens in a variety of stages of characterization, including proteins with molecular weights of 64 kd (non-GAD 64 kd autoantigen[7]), 155 kd,[8,9] 52 kd,[10] 37–38 kd.[7,11] Finally a number of other known molecules have been associated with type I diabetes but their association with type I diabetes has either not been evaluated in man, has not been substantiated, or follow-up studies have not been published, including anti-bovine serum albumin antibodies (anti-BSA),[12] anti-insulin receptor antibodies,[13] antibodies to heat shock proteins,[14,15] antibodies to jun-B,[16] and antibodies to a series of autoantigens identified by screening islet libraries. Finally, a subset of autoantibodies termed anti-islet cell surface antibodies are currently rarely measured as most recent studies have failed to demonstrate disease specificity.[17]

It is likely that anti-islet autoantibodies do not directly contribute to the beta cell destruction that leads to type I diabetes. The most cogent evidence of lack of direct damage by autoantibodies is the lack of diabetes in infants born to ICA-positive mothers, or women who develop type I diabetes during pregnancy. Autoantibodies (ICA, anti-insulin, and anti-GAD autoantibodies) are readily detected in the serum of infants of such antibody-positive mothers in the absence of diabetes in the child.

Studies by groups associated with Blizzard, Nerup, and Irvine in the early 1970s demonstrated that type I diabetes was specifically associated with idiopathic Addison's disease.[18] This was in contrast to tuberculous Addison's disease. Idiopathic Addison's disease with lymphocytic infiltrates and destruction of the adrenal cortex was considered an organ-specific autoimmune disorder. In addition, insulitis in the pancreatic islets of new-onset diabetic patients who died shortly after diagnosis was reported. These two findings and discovery of human leukocyte (HLA) alleles associated with type I but not type II diabetes led to the hypothesis that in a subset of patients with type I diabetes, the disease resulted from autoimmune beta cell destruction. This same patient population, so important for recognizing the association of type I diabetes with autoimmunity, was instrumental in the discovery of cytoplasmic islet cell autoantibodies.[19] Patients with polyendocrine autoimmunity had high titers of antibodies that reacted with frozen sections of human pancreas. As is currently recognized, such patients with type I diabetes have ICAs that frequently persist for decades, in contrast to the majority of patients with type I diabetes where the ICA autoantibodies usually disappear within 5 years. The discovery of cytoplasmic islet cell antibodies in this population facilitated their identification in patients with the more common form of type I diabetes. Nevertheless, the utilization of a poorly standardized immunohistochemical test for autoantibodies dependent upon human pancreas obtained at the time of cadaveric donation (namely the ICA test) has led to a continuing debate as to whether such antibodies are predictive of diabetes in the general population and whether such antibodies frequently appear and disappear in relatives of patients with type I diabetes.[20,21]

Islet Cell Autoantibodies (ICAs)

Since the discovery of ICAs multiple workshops have been held and a Proficiency Testing Service established for laboratories measuring cytoplasmic islet cell autoantibodies.[22] The International Diabetes Workshop (IDW) workshops rapidly demonstrated that there existed remarkable variation between laboratories in terms of sera that they called ICA positive. A standard for ICA was established utilizing dilutions of sera and the units assigned were termed JDF units (named for the Juvenile Diabetes Foundation, which sponsored the meetings). With such a standard, differences in assay sensitivity could be rationalized and it became apparent that greater than 20 JDF units of cytoplasmic islet cell autoantibodies were highly predictive of diabetes among first-degree relatives. Laboratories attempting to measure cytoplasmic islet cell autoantibodies are strongly encouraged to take part in a proficiency service. Many laboratories throughout the world can achieve 100% specificity and sensitivity in the small panel of sera sent "blinded" to laboratories at regular intervals, but even as recently as the last proficiency exchange many laboratories had unacceptable sensitivity and specificity. Noel MacLaren at the University of Florida at Gainesville can be contacted for information concerning the IDW proficiency service.

Given the difficulty of the ICA test and its variability between laboratories, we give relatively little credence to reports of frequent fluctuation of these antibodies in prediabetics and welcome the development of biochemically based autoantibody assays. A major question relative to the development of such assays involves considerations as to what are the autoantigens recognized by islet cell autoantibody positive sera. The crudeness of the ICA test should be appreciated. Current ICA testing measures greater binding of immunoglobulin to islet versus acinar pancreas. Thus any antigen that is in greater density within islets, or that for a variety of reasons survives the preparation of frozen sections of pancreas better within islets than within acinar pancreas, may be recognized by antibodies and contribute to ICA positivity. Despite this caveat, in appropriate populations high titers of ICA are a very important risk factor for the development of type I diabetes.[82] Recently, prognostically significant heterogeneity of ICA has been appreciated and there exist first-degree relatives of patients with type I diabetes or patients with polyendocrine autoimmunity with high titers of ICA with a very low risk of progression to overt diabetes.[23,24]

To date, three classes of autoantigens have been defined that contribute to the ICA positivity found in relatives of patients with type I diabetes and among polyendocrine autoimmune patients (Table 10.1). The best-characterized subset of ICA autoantibodies is unusual (high titers and unique determinants) anti-GAD autoantibodies.[23,24] Such antibodies appear to be present in a small minority of individuals actually developing type I diabetes but are present in a significant proportion of ICA-positive relatives or polyendocrine patients followed for more than 5 years without developing diabetes. Such ICA antibodies have been termed restricted/selective in that they fail to react with mouse islets and give a beta cell–specific pattern of staining. These ICA antibodies can be absorbed with GAD and are similar to the ICA antibodies found in patients with stiff-man syndrome.

The other defined antigens accounting for a subset of ICA staining appear to be antibodies reacting with ICA512/IA-2 and glycolipids and may represent the bulk of ICA reactivity in individuals progressing to diabetes.[6,25] It is also likely that the above two sets of autoantigens do not account for all ICA reactivity and in particular there exist human-specific antibodies that fail to react with mouse and rat pancreas (Table 10.1) and that are not absorbed by GAD or ganglioslides.

Sequenced Autoantigens

Glutamic Acid Decarboxylase (GAD)

The path to discovery that anti-GAD autoantibodies accounted for an important component of anti-64 kd autoantibodies and a subset of ICA began with the discovery that patients with stiff-man syndrome expressed

Table 10.1. Heterogeneity of Cytoplasmic ICA Autoantibodies

	Species	*Absorbed GAD*	*Absorbed Gangliosides*	*Diabetes Risk*
Restricted/Selective	$Human^+/Rat^+/Mouse^-$	Yes	No	Low
Non-restricted	$Human^+/Rat^+/Mouse^+$	No	Subset	High
Human Specific	$Human^+/Rat^-/Mouse^-$	No	No	High

autoantibodies that gave rise to ICA staining and high titers of anti-GAD autoantibodies.[26] Glutamic acid decarboxylase (GAD) is the enzyme responsible for GABA synthesis within the central nervous system and within islet cells. In human islets, GAD is expressed within both beta cells and non-beta cells.[27,28] In that only the beta cells are destroyed in man, and insulitis in man and animal models disappears from islets once all the beta cells are destroyed, it is possible that anti-GAD autoantibodies and the immune response to GAD is of secondary rather than of primary pathogenic importance.[29] In addition to islets, the two forms of GAD, termed GAD65 and GAD67, are synthesized in testes, ovary, and neurons.[30] The anti-GAD autoantibodies of patients with stiff-man syndrome (SMS) (a rare neurological disorder characterized by spasms of muscular rigidity) were unusual in that they stained fixed sections of the brain, reacted on Western blots with purified GAD, and gave visible ICA staining of islets.[26] A number of years previously, Baekkeskov and coworkers[31,32] had described anti-64 kd autoantibodies utilizing an immunopreciptation assay of metabolically labeled islet cells. Although a high percentage of patients with new-onset diabetes had anti-GAD autoantibodies with this assay, their antibodies do not Western blot GAD or show immunohistochemical reactivity with neurons. Furthermore, anti-GAD stiff-man antibodies recognized different epitopes than the anti-GAD antibodies usually found in new-onset diabetic patients.[83] In 1990, the groups of DeCamilli and Baekkeskov[2] jointly discovered that the bulk of anti-64 kd autoantibodies reacted at low titer (relative to stiff-man syndrome antibodies) with GAD and that a small subset of the anti-GAD autoantibodies of new-onset diabetics were similar to anti-GAD stiff-man syndrome antibodies. In 1991, Gianani and coworkers[23] (for relatives of patients with type I diabetes) and Genovese and coworkers[24] (for polyendocrine patients) discovered that individuals with high titers of anti-GAD antibodies reacted on sections and Western blot similar to SMS patient anti-GAD antibodies. These antibodies were termed "restricted" ICA or "selective" ICA[23,24] in that the antibodies failed to react with islets of mouse pancreas and on rat islets stained only beta cells. This restricted reactivity is apparently due to the almost eight-fold less expression of GAD by mouse islets.[33] When ICA reactivity is due solely to autoantibodies reacting with GAD, absorption of sera with affinity purified GAD, recombinantly produced GAD, or absorption with a brain extract can be used to identify such antibodies (Table 10.1).[24,34] In studies utilizing brain extracts, the specificity for GAD absorption is usually evaluated by preclearing the extract with a monoclonal anti-GAD antibody.[35] Utilization of beta cell–specific staining to aid in identification of restricted ICA is a problem with human pancreas in that GAD is expressed by a subset of non-beta cells of human pancreas.[27] In contrast, within rat islets GAD expression is beta cell specific.

Several different radioassays for anti-GAD autoantibodies have been developed and the first International Diabetes Workshop (IDW) for measuring such antibodies was held. Four formats for determining anti-GAD autoantibodies include (1) determination of antibody precipitation of GAD enzymatic activity,[36] (2) radioassays utilizing affinity purified porcine brain GAD that has been labeled with I^{125}, (3) radioassays utilizing endogenously labeled GAD produced by in vitro transcription and translation of GAD cDNA,[37] and (4) ELISA assay formats. These assay formats are likely to give very different results depending upon the population studied. In particular, the immunenzymatic assay appears to be less sensitive than either radioassay. We have initial data that the two radioassay formats give very different results. With the affinity purified porcine GAD radioassay we have utilized, a large proportion (approaching 50%) of first-degree relatives less than age 10 express anti-GAD autoantibodies exceeding normal age-matched controls.[38] Less than 5% of first-degree relatives of patients with type I diabetes progress to overt diabetes. In contrast to anti-GAD autoantibodies measured with I^{125}-porcine GAD, a radioassay utilizing in vitro translated human GAD detects antibodies in less than 10% of ICA-negative relatives and is highly correlated with diabetes risk.

A major difference between the two radioassay formats may relate to the quantity of GAD in the assay and therefore the assay with in vitro translated GAD may only measure high-affinity autoantibodies. Both radioassays appear to give similar percentages of positives in normal controls (<2%) and for new-onset and prediabetic individuals (approximately 70%). Thus it is likely that simply for prediction, in vitro translated GAD assay formats would give a much higher positive predictive value for future diabetes among first-degree relatives of patients with type I diabetes than assays utilizing affinity purified GAD. These generalizations require further study and international standardization.

The quantitation of anti-GAD autoantibodies can also aid in the detection of extremely high titers of such antibodies associated with restricted ICA. The highest levels of anti-GAD autoantibodies that we have observed among ICA-positive relatives occur in relatives with restricted ICA independent of the GAD autoantibody assay utilized.

Among ICA-positive first-degree relatives of a patient with type I diabetes, the levels of anti-GAD autoantibodies are remarkably constant with up to a decade of prospective evaluation. Such extremely high levels of anti-GAD autoantibodies are rarely associated with progression to diabetes. It is noteworthy that Harrison and coworkers[39] have recently reported that there is an inverse correlation between levels of GAD autoantibodies and a T cell proliferative response to GAD. Thus it is hypothesized that high levels of GAD autoantibodies may be associated with a diminished anti-islet T cell response (Th 1 rather than Th2) and therefore less or no beta cell destruction.

Non-GAD 64kd Autoantigen (not yet sequenced)

Following the identification that a major component of the 64 kd antigen is GAD,[2] many groups reported an association between type I diabetes and anti-GAD antibodies. Evidence for heterogeneity of anti-64 kd autoantibodies came from the work of Christie,[36] who found that different tryptic fragments were generated after mild trypsinization of 64 kd molecule(s). In particular, precipitation of human islets with sera from nondiabetic polyglandular failure individuals, followed by trypsinization, yielded a 50 kd fragment whereas a 38–40 kd fragment was precipitated by new-onset and prediabetic sera. Of note, mild trypsinization of the GAD molecule yields a 50 kd fragment. Several reports[24,36] indicated that autoantibodies to the 37–38 kd fragment had a higher positive predictive value for diabetes than anti-GAD antibodies. It appears that there exist two different 64 kd autoantigens in human islets, one being GAD and another molecule that after trysinization yields a fragment of 37–40 kd. Recently Christie reported that the 37 kd fragment is related to the protein tyrosine phosphatase IA-2 (ICA512).[84]

Glycolipid Autoantigens

The initial studies suggesting that antibodies directed against islet glycolipids may be a component of anti-islet autoantibodies came from evaluation of monoclonal antibodies that reacted with neuronal gangliosides and that also react with islets. Monoclonal antibodies A2B5,[40] 3G5,[41] R2D6,[42] and tetanus toxin all react with complex gangliosides and all give an ICA pattern of staining that involves all cells within islets. In contrast to anti-islet monoclonal antibodies that react with proteins (eg, HISL19,[43] 4F2[44]), the above anti-ganglioside antibodies were not species specific. In that gangliosides are composed of a ceramide group connected to a complex polysaccharide with at least one sialic acid group, gangliosides are amphiphilic. Thus, organic solvents such as methanol remove gangliosides from tissue sections, while gangliosides are stable to nonpolar solvents such as acetone. Stability to acetone but removal by methanol was a quality found for most ICA. Gangliosides can readily be extracted from tissues with organic solvents and then separated from nonpolar lipids by partitioning with chloroform. Extraction of human pancreas followed by the above Folch partition, followed by chromatography that separates gangliosides based on their hydrophobicity (thin-layer chromatography, TLC) or number of sialic acid residues (DEAE chromatography) allowed the isolation of ganglioside preparations that, when incubated with ICA-positive sera, removed all reactivity.[25] It is noteworthy that the absorption assay utilized mouse pancreas.[25] It is likely (in retrospect) that the choice of mouse pancreas allowed absorption to be demonstrated even if sera contained high-titer anti-GAD autoantibodies that are not absorbed by glycolipid preparations (and that do not give ICA-positive staining with mouse islets; eg, restricted ICA).

Which glycolipids are autoantigens and which are the target autoantigens for ICA? Three candidate molecules are GT3,[5] sulphatides,[45] and what has been termed a GM2-1[46] ganglioside (on thin-layer chromatography it has a mobility between GM2 and GM1 standards). Answers to the above questions will almost by necessity lead to the development of a biochemical assay for anti-glycolipid autoantibodies to aid in the prediction of type I diabetes. Buschard and coworkers have reported in abstract form that sulphatides may be a relevant autoantigen as they detect anti-sulphatide antibodies (utilizing immunochemical detection of the staining of sulphatides following thin-layer chromatography) in the majority of patients with recent-onset diabetes.[45] Marcus and coworkers, utilizing a liposome-based assay, detected antibodies to GT3.[5] Finally, Dotta and coworkers have analyzed islets of man[47] and NOD mice for gangliosides. They have isolated and sequenced a molecule termed GM2-1[6,85] isolated from human pancreas that contains a terminal sialic acid residue. In addition, they have developed a TLC-based assay for autoantibodies reacting with GM2-1 and find the majority of prediabetics express antibodies reacting with this molecule.[5] Isolation and/or synthesis of large quantities of GM2-1 should allow the development of a standardized assay for autoantibodies and the direct testing by absorption of the frequency of antibodies to this molecule.

Insulin

Insulin is a 51–amino acid disulphide-linked heterodimer that is specifically produced by beta cells of islets. To date it is the only known beta cell–specific autoantigen within human islets (all other putative autoantigens are produced in man by non-beta cells). There is a possibility that insulin is transiently and at extremely low concentrations produced within the thymus. Transgenic mice with the insulin promoter coupled to noninsulin proteins indicate that such thymic transcription of the insulin gene is possible. Insulin is produced as a preprohormone that is processed to proinsulin and then, with removal of a connecting peptide (C peptide), to mature insulin. Processing occurs within beta cell secretory granules, where insulin is packaged in a crystal form. Equimolar concentrations of insulin and C peptide are secreted by beta cells.

In the 1950s, Berson and Yallow developed the first radioimmunoassay utilizing sera with insulin antibodies from patients treated with bovine insulin.[48] Bovine insulin differs from human insulin at 3 of 51 amino acids and porcine insulin differs from human insulin by one amino acid (at the terminus of the B chain). For most patients treated with subcutaneous insulin, the presence of anti-insulin antibodies does not interfere with insulin therapy. A subset of insulin-treated patients with extremely high levels of insulin antibodies are insulin resistant. For such patients the species of insulin used for therapy is usually changed (eg, from bovine to human insulin) or ultimately therapy with sulfated insulin is attempted.[49] Anti-insulin antibodies during pregnancy may facilitate transplacental passage of animal insulins and can be correlated with fetal macrosomia.[50]

The production of antibodies to animal insulins was not unexpected. It was, however, discovered that individuals treated with human insulin also produce anti-human insulin antibodies (though at a lower concentration).[51] The development of anti-insulin antibodies following subcutaneous therapy with human recombinant insulin has been ascribed to possible presence of "denatured" insulin molecules. It is, however, very likely that most self proteins when administered subcutaneously, especially in a depot form (eg, complexed with the positively charged protein (neutral protein Hagedorn, NPH), or zinc, as in the two most common pharmacologic long-acting insulin preparations), will induce anti-insulin antibodies. Antibodies also develop following therapy with a number of other recombinant proteins including human growth hormone and factor VIII. To test the generality of production of insulin antibodies following subcutaneous insulin administration, we transplanted a pituitary cell line producing rat insulin (which has the same sequence as mouse insulin) into non-histocompatible mice and rats. With rejection of the tissue, anti-insulin "autoantibodies" were induced.[52]

The first reports of spontaneous anti-insulin autoantibodies in man originated from Japan. A small but significant number of patients, when treated with methimazole for Graves's thyroid autoimmunity, develop high levels of anti-insulin antibodies.[53] Autoimmunity was almost exclusively restricted to individuals with HLA DR4.[54] Such antibodies, for reasons that are not clearly defined, are associated with spontaneous hypoglycemia rather than insulin resistance. It is hypothesized that these anti-insulin antibodies release insulin in a non-regulated manner and thus induce hypoglycemia. Recently the epitope recognized by a monoclonal antibody derived from a patient has been characterized and was reported to involve amino acid B3. In that many of these patients have been reported to have antibodies that distinguish human from bovine insulin, the antibodies also apparently recognize determinants influenced by the A8 through A10 loop of insulin.

In 1983 Palmer and coworkers[51] discovered the presence of anti-insulin antibodies in patients with new-onset type I diabetes, prior to the administration of exogenous insulin therapy. Subsequently a large number of studies have demonstrated that anti-insulin antibodies are present for years before the development of type I diabetes.[55] Initially, two different assay formats were utilized to detect such antibodies (an ELISA format with insulin immobilized on plates and fluid phase radioassays). The two different formats gave very different results relative to the positive predictive value for development of type I diabetes. A series of international workshops and sera exchanges led to the observation that the two formats measure different antibodies, and that only the antibodies detected with the radioassay formats were associated with risk for type I diabetes.[1] Both assay formats detected antibodies following insulin therapy and rarely were positive in normal controls.

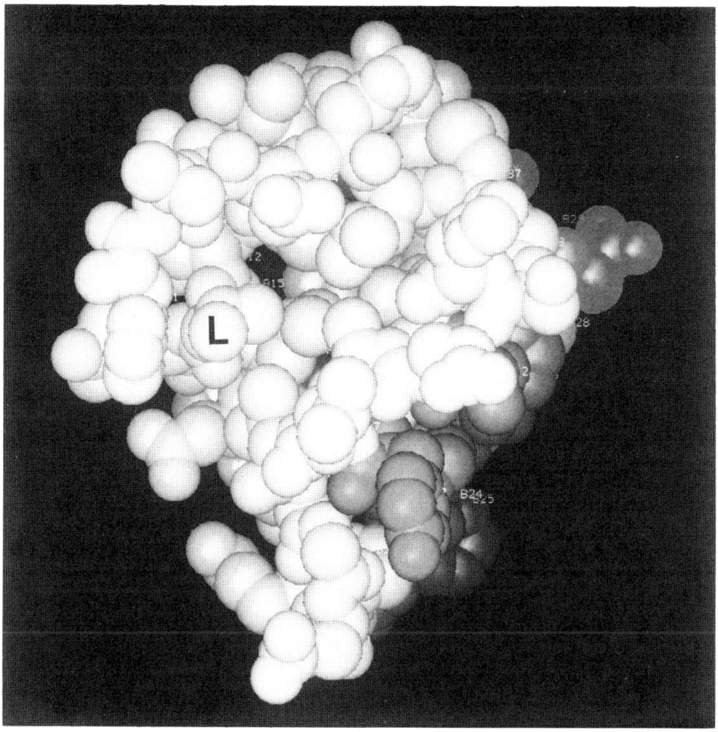

Figure 10.1. Three-dimensional representation of insulin, with the leucine at A13 highlighted (*L*) and receptor binding region darkened.

As more has been learned concerning insulin autoantibodies, the inability of standard ELISA assays to detect disease-relevant antibodies is understandable. In particular, the anti-insulin autoantibodies associated with diabetes risk are all of extremely high affinity and, most important, of very low capacity (10^{-12} M), making their detection with plate-binding assays problematic.[56] The epitope of the insulin molecule recognized with fluid phase assays appears to be homogeneous.[57] In particular, the antibodies from all antibody-positive relatives we have studied react with a conformational epitope (do not react with either the A or B chain) and react equally well with insulin and proinsulin. To date, all insulin autoantibodies of at-risk relatives react with des B23 to B30 insulin lacking the terminal eight amino acids of the B chain. Des B23 to B30 insulin fails to bind to the insulin receptor. Figure 10.1 illustrates the three-dimensional structure of insulin with the A13 leucine and receptor binding region highlighted. The A13 leucine is in the base of a pocket, and if this leucine is replaced by a tryptophan that extends out of the pocket, insulin autoantibody reactivity is abrogated. The reason for this marked specificity of insulin autoantibodies reacting with the face opposite the insulin-binding domain is unknown. It is, however, very likely that the antibody response to insulin is "antigen driven," giving rise to high-affinity autoantibodies. Insulin

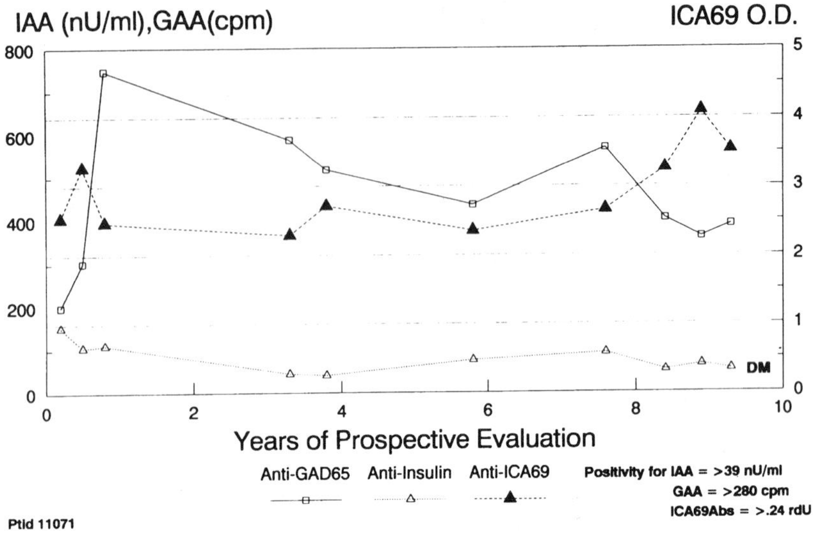

Figure 10.2. Levels of GAD, anti-insulin and anti-ICA69 autoantibodies in a first-degree relative with ten years of prospective evaluation prior to diabetes onset. Both ICA69 and anti-insulin autoantibodies were positive from the first measurement and remained always positive. GAD autoantibodies were negative at the first determination but thereafter remained positive.

may react with B cells while bound to insulin receptors, either of neighboring immunocytes or perhaps following its transport on insulin receptors through the endothelium. The ability to produce insulin analogues that are recognized by insulin autoantibodies but not by the insulin receptor suggests that one can selectively target B cells producing such antibodies. Whether elimination of such B cells which are probably extremely efficient at presenting insulin to T cells, would influence beta cell destruction is unknown.

Levels of insulin autoantibodies, similar to GAD autoantibodies, appear to be regulated at different levels over long periods of time in prediabetic first-degree relatives (Figure 10.2). The levels of antibodies correlate inversely with the age at which type I diabetes develops. Thus levels greater than 2000 nU/ml are almost exclusively found in patients who progress to type I diabetes prior to age 5, and less than half of individuals developing type I diabetes after age 15 have levels of anti-insulin autoantibodies distinguished from controls. The levels of such antibodies are to a major extent genetically influenced, are associated with DR4,[55] and are also associated with other haplotypes with DQA1 alleles of lineage 2, DQA1*0102, 0201, 0301, 0401.[58] Presence of anti-insulin autoantibodies and their levels appear to be associated with such lineage 2 alleles in a dominant manner. In particular, individuals developing type I diabetes who are homozygous for DQA1*0501/DQB1*0201 (DR3 homozygotes) either are negative for anti-insulin autoantibodies or have very low levels. There are suggestive data that the levels of anti-insulin autoantibodies among ICA-positive first-degree relatives correlate with the rate at which individuals progress to overt diabetes.[55,59] Relatives, however, who only express anti-insulin autoantibodies infrequently progress to overt diabetes. A high proportion of such anti-insulin autoantibody-positive, ICA-negative relatives under the age of 10 convert to ICA positivity.

ICA69

Pietropaolo and coworkers identified a novel islet protein termed ICA69[60] through the screening of a lambda gt11 human islet expression library with ICA-positive sera. This protein, which on SDS gel migrates at 69 kd, has been sequenced and found to have a molecular mass of 54,600 (the aberrant gel migration is probably explained by the presence of several highly charged regions in the molecule, as ICA69 is not glycosylated).

ICA69 is present, at least at the level of messenger RNA, in brain, lung, kidney, and heart, with high levels in islets and other neuroendocrine tissues. In the rat, ICA69 is beta cell specific. The subcellular localization and the function of ICA69 remain to be elucidated.

ICA69 is identical in sequence to the cow's milk–related protein p69 described by Dosch and coworkers.[61] It has been reported that diabetic individuals have antibodies to bovine serum albumin and there are a number of epidemiological studies indicating that the neonatal ingestion of cow's milk increases the development of type I diabetes. ICA69 and bovine serum albumin have two short regions (five amino acids) of identity and in the region of the ABBOS albumin peptide (potential T cell epitope), four of nine amino acids are identical. Such identity may be enough to stimulate cross-reactive T cell clones.

In the current assay format, antibodies to ICA69 are measured by Western blot utilizing recombinant ICA69. The Western blot assay format relative to radioassays for antibodies reacting with insulin, GAD65, and ICA512 is inadequate, with more than 5% of normal controls reacting on Western blots. Anti-ICA69 autoantibodies are clearly diabetes-related autoantibodies, but are present also in rheumatoid arthritis patients.[85] Further studies are needed to elucidate the role of this molecule in the pathogenesis of type I diabetes. A recent report by Atkinson and coworkers questions the association with type I diabetes of anti-albumin antibodies and of T cell responses to albumin.[62]

Carboxypeptidase H

Carboxypeptidase H is another autoantigen discovered by the screening of islet expression libraries with prediabetic sera. Within islets, carboxypeptidase H[3] cleaves carboxyterminal amino acids during the processing of proinsulin to insulin. This molecule is not islet specific, being present also in bovine adrenal, pituitary, and kidney.[63] In beta cells, carboxypeptidase H is localized in the insulin secretory granule, where it exists both in a membrane bound (52 kd) and soluble form (50 kd). Carboxypeptidase H is probably the most abundant islet protein after proinsulin-insulin. A radioassay or an ELISA for anti-carboxypeptidase antibodies has not yet been developed. In the original assay format utilizing reactivity with recombinant Escherichia coli plaques, one of four prediabetics had anti–carboxypeptidase H antibodies.

ICA512/IA-2

Screening a lambda gt11 library with sera from newly diagnosed IDDM patients, Rabin and coworkers[72,86] identified two islet autoantigens named ICA12 and ICA512. Five out of 12 diabetic sera recognized the ICA12 protein in a Western blot format, 10 of 12 sera recognized the protein ICA512, and 0 of 13 nondiabetic sera tested recognized either antigen.

We have recently developed a radioassay utilizing a lambda gt11 clone of ICA512.[87] This radioassay has high specificity and moderate sensitivity. Approximately 40% of individuals developing type I diabetes express autoantibodies reacting with ICA512 versus less than 1% of 200 control individuals. The radioassay format is identical to that employed with GAD65 and utilizes in vitro transcribed and translated ICA512. ICA512 is related to a molecule termed IA-2,[88] and it is possible that constructs with additional C-terminal sequences will enhance sensitivity. We currently employ three radioassays for anti-islet autoantibodies, insulin, GAD65, and ICA512. One or the other of the three autoantibodies (with cutoffs set at the 99th percentile) is positive in 98% of prediabetic individuals. Two or more autoantibodies are present in approximately 80% of prediabetic individuals. Given such high sensitivity and specificity, we currently utilize such radioassays and are abandoning the use of cytoplasmic ICA testing for general screening.

Partially Characterized Autoantigens

52 kd

A 52 kd antigen distinct from carboxypeptidase has been identified by Western blotting of human islet extracts with diabetic sera.[10] Interestingly, this antigen that appears to be islet cell–specific shares an antigenic determinant with the protein PC2, a component of the rubella virus capsid. The rubella virus is as yet the only virus that has been clearly associated with development of diabetes and only congenital rubella infection is associated with diabetes. The 52 kd antigen appears to be expressed within beta cell granules[64] and with future characterization may contribute to detection of anti-islet autoimmunity.

37–38 kd

A number of groups have reported antibodies to 38 kd molecules in patients with type I diabetes and their first-degree relatives. In the original description of antibodies precipitating the 64 kd molecule form islets, it was shown that some sera also precipitated a 38 kd molecule. Honeymann and coworkers[16] identified a 38 kd autoantigen as the nuclear transcription protein jun-B from an islet expression library. The relevance of this antigen to autoantibodies of prediabetics is unclear. An additional 38 kd molecule has been described by Pak and coworkers.[65] Following their observation that some new-onset diabetic patients have cytomegalovirus infection, they immunized BALB/c mice with cytomegalovirus and obtained islet-reactive monoclonal antibodies that by Western blot recognize a 38 kd human islet protein.

Roep and coworkers[11] have identified a 38 kd islet granule autoantigen to which T cells react. The relationship between this antigen recognized by T cells and autoantibodies to 38 kd molecules is unknown.

155 kd

In 1990, McEvoy and coworkers[8] used a novel method to detect diabetes-associated autoantigens. They developed a panel of mouse monoclonal antibodies reacting with the rat insulinoma cell line RIN5F and displaced the binding of the monoclonals to the tumor cells with diabetic sera. The binding of one of these monoclonals, termed 1A2, was selectively displaced by sera from diabetic children. The 1A2 monoclonal binds specifically to the insulinoma cell line RIN5F but not to other rat or human tissues. In a subsequent communication,[9] the authors reported that monoclonal 1A2 recognizes by Western blot a 150 kd membrane-bound protein DAP1 (diabetes associated protein 1). Several sera from IDDM patients also identified a 150 kd band by Western blotting of rat brain homogenates. Using an assay based on displacement of the radiolabeled monoclonal binding to rat insulinoma cells, 159 of 169 sera of children with IDDM versus 10 of 351 age-matched control sera were positive for autoantibodies to DAP1. Autoantibodies to this antigen are, however, also present in a large percentage of nondiabetic first-degree relatives (> 60%).

Other Autoantigens

Reports from Elias and coworkers[66] suggested a role for T cell clones reacting to the heat shock protein (HSP) 65 in the pathogenesis of diabetes in the NOD mouse. In particular, these authors identified a peptide within the sequence of the human HSP that was recognized by T cell clones that could transfer a transient form of diabetes and hyperglycemia.[67] The administration of irradiation-attenuated HSP-specific T cells, or of the HSP peptide, prevented diabetes in the NOD mouse. Despite initial reports,[68] HSP65 is apparently not an autoantigen of humoral autoimmunity in man.[69]

In 1990, Johnson and coworkers[70] suggested that an islet-specific glucose transporter is an autoantigen in type I diabetes. The evidence supporting this conclusion derived from the ability of IgG fractions from diabetic patients to inhibit glucose uptake from rat islet cells. This inhibitory activity could be removed by incubation of the IgG fraction with islet cell and hepatocyte membranes (which express two types of glucose transporter, GLUT-1 and GLUT-2), but not with erythrocytes or brush border membranes (which express only GLUT-2). Sera from 26 of 27 patients with IDDM inhibited the rat islet glucose uptake versus 0 of 5 sera from patients with NIDDM. Interestingly, the uptake of L-leucine was not affected by the IgG fractions. Though no direct biochemical data are provided for reaction of antibodies with GLUT-2, a recent publication indicates that introduction of the GLUT-2 gene into cell lines results in detection of surface autoantibodies,[71] implying that GLUT-2 is recognized by autoantibodies of diabetic patients.

T Cell Reactivity

Some of the target molecules of autoantibodies described in this chapter are also able to drive specific proliferation of T cells from patients with type I diabetes or from ICA-positive individuals. Atkinson and coworkers[73,89] studied the reactivity of peripheral blood mononuclear cells to recombinant glutamic acid decarboxylase in newly diagnosed IDDM patients, ICA-positive and ICA-negative relatives of individuals with IDDM, and in healthy controls. A higher proportion of subjects give a positive proliferative response to GAD among the newly diagnosed patients than among the controls (67% versus 0%). Interestingly, nondiabetic ICA-positive relatives were also more likely to express T cell reactivity to GAD (63% versus 11%). Harrison and coworkers[74] reported proliferation of peripheral blood T cells in presence of the central region of GAD67 (aa 208-404) in 38% of newly diagnosed IDDM patients and in 41% of ICA-positive relatives (>20 JDF units). Only 4% of HLA-matched controls responded to GAD67. In a subsequent report, Harrison and coworkers[39] described an inverse relationship between humoral and cellular immunity to glutamic acid decarboxylase, suggesting that ICA-positive relatives who have increased T cell reactivity to GAD (and lower titer of anti-GAD antibody) represent a group with higher diabetes risk.

Assays for reactivity of peripheral blood lymphocytes with GAD give relatively low stimulation indices.[39,73] In the NOD mouse, utilizing spleen cells, Kaufman and coworkers[75] and Tisch and coworkers[76] report that T cell proliferative responses to GAD precede responses to other antigens such as insulin. The stimulation indices again are very low, and few T cell clones to GAD have been derived. In addition, none of the standard NOD T cell clones that are able to transfer diabetes react with GAD (see Chapter 4).

Dosch and coworkers[77] have reported that T cells from new-onset diabetic children proliferate in the presence of the "ABBOS peptide," a bovine albumin-specific region that has homology with the previously described islet molecule p69, and it is also a target of autoantibodies in IDDM. However, a study by Atkinson and coworkers[78] failed to confirm these results. Atkinson and coworkers speculate that anti-BSA autoantibodies are a marker of autoimmunity rather than a specific marker for type I diabetes.

Roep[79] reported that cell lines from newly diagnosed patients selectively respond to insulin secretory granule proteins. Such a response was identified in 14 diabetes-derived cell lines and in only two cell lines of controls. Interestingly, two nondiabetic ICA-positive individuals produced T cell lines responsive to insulin granule proteins. A 38 kd[29] insulin secretory granule membrane protein was eluted from gels after electrophoresis of insulin secretory granule membranes. Stimulation of insulin granule–responsive T cell lines with this protein generated a response in 80% of the lines tested.[80] Reactivity to this protein was restricted to IDDM patients and to an ICA-positive individual.

T cell proliferative responses to insulin are present utilizing peripheral blood of prediabetics or splenocytes of NOD mice, but again stimulation indices are low.[81] In contrast, Wegmann and coworkers have recently discovered that a large percentage of T cells infiltrating islets of NOD mice strongly proliferate to insulin and a B-chain peptide of insulin.[82] In contrast, a minimal response of splenocytes to insulin is found. A subset of these T cell clones are able to transfer diabetes into immunodeficient NOD mice and thus are sufficient for disease pathogenesis. A response to insulin is seen as early as 4 weeks of age. This study in NOD mice, where islets are available for analysis, highlights a potential difficulty of studies in man utilizing peripheral lymphocytes.

Conclusions

During the past 2 years, investigators have begun to define a growing family of islet autoantigens recognized by autoantibodies of prediabetics. The ability to produce many of the antigens with recombinant technology (insulin, GAD, ICA512) will facilitate the prediction of type I diabetes. In addition, availability of such autoantigens will be important to elucidate the pathogenesis of type I diabetes. It is likely that such a large number of autoantibodies is secondary to beta cell destruction and the presentation of normal antigens in an inflammatory environment. Nevertheless, studies in the NOD mouse suggest that influencing the immune response to several autoantigens (eg, oral insulin, intravenous GAD, subcutaneous insulin) will prevent diabetes. At present, the primacy in disease pathogenesis of any of the defined autoantigens is unknown. Transgenic expression and deletion of the expression of selected antigens, combined with studies of T cell clones reactive to specific antigens, should aid in understanding the role of specific molecules as targets determining beta cell destruction.

Despite uncertainty about pathogenic importance, the ability to biochemically detect a series of autoantigens will greatly facilitate the prediction of type I diabetes[90] (Fig. 10.3). Utilizing only three radioassays for autoantibodies, insulin, in vitro translated human GAD, and ICA512, 98% of

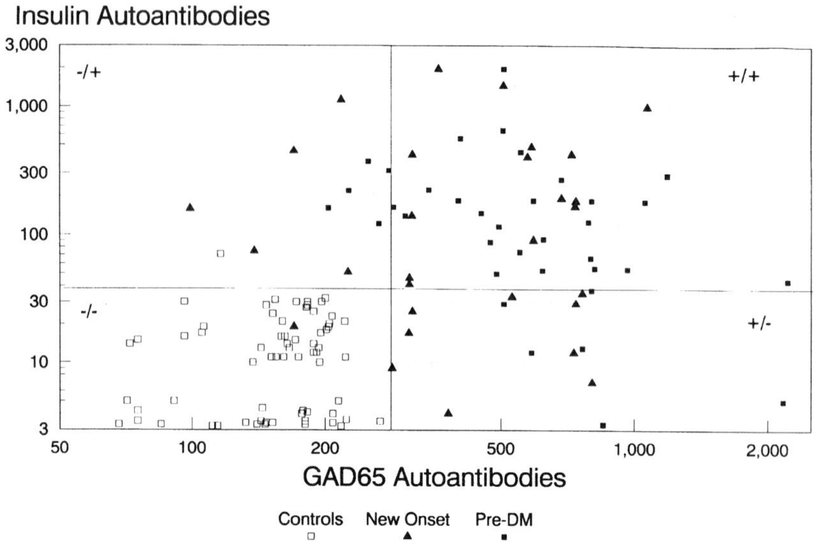

Figure 10.3. GAD and insulin autoantibodies on a log scale for normal controls, relatives followed to diabetes, and new onset prediabetics. All but one prediabetic were positive for one of these two autoantibodies, and this one relative had anti-ICA69 autoantibodies.

prediabetic or recent-onset diabetic individuals express one or more antibodies (versus only 3 out of 100 controls). Eighty percent express two or more autoantibodies, versus no controls. Twenty-five percent of diabetics or prediabetics express all three of the above autoantibodies. The expression of autoantibodies assorts independently in prediabetic individuals and thus, by utilizing the three assays, a high positive predictive value for disease is possible while retaining disease sensitivity. Such biochemical screening will likely have its largest impact for the prediction of type I diabetes in the general population where the positive predictive value of ICA positivity is less than 10%, while presence of two or more of the three autoantibodies should give positive predictive values greater than 70%. Screening of the general population for diabetes risk is likely to be of major importance if trials for the prevention of type I diabetes among first-degree relatives are successful. Approximately 90% of individuals who develop type I diabetes have no first-degree relatives with the disease and thus such screening may be essential for the large-scale prevention of type I diabetes.

References

1. Greenbaum C, Palmer JP, Kuglin B, Kolb H, and Participating Laboratories. Insulin autoantibodies measured by radioimmunoassay methodology are more related

to insulin-dependent diabetes mellitus than those measured by enzyme-linked immunosorbent assay: results of the Fourth International Workshop on the Standardization of Insulin Autoantibody Measurement. *J Clin Endocrinol Metab.* 1992; 74:1040–1044.

2. Baekkeskov S, Aanstoot H, Christgau S, et al. Identification of the 64K autoantigen in insulin dependent diabetes as the GABA-synthesizing enzyme glutamic acid decarboxylase. *Nature.* 1990; 347:151–156.
3. Castano L, Russo E, Zhou L, Lipes MA, Eisenbarth GS. Identification and cloning of a granule autoantigen (carboxypeptidase H) associated with type I diabetes. *J Clin Endocrinol Metab.* 1991; 73:1197–1201.
4. Pietropaolo M, Castano L, Babu S, et al. Islet cell autoantigen 69 kDa (ICA69): molecular cloning and characterization of a novel diabetes associated autoantigen. *J Clin Invest.* 1993; 92:359–371.
5. Gillard BK, Thomas JW, Nell LJ, Marcus DM. Antibodies against ganglioside GT3 in the sera of patients with type I diabetes mellitus. *J Immunol Methods.* 1989; 142:3826–3832.
6. Dotta F, Previti M, Tiberti C, Lenti L, Pugliese G, DiMario U. Identification of the GM2-1 islet ganglioside: similarities with a major neuronal autoantigen. *Diabetes.* 1992; 41:365A. Abstract.
7. Christie MR, Hollands JA, Brown TJ, Michelsen BK, Delovitch TL. Detection of pancreatic islet 64,000 Mr autoantigens in insulin-dependent diabetes distinct from glutamate decarboxylase. *J Clin Invest.* 1993; 22:240–248.
8. Thomas NM, Ginsberg-Fellner F, Mcevoy RC. Strong association between diabetes and displacement of mouse anti-rat insulinoma cell monoclonal antibody by human serum in vitro. *Diabetes.* 1990; 39:1203–1211.
9. Pan Y-X, Thomas NM, Mcevoy RC. Purification and partial characterization of 160 kD and 155 kD B cell membrane antigens detected by MAb 1A2. *Autoimmunity.* 1993; 15(suppl):77A. Abstract.
10. Karounos DG, Wolinsky JS, Thomas JW. Monoclonal antibody to rubella virus capsid protein recognizes a B-cell antigen. *J Immunol.* 1993; 150:3080–3085.
11. Roep BO, Kallan AA, Hazenbos WLW, et al. T-cell reactivity to 38kD insulin-secretory-granule protein in patients with recent-onset type 1 diabetes. *Lancet.* 1991; 337:1439–1441.
12. Karjalainen J, Martin JM, Knip M, et al. A bovine albumin peptide as a possible trigger of insulin-dependent diabetes mellitus. *N Engl J Med.* 1992; 327:302–307.
13. Elias D, Cohen I, Shechter Y, Spirer Z, Golander A. Antibodies to insulin receptor followed by anti-idiotype. *Diabetes.* ; 1987:36–348#354.
14. Georgopoulos C, McFarland H. Heat shock proteins in multiple sclerosis and other autoimmune diseases. *Immunol Today.* 1993; 14:373–375.
15. Atkinson MA, Maclaren NK, Scharp DW. No evidence for HSP65 in insulin dependent diabetes. *Lancet.* 1990; 337:263–264.
16. Honeyman mc, Cram DS, Harrison LC. Transcription factor jun-B is target of autoreactive T-cells in IDDM. *Diabetes.* 1993; 42:626–630.
17. Lernmark A, Freedman ZR, Hofmann C, et al. Islet-cell-surface antibodies in juvenile diabetes mellitus. *N Engl J Med.* 1978; 299:375–380.
18. Nerup J. Addison's disease—clinical studies: a report of 108 cases. *Acta Endocrinol.* 1974; 76:127–141.
19. Bottazzo GF, Florin-Christensen A, Donniach D. Islet cell antibodies in diabetes mellitus with autoimmune polyendrocrine deficiencies. *Lancet.* 1974; 2:1279–1283.

20. Eizirik DL, Sandler S, Palmer JP. Repair of pancreatic B-cells: a relevant phenomenon in early IDDM? *Diabetes.* 1993; 42:1383–1391.
21. Thai A-C, Eisenbarth GS. Natural history of IDDM. *Diabetes Rev.* 1993; 1:1–14.
22. Greenbaum CJ, Palmer JP, Nagataki S, et al. Improved specificity of ICA assays in the Fourth International Immunology of Diabetes Exchange Workshop. *Diabetes.* 1992; 41:1570–1574.
23. Gianani R, Pugliese A, Bonner-Weir S, et al. Prognostically significant heterogeneity of cytoplasmic islet cell antibodies in relatives of patients with type I diabetes. *Diabetes.*1992; 41:347–353.
24. Genovese S, Bonifacio E, McNally JM, et al. Distinct cytoplasmic islet cell antibodies with different risks for type I (insulin-dependent) diabetes mellitus. *Diabetologia.* 1992; 35:385–388.
25. Colman PG, Nayak RC, Campbell IL, Eisenbarth GS. Binding of cytoplasmic islet cell antibodies is blocked by human pancreatic glycolipid extracts. *Diabetes.* 1988; 37:645–652.
26. Solimena M, Folli F, Denis-Donini S, et al. Autoantibodies to glutamic acid decarboxylase in a patient with stiffman syndrome, epilepsy, and type I diabetes mellitus. *N Engl J Med.* 1988; 318:1012–1020.
27. Petersen JS, Russel S, Marshall MO, et al. Differential expression of glutamic acid decarboxylase in rat and human islets. *Diabetes.* 1993; 42:484–495.
28. Richter W, Shi Y, Baekkeskov S. Autoreactive epitopes defined by diabetes-associated human monoclonal antibodies are localized in the middle and C-terminal domains of the smaller form of glutamic decarboxylase. *Proc Natl Acad Sci U S A.* 1993; 90:2832–2836.
29. Eisenbarth GS. Mouse or man: is GAD the cause of type I diabetes? *Diabetes Care.* 1994; 17:605–607.
30. Erdo SL, Wolff JR. Gamma-aminobutyric acid outside the mammalian brain. *J Neurochem.* 1990; 54:363–372.
31. Christie M, Landin-Ollson M, Sundkvist G, Dahlquist G, Lernmark A, Baekkeskov S. Antibodies to a Mr-64,000 islet cell protein in Swedish children with newly diagnosed Type I (insulin-dependent) diabetes. *Diabetologia.* 1988; 31:597–602.
32. Baekkeskov S, Landin M, Kristensen JK, et al. Antibodies to a 64,000 M, human islet cell antigen precede the clinical onset of insulin dependent diabetes. *J Clin Invest.* 1987; 79:926–934.
33. Kim J, Richter W, Aanstoot HJ, et al. Differential expression of GAD65 and GAD67 in human, rat and mouse pancreatic islets. *Diabetes.* 1993; 42:1799–1808.
34. Gianani R, Jackson R, Eisenbarth GS. Evidence that the autoantigen of restricted ICA is GAD. *Diabetes Res Clin Pract.* 1991; 14(suppl 1):S13. Abstract.
35. Reich E, Scaringe D, Yabi J, Sherwin RS, Janeway CA. Prevention of diabetes in NOD mice by injection of autoreactive T-lymphocytes. *Diabetes.* 1989; 38:1647–1651.
36. Christie MR, Richard YM, Tun RYM, et al. Antibodies to GAD and tryptic fragments of islet 64K antigen as distinct markers for development of IDDM: studies with identical twins. *Diabetes.* 1992; 41:782–787.
37. Velloso LA, Kampe O, Hallberg A, Christmanson L, Betsholtz C, Karlsson FA. Demonstration of GAD-65 as the main immunogenic isoform of glutamate decarboxylase in type I diabetes and determination of autoantibodies using a radioligand produced by eukaryotic expression. *J Clin Invest.* 1993; 91:2084–2090.
38. Gianani R, Yu L, Eisenbarth GS. Inverse relationship between levels of GAD

autoantibodies, insulin autoantibodies and progression to type I diabetes. *Autoimmunity.* 1993; Abstract.

39. Harrison LC, Honeyman MC, DeAizpurua HJ, et al. Inverse relation between humoral and cellular immunity to glutamic acid decarboxylase in subjects at risk of insulin-dependent diabetes. *Lancet.* 1993; 341:1365–1369.
40. Kundu SK, Pleatman MA, Redixine WA, Boyd AE, Marcus DM. Binding of monoclonal antibody A2B5 to gangliosides. *Biochem Biophys Res Commun.* 1983; 116(3):836–842.
41. Nayak RC, Attawia NA, Cahill CJ, King GL, Ohashi O, Moromisato R. Expression of a monoclonal antibody (3G5) defined ganglioside antigen in renal cortex. *Kidney Int.* 1992; 41:1638–1645.
42. Alejandro R, Shienvold FL, Hajek SAV, Pierce M, Paul R, Mintz DH. A ganglioside antigen on the rat pancreatic B cell surface identified by monoclonal antibody R2D6. *J Clin Invest.* 1984; 74:25–38.
43. Srikanta S, Krisch K, Eisenbarth GS. Islet cell protein defined by monoclonal islet cell antibody HISL-19. *Diabetes.* 1986; 35:300–305.
44. Srikanta S, Telen M, Pisillico JT, et al. Monoclonal antibodies to a human islet cell surface glycoprotein: 4F2 and LC7-2. *Endocrinology.* 1987; 120:2240–2244.
45. Buschard K, Josefsen K, Horn T, Larsen S, Fredman P. Sulphatide and anti-sulphatide antibodies in type I diabetes mellitus. *Diabetes.* 1993; 42(suppl 1):5A. Abstract.
46. Dotta F, Gianani R, Dionisi S, Tiberti C, Eisenbarth GS, DiMario U. Expression of anti-GM2-1 islet ganglioside antibodies in ICA+ relatives of type I diabetics. *Autoimmunity.* 1993; 15(suppl):70. Abstract.
47. Dotta F, Colman PG, Nayak RC, et al. Ganglioside expression in human pancreatic islets. *Diabetes.* 1989; 38:1478–1483.
48. Berson SA, Yallow RS. Quantitative aspects of the reaction between insulin and insulin-binding antibody. *J Clin Invest.* 1959; 38:1996–2016.
49. Davidson JK, DeBra DW. Immunologic insulin resistance. *Diabetes.* 1978; 27(3):307–318.
50. Menon RK, Cohen RM, Sperling MA, Gutfield Ws, Mimouni F, Khoury JC. Transplacental passage of insulin in pregnant women with insulin dependent diabetes mellitus. *N Engl J Med.* 1990; 323:309–315.
51. Palmer JP, Asplin CM, Clemons P, et al. Insulin antibodies in insulin-dependent diabetics before insulin treatment. *Science.* 1983; 222:1337–1339.
52. Ziegler AG, Vardi P, Gross DJ, et al. Production of insulin antibodies by mice rejecting insulin transfected cells. *J Autoimmunity.* 1989; 2:733–737.
53. Hirata Y, Tominaga M, Ito J, Noguchi A. Spontaneous hypoglycaemia with insulin autoimmunity in Graves' disease. *Ann Intern Med.* 1974; 81:214–218.
54. Uchigata Y, Kuwata S, Tsushima T, et al. Patients with Graves' disease who developed insulin autoimmune syndrome (Hirata disease) possess HLA-Bw62/Cw4/DR4 carrying DRB1*0406. *J Clin Endocrinol Metab.* 1993; 77:249–254.
55. Ziegler AG, Ziegler R, Vardi P, Jackson RA, Soeldner JS, Eisenbarth GS. Life table analysis of progression to diabetes of anti-insulin autoantibody-positive relatives of individuals with type I diabetes. *Diabetes.* 1989; 38:1320–1325.
56. Kariv I, Greenbaum CJ, Palmer JP, Kuglin B, Kolb H. Insulin autoantibodies measured by radioimmunoassay methodology are more related to insulin-dependent diabetes mellitus than those measured by enzyme-linked immunoabsorbent assay: results of the Fourth International Workshop on the

Standardization of Insulin Autoantibody Measurement. *J Clin Endocrinol Metab.* 1992; 74(5):1040–1044.

57. Castano L, Ziegler A, Ziegler R, Shoelson S, Eisenbarth GS. Characterization of insulin autoantibodies in relatives of patients with insulin-dependent mellitus. *Diabetes.* 1993; 42:1202–1209.
58. Pugliese A, Bugawan T, Moromisato R, et al. Two subsets of HLA-DQA1 alleles mark phenotypic variation in levels of insulin autoantibodies in first degree relatives at risk for insulin-dependent diabetes. *J Clin Invest.* 1994; 93:2447–2452.
59. Vardi P, Ziegler AG, Matthews JH, et al. Concentration of insulin autoantibodies at onset of type I diabetes: inverse log-linear correlation with age. *Diabetes Care.* 1988; 11:736–739.
60. Shehada N, Calcinaro F, Lafferty KJ. Oxygen radicals inhibit insulin secretion from freshly isolated human islets. *Diabetes.* 1992; 41:160A.
61. Miller JFAP, Morahan G, Allison J, Bhathal PS, Cox KO. T-cell tolerance in transgenic mice expressing major histocompatibility class I molecules in defined tissues. *Immunol Rev.* 1989; 107:109–123.
62. Atkinson MA, Bowman MA, Kuo-Jang K, Campbell L, Dush L, Shah SC, Smell O, Maclaren NK. Lack of immune responsiveness to bovine serum albumin in insulin-dependent diabetes. *N Engl J Med.* 1993; 329:1853–1858.
63. Davidson HW, Hutton JC. The insulin-secretory-granule carboxypeptidase H. *Biochem J.* 1993; 245:575–582.
64. Karounos DG, Simmerman L, Hickman SL, Jacob RJ. Identification of the p52-rubella related autoantigen as an insulin secretory granule protein. *Diabetes.* 1993; 42(suppl 1):221A. Abstract.
65. Pak CY, Cha CY, Rajotte RV, McArthur RG, Yoon YW. Human pancreatic islet cell specific 38 kilodalton autoantigen identified by cytomegalovirus-induced monoclonal islet cell autoantibody. *Diabetologia.* 1990; 33:569–572.
66. Elias D, Reshef T, Birk OS, Zee R, Walker MD, Cohen IR. Vaccination against autoimmune mouse diabetes with a T-cell epitope of the human 65-kDa heat shock protein. *Proc Natl Acad Sci U S A.* 1991; 88:3088–3091.
67. Elias D, Markowits D, Reshef T, Van der Zee R, Coen IR. Induction and therapy of autoimmune diabetes in the non-obese diabetic mouse by a 65kd heat shock protein. *Proc Natl Acad Sci U S A.* 1991; 88:3088–3091.
68. Jones DB, Hunter NR, Duff GW. Heat-shock protein 65 as a B cell antigen of insulin-dependent diabetes. *Lancet.* 1990; 336:583–585.
69. Atkinson M, Holmes LH, Scharp DW, Lacy PE, Maclaren NK. No evidence for serological autoimmunity to islet cell heat shock proteins in insulin dependent diabetes. *J Clin Invest.* 1991; 87:721–724.
70. Johnson TH, Crider BP, McCorkle K, Alford M, Unger RH. Inhibition of glucose transport into rat islet cells by immunoglobulins from patients with new-onset insulin-dependent diabetes mellitus. *N Engl J Med.* 1990; 322:653–659.
71. Inman LR, McAllister CT, Chen L, et al. Autoantibodies to the GLUT-2 glucose transporter of B cells in insulin-dependent diabetes mellitus of recent onset. *Proc Natl Acad Sci U S A.* 1993; 90:1281–1284.
72. Rabin DU, Pleasic SM, Palmer-Crocker R, Shapiro JA. Cloning and expression of IDDM-specific human autoantigens. *Diabetes.* 1992; 41:183–186.
73. Atkinson MA, Kaufman DL, Campbell L, et al. Response of peripheral-blood mononuclear cells to glutamate decarboxylase in insulin-dependent diabetes. *Lancet.* 1992; 339:458–459.
74. Harrison LC, Chu SX, DeAizpurua HJ, Graham M, Honeyman MC, Colman PG.

Islet-reactive T cells are a marker of preclinical insulin-dependent diabetes. *J Clin Invest.* 1992; 89:1161–1165.

75. Kaufman DL, Clare-Salzler M, Tian J, et al. Spontaneous loss of T-cell tolerance to glutamic acid decarboxylase in murine insulin-dependent diabetes. *Nature.* 1993; 366:69–72.

76. Tisch R, Yang X-D, Singer SM, Liblau RS, Fugger L, McDevitt HO. Immune response to glutamic acid decarboxylase correlates with insulitis in nonobese diabetic mice. *Nature.* 1993; 366:72–75.

77. Karjalainen J, Cheung R, Vandermeulen JM, et al. T cell proliferation response against bovine albumin (BSA) follows the natural course and is restricted to the linear ABBOS sequence in insulin-dependent diabetes mellitus. *Autoimmunity.* 1993; 15(suppl):62A. Abstract.

78. Atkinson MA, Bowman MA, Kuo-Jang K, et al. Lack of immune responsiveness to bovine serum albumin in insulin-dependent diabetes. *N Engl J Med.* 1993; 329:1853–1858.

79. Roep BO, Arden SD, deVries RP, Hutton JC. T-cell clones from a type-1 diabetes patient respond to insulin secretory granule proteins. *Nature.* 1990; 345:632–634.

80. Van Vliet E, Roep BO, Meulenbroek L, Jan Bruining G, De Vries RRP. Human T cell clones with specificity for insulinoma cell antigens. *Eur J Immunol.* 1989; 19:213–216.

81. Keller RJ. Cellular immunity to human insulin in prediabetic individuals. *J Autoimmunity.* 1990; 3:321–327.

82. Bonifacio E, Genovese S, Braghi S, Bazzigaluppi E, Lampasona V, Bingley PJ, Rogge L, Pastore MR, Bognetti E, Bottazzo GF, Gale EAM, Bosi E. Islet autoantibody markers in IDDM: risk assessment strategies yielding high sensitivity. *Diabetologia.* 1995; 38:816–822.

83. Bjork E, Velloso LA, Kampe O, Karlsson F. GAD autoantibodies in IDDM, stiff-man syndrome and autoimmune polyendocrine type I recognize different epitopes. *Diabetes.* 1994; 43:161–165.

84. Payton MA, Hawkes CD, Christie MR. Relationship of the 37,000- and 40,000-MR trypic fragments of islet antigens in insulin-dependent diabetes to the protein tyrosine phosphatase-like molecule IA-2 (ICA512). *J Clin Invest.* 1995; 96:1506–1511.

85. Dotta F, Previti M, Lenti L, Dionisi S, Casetta B, D'Erme M, Eisenbarth GS, DiMario U. GM2-1 pancreatic islet ganglioside: identification and characterization of a novel islet-specific molecule. *Diabetologia.* 1995 (in press).

86. Rabin DU, Pleasic SM, Shapiro JA, Yoo-Warren H, Oles J, Hicks JM, Goldstein DE, Rae PMM. Islet cell antigen 512 is a diabetes-specific islet autoantigen related to protein tyrosine phosphatase. *J Immunol.* 1994; 152:3183–3187.

87. Gianani R, Rabin DU, Verge CF, Yu L, Babu S, Pietropaolo M, Eisenbarth GS. ICA512 autoantibody radioassay. *Diabetes.* 1995 (in press).

88. Lan MS, Lu JIA, Goto Y, Notkins AL. Molecular cloning and identification of a receptor-type protein tyrosine phosphatase, IA-2, from human insulinoma. *DNA and Cell Biol.* 1994; 13:505–514.

89. Atkinson MA, Bowman MA, Campbell L, Darrow BL, Kaufman DL, Maclaren NK. Cellular immunity to a determinant common to glutamate decarboxylase and Coxsackie virus in insulin-dependent diabetes. *J Clin Invest.* 1994; 94:2125–2129.

11

Prediction of Type I Diabetes: The Natural History of the Prediabetic Period

Charles F. Verge
George S. Eisenbarth

The importance of understanding the natural history of prediabetes lies in the development of prevention strategies. Randomized clinical intervention trials are now beginning and they rely on the accurate identification of individuals who are at high risk of progression to diabetes. This is essential to ensure that trials will have sufficient statistical power to detect a given effect of the intervention (if it exists) within the time available for the study.[1] Such understanding is also needed to avoid exposing those who will not develop diabetes to the risk of adverse effects of the intervention. In addition, it is likely that an intervention will be more effective if given early, while many beta cells remain intact. This will require the development of more sensitive and specific methods to detect autoimmune beta cell destruction in its earliest stages.

The first-degree relatives of individuals with type I diabetes have approximately 5% risk of also developing the disease. Longitudinal studies of autoantibody-positive relatives have provided a wealth of information on the natural history of autoimmunity during the prehyperglycemic phase of the disease (prediabetes). They have established the predictive value of age,[2] islet cell antibodies (ICAs),[3] first-phase insulin release (FPIR),[4] and human leukocyte (HLA) haplotypes.[5] Increasingly, combinations of markers are being used to better define the risk of diabetes. Prediction is not absolute, but can be expressed as a percentage risk of developing diabetes within a given time period. This chapter will review predictive factors currently in use and discuss some of the unanswered question on the natural history of prediabetes.

Predictive Factors in Relatives

Riley and coworkers reported on the University of Florida, Gainesville, family study in 1990.[2] At that time 3413 first-degree relatives had been screened for ICA, of whom 3.3% were positive. Positive sera were defined as those with 10 or more Juvenile Diabetes Foundation (JDF) units. ICAs were more frequent among the siblings of diabetic probands than among parents. They were also more frequent among relatives from multiplex families and among relatives less than 20 years old. After a maximum follow-up of 10 years (median 3.5 years), 40 relatives developed type I diabetes. The risk of diabetes was significantly higher in relatives with ICAs of 20 or more JDF units at the time of initial screening, those aged under 10 years (at initial screening), and those from multiplex families. Each of these risk factors was independent of the others. The presence of IAA was not an independent risk factor, after allowing for ICA. However, a later report with further follow-up came to the opposite conclusion, with evidence that IAA adds independently to prediction.[6] The presence of ICA in titers of less than 20 JDF units did not confer significantly increased risk of diabetes, but increasing titers above this level were associated with progressively increasing risk. Nevertheless, one third of the relatives progressing to diabetes were ICA negative on the first test and, of these, 62% remained ICA negative at the onset of diabetes.

The Bart's-Windsor family study, conducted in England from 1978 onwards, also found that higher ICA titer was associated with shorter diabetes-free survival.[3] Seven hundred and nineteen first-degree relatives were followed for up to 10.5 years. ICAs were tested every 4 to 6 months, using a sensitive assay with a detection limit of 4 JDF units. Detectable ICAs were found in the sera of 3.3% of the relatives at initial testing, compared with 2.2% of 540 healthy child and adult controls. However, only one control had ICA of 20 or more JDF units, compared with 10 relatives. ICAs were detected in an additional 14 relatives on follow-up samples and the follow-up time for survival analysis was calculated from the time of ICA detection. With increasing ICA cutoff the positive predictive value for future diabetes rose, and the sensitivity fell. The risk of diabetes within 10 years associated with ICAs of 80 or more JDF units, was 100% (95% confidence interval: 52%–100%). In comparison, ICAs of 20 or more JDF units were associated with a 73% risk (95% confidence interval: 45%–100%), and ICAs of 4 or more JDF units with a 40% risk (95% confidence interval: 23%–57%).

Data from the Joslin Diabetes Center family study indicate that impaired FPIR is an additional risk factor.[4] Thirty-five first-degree relatives with high-titer ICAs ($\geq$40 JDF units) underwent serial intravenous glucose tolerance testing (IVGTT). The age of the subjects ranged from 2.6 to 66 years, the mean follow-up was 3.6 years from the first test, and 18 progressed to overt diabetes. The FPIR was calculated as the sum of the 1- and 3-minute insulin levels after a standard bolus of intravenous glucose (0.5 g per kg body weight, infused as a 20%–25% solution over 2 to 4 minutes). Percentiles for the FPIR were determined in 225 healthy, nonobese, control subjects. Even in control subjects the

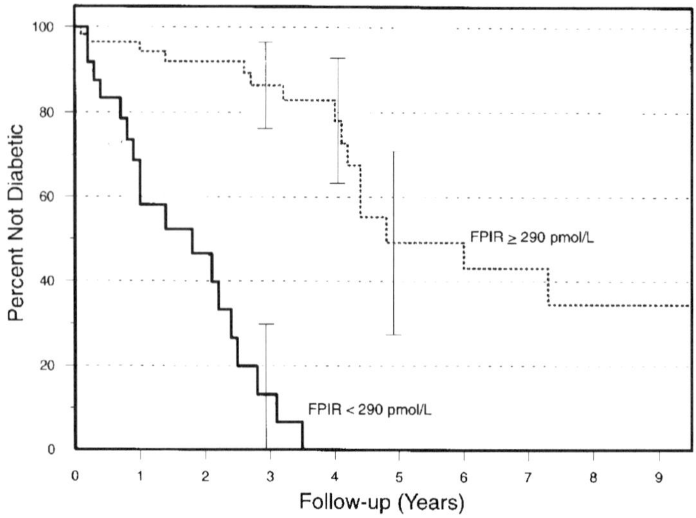

		0	1	2	3	4	5	6	7	8	9
FPIR ≥ 290 pmol/L	n = 55		46	38	27	17	8	8	6	4	3
FPIR < 290 pmol/L	n = 24		13	7	2	0					

Figure 11.1. Survival analysis of the progression to diabetes in ICA-positive first-degree relatives followed in the Joslin family study. The relatives were subdivided by the FPIR on the earliest IVGTT performed, above or below the first percentile (48 mU/L or 290 pmol/L). Error bars show the 95% confidence intervals for survival estimates. Survival was significantly different between the two groups (p<0.0001, log-rank test). Reproduced with permission from: Eisenbarth GS, et al, *Diabetes*, 1993; 42:941–947. Copyright © **1993 by the American Diabetes Association.**

FPIR showed wide within-subject variation (discussed in detail below). Nevertheless, relatives with an initial FPIR below the first percentile (48 mU/l) had significantly reduced diabetes-free survival. Importantly, the presence of FPIR below the first percentile did not signify that diabetes was already present. For most of the relatives, oral glucose tolerance tests (OGTT) were also performed during follow-up to detect asymptomatic diabetes. For the survival analysis, the onset of diabetes was defined by a diabetic OGTT or the occurrence of symptomatic hyperglycemia, whichever came first. The average time from the discovery of FPIR below the first percentile to the onset of diabetes was 1.8 years.

Updated data from the Joslin family study, with longer follow-up and larger numbers of relatives, have confirmed these findings (Fig. 11.1). Among 79 relatives with high-titer ICAs (≥40 JDF units), those with FPIR below the first percentile on the first test had a 3-year diabetes-free survival of 13% (95% confidence interval: 0%–30%) compared with 78% (95% confidence interval: 63%–93%) for the group with higher FPIR.[1] Studies at the Barbara Davis Center have confirmed the predictive value of FPIR measurements.[7]

Data from the Joslin study also suggest that IAA add to the prediction of type I diabetes, but with a weaker effect than ICA.[8] Forty-two ICA-positive

($\geq$20 JDF units) relatives and 1670 ICA-negative relatives (representing a subset of all relatives found to be ICA negative) were tested for IAA. Among the ICA-negative relatives, 2.7% were IAA positive, whereas among ICA-positive relatives, 45% were IAA positive. IAA alone had less predictive value than ICA, but the combination of IAA and ICA was useful. The risk of diabetes within 5 years was 17% for the IAA-positive/ICA-negative group, increasing to 42% for the ICA-positive/IAA-negative group and to 77% for double autoantibody positive relatives.

Accounting for ICA subtypes also improves the predictive value of ICA. The restricted ICA subtype, defined according to the pattern of staining on pancreatic sections, confers a significantly lower risk of progression to diabetes than the nonrestricted subtype[9] (Chapter 10) and is associated with the protective DQB1*0602 allele (Chapter 7). Preabsorption of sera with glutamate decarboxylase (GAD) blocks the ICA staining of restricted ICA-positive sera[10] and reduces the ICA staining of most non-restricted ICA-positive sera.[11] This suggests that restricted ICA are due to antibodies directed against a single antigen (GAD).

The identification of the other antigens responsible for ICA staining and the measurement of multiple antibodies against different biochemically defined antigens is likely to further improve the accuracy of prediction. The ICA assay is difficult to standardize, is labor intensive, and requires human pancreas. At the Barbara Davis Center, we utilize a combination of three assays employing recombinant antigen (IAA, anti-GAD, and anti-ICA512[12]) in addition to ICA. The ICA assay provides only marginal additional information, compared with the combination of defined-antigen assays. Relatives expressing two or more of IAA, anti-GAD, and anti-ICA512 have an overall risk of diabetes within 5 years of more than 68% by life table analysis. Once these three antibodies are considered, the presence or absence of ICA does not influence this risk. However, the addition of intravenous glucose tolerance testing does improve prediction of the time to overt diabetes. Among relatives with two or more antibodies, those with an FPIR less than the first percentile have a 50% risk of diabetes within 1 year; those with higher FPIR have a 50% risk within 3 years.

Genetic factors should also be considered in assessing diabetes risk. Deschamps and coworkers examined the predictive value of HLA typing in a study of 536 siblings of diabetic probands in France.[5] The risk of type I diabetes after 8 years, estimated by life table analysis, was 10% for siblings who were HLA identical with the proband, 3%–4% for siblings with either DR3 or DR4, and 16% for those with DR3/DR4. This compares with 56% for those with ICA greater than 4 JDF units and 70% for those with the combination of ICA and the highest risk HLA type, DR3/DR4. In other studies, molecular typing has revealed that the HLA haplotype DQA1*0102, DQB1*0602 confers strong protection from type I diabetes, in a dominant fashion (Chapter 7). In our experience, autoantibody-positive relatives with this haplotype have a very low risk of progression to diabetes[169] and usually express only a single autoantibody, namely anti-GAD, although a few also express IAA.

Prediction in the General Population

It is likely that genetic typing will have an even greater impact on assessing diabetes risk in the general population. Most studies of prediabetic subjects have involved the screening of first-degree relatives of diabetic probands, rather than the general population. However, less than 10% of new cases of type I diabetes have an affected relative, so the general population will need to be screened eventually if an effective intervention is to have a major impact. Screening the general population is likely to be more difficult than screening relatives. Bayes' theorem states that a screening test will have a lower positive predictive value in the general population than in a selected group with a higher prevalence of disease, such as first-degree relatives. One approach toward solving this problem is to screen the general population with markers of genetic susceptibility first, followed by autoantibody testing of susceptible individuals. For example, among the general population approximately 2% of individuals express both DR3 and DR4. Of this subgroup, approximately 6% will develop type I diabetes, similar to the risk among first-degree relatives.

Unexpectedly, studies performed in Florida suggest that ICA have a predictive value in the general population similar to that in relatives.[13] In contrast, studies in England suggest that ICA will have a lower positive predictive value in the general population. The prevalence of ICAs of 20 or more JDF units was only two to three times higher in siblings than in the general population, compared with a 13 times greater risk of diabetes in the siblings.[14] Many population studies have been initiated (Table 11.1) but, with relatively short follow-up at the present time, the number of subjects progressing to diabetes may be too few to accurately determine the positive predictive value of ICA and other markers.

At What Stage in Life is Beta Cell Autoimmunity Initiated, What Is the Initial Target Antigen, and in What Sequence Do Different Autoantibodies Appear?

Studies in first-degree relatives have detected evidence of beta cell autoimmunity many years before clinical presentation with overt hyperglycemia.[2,3,15] However, the existence of young infants with type I diabetes indicates that beta cell destruction may also occur rapidly in some individuals. A plausible hypothesis is that beta cell autoimmunity begins early in life, with variation in the age at onset of overt diabetes explained by differences in the rate of beta cell destruction from one individual to another. In support of this hypothesis, a major peak in the incidence of type I diabetes occurs during early adolescence in nearly all populations studied.[16]

After the age of about 15 years, measuring the incidence of type I diabetes is complicated by the misclassification of some patients as type II diabetics. Nevertheless, it has been estimated that at least 37% of type I diabetes occurs after the age of 19 years and 15% after the age of 30 years.[17]

Table 11.1. The Prevalence of Islet Cell Antibodies (ICA) among Schoolchildren in the General Population of Different Countries Compared with Incidence of Type I Diabetes

Country	*Age Range*	*Number Screened*	*Prevalence of ICA*	*Cutoff (JDF units)*	*Incidence[a] of Type I Diabetes*	*References*
Japan	7–18	473	0.4%	—	2.0	75, 152
Germany	6–21	4,287	1.05%	≥5	7.0	153, 154
			0.4%	≥20		
France	6–17	8,363	1.79%	≥4.5	7.1	118, 155
			0.2%	≥24		
Netherlands	5–19	4,806	0.42%	≥0.6	11.0	156, 157
Spain	14–17	2,291	0.35%	≥5	11.3	158, 159
New Zealand	5–7	20,000	1.2%	≥10	12.8	160, 161
USA						
Florida	5–18	9,696	0.59%	≥10	13.7[b]	13, 162, 163
Washington State	12–18	3,992	1.7%	≥1		
Australia	4–18	1,900	0.68%	≥20	14.5	67, 164
England	9–13	2,925	2.8%	≥4	15.6	14, 165
			0.8%	≥20		
Sweden	0–14	420	3%	≥5	23.6	65, 166
Finland	3–18	1,212	4.1%	≥3	35.3	117, 167

[a]Per 100,000 per year in the 0–14 age group.
[b]Incidence in Pennsylvania.

New cases of type I diabetes presenting in adult life tend to have a longer duration of symptoms before diagnosis and higher C peptide levels remaining at diagnosis compared with those presenting in childhood,[18] suggesting a slower rate of beta cell destruction. "Slow onset" type I diabetes, presenting in late adult life, may be diagnosed initially as type II diabetes. Tuomi and coworkers studied 102 adults who were treated for type II diabetes, of whom one third had low stimulated C peptide levels and two thirds had normal levels.[19] Of the group with low C peptide, 76% were positive for anti-GAD (similar to the frequency among children with newly diagnosed type I diabetes). In comparison, only 12% of the group with normal C peptide were positive for anti-GAD.

Defining the sequence in which immunological abnormalities appear is of great interest because the autoantigen against which antibodies are first produced is likely to be involved in the initiation of beta cell autoimmunity. Other autoantibodies that appear later may be less important, although useful as markers of diabetes risk. Such secondary autoantibodies may arise from the presentation of autoantigens that are normally isolated from the immune system, or from their presentation in association with beta cells undergoing autoimmune attack. As an example of this, IAA may appear in normal mice during the immune destruction of transplanted histo-incompatible non-islet cells that have been genetically engineered to express insulin.[20]

Most of the at-risk relatives followed to date were initially identified by testing for autoantibodies. It is unknown how long autoantibodies were present in these individuals before they were discovered. However, studies by Pilcher and Elliott in New Zealand suggest that ICAs develop early in childhood and are usually preceded by IAA.[21] In these studies 666 first-degree relatives, aged less than 20 years and initially ICA negative (<10 JDF units), were followed longitudinally. Those aged under 5 years were retested annually, with older subjects retested every 3 to 5 years. Sixteen (2.4%) became ICA positive during follow-up, with seroconversion occurring at an average age of 3.2 years, ranging from 1.6 to 7.1 years. All except the two oldest seroconverters were IAA positive at the time of seroconversion and the appearance of IAA was documented to precede ICA in 6 (46%) of 13 seroconverters who could be retrospectively checked for IAA.

A cohort of infants of mothers with type I or gestational diabetes has been studied by Ziegler and coworkers in Germany.[22] Preliminary data from this study also indicate that autoantibodies may appear very early in life, with IAAs appearing first. A high frequency of both IAAs and ICAs was found in cord blood samples. This was attributable to transplacental passage of maternal IgG and to falsely positive IAA results (that may be obtained in up to one half of cord blood samples from normal pregnancies).[23] However, by 9 months of age all became ICA negative and only 3 of 90 infants remained IAA positive. By 2 years of age, one of these infants became IAA negative, two remained IAA positive, and another child became persistently IAA positive for the first time. ICA, with or without anti-GAD,[24] appeared after IAA in all three persistently IAA-positive children.

Both insulin and GAD have been suggested as candidates for the initiating antigen but another (unidentified) autoantigen could be responsible. Neither IAA nor anti-GAD is universally present among patients with newly diagnosed type I diabetes.[25–31] GAD is an antigen recognized by the ICA assay,[10] so the findings in very young children discussed above favor insulin as an initiating autoantigen rather than GAD. However, only small numbers have been studied so far and it should be recognized that the assay for ICA by indirect immunofluorescence is likely to have lower sensitivity than the radioassay for IAA. Biochemical characterization of the antigens responsible for ICA[10,32] will allow the development of more precise assays for these sera. A study in Colorado is screening newborn infants from the general population for genetic risk markers and following from birth those with the high-risk HLA genotype DR3/DR4 (M. Rewers, personal communication).

Several other observations provide circumstantial evidence for insulin as an initiating autoantigen. Insulin is the only antigen unique to the beta cell and it is present on the cell surface.[33,34] In contrast, GAD is also present in alpha cells,[35] which are not destroyed,[36] and insulitis disappears when all insulin-containing cells have been destroyed.[37] IAAs occur with greater frequency and at higher levels in younger newly diagnosed patients[26,38–40] and the level of IAA appears to correlate with the rate of beta cell destruction in prediabetic individuals.[41] When 29 patients were studied, their IAAs recognized the same epitope.[42] Treatment with insulin during the prediabetic period may provide protection from diabetes in nonobese diabetic (NOD) mice, when given either orally[43] or parenterally.[44] This protection is afforded by the B chain alone,[44] which lacks metabolic function. Furthermore, insulin-like growth factor 1 (IGF-1), given in doses with equivalent hypoglycemic effects, confers no protection against diabetes.[45] These findings suggest that the protective effect of insulin is not merely due to its metabolic effects inducing a state of "beta cell rest," associated with reduced expression of autoantigens. Rather, they imply that protection may result from the induction of immunological tolerance. Preliminary results in prediabetic humans also suggest a protective effect of parenteral insulin administration[46] and a nationwide randomized trial is now beginning in the United States.

Among ICA-positive first-degree relatives, those with restricted ICAs[10] (that can be abolished by pre-incubation of the serum with GAD) have a significantly lower risk of progression to diabetes.[9] This suggests that the loss of tolerance to GAD alone may not predict eventual diabetes, although restricted ICAs appear to recognize a different GAD epitope from other anti-GAD antibodies.[47]

In contrast, two recent studies in the NOD mouse suggest that the loss of tolerance to GAD may be the initiating event, followed by a sequential loss of tolerance to other beta cell autoantigens.[48,49] Kaufman and coworkers[48] studied the proliferative responses of T cells from NOD mice to a panel of autoantigens and control antigens, from birth to 28 weeks of age. The reactivity of splenocytes (not islet T cells) was studied. The first response (at 4 weeks of age) was to GAD, followed by the addition of responses to heat shock protein (at 6 weeks), carboxypeptidase H (at 8 weeks), and insulin (at 12–15 weeks). The GAD response was initially to a single epitope, but, with time, this broadened to involve several epitopes. Tisch and coworkers[49] obtained similar results (but did not study responses to insulin), with the additional finding of a sequential appearance of autoantibodies in parallel with the T cell responses. Intravenous[48] or intrathymic[49] injection of GAD causes a marked reduction in the T cell response. Significantly, Kaufman and coworkers found that treatment with intravenous heat shock protein caused T cell tolerance to heat shock protein alone, whereas intravenous GAD produced tolerance to all of the autoantigens studied.[48] The effects of tolerization with insulin were not determined in these experiments.

These findings, utilizing NOD spleen cells, support a primary role for GAD in the initiation of beta cell autoimmunity. In contrast, studies of T cells isolated from NOD islets reveal little response to GAD but a strong response to insulin in proliferation assays. In limiting dilution assays, 5%–20% of islet T cells respond to insulin. These insulin-responsive T cells can accelerate the development of diabetes when injected back into young NOD mice (D. Wegman, personal communication).

It is likely that other autoantigens involved in early events remain to be discovered. Gelber and coworkers studied the proliferative response of peripheral T cells from young female NOD mice to extracts of beta cells.[50] Responsive T cells were present prior to any detectable insulitis and these early T cells recognized multiple different antigens (determined by fractionation of the extracts). However, none of these were known antigens (GAD, insulin, ICA69, heat shock protein, carboxypeptidase H, or peripherin).

Are Environmental Factors Important, Either in the Initiation of Beta Cell Autoimmunity or in Modulating the Process Once It Has Begun?

The diabetes susceptibility genes identified so far are present in a high proportion of the general population, indicating that they are not sufficient to cause the disease. Furthermore, the concordance rate observed in HLA-identical siblings is lower than that in identical twins,[5,51,52,168] suggesting that other important loci remain to be discovered. As Type I diabetes is associated with other autoimmune diseases,[53,54] it is likely that at least some of the important genes will not be specific to type I diabetes but also involved in the susceptibility to these other autoimmune diseases.

Despite the importance of genetic factors, the low concordance rate (<40%) seen in identical twins[51,52,168] implies a critical role for nongenetic factors. Several mechanisms could account for such discordance, including the random rearrangement of antigen receptor genes during the differentiation of T lymphocytes,[55] somatic mutation, and environmental factors. Epidemiological studies with validated case ascertainment support a role for environmental factors. A rising incidence of type I diabetes over time, too rapid to be explained by an increase in the frequency of diabetogenic genes in the population, has been reported in several European countries.[56–62] In addition, increased rates have been observed in migrant populations compared with their countries of origin.[63,64]

An environmental factor could be involved either by initiating autoimmunity or by altering its progression, once established. There is a seasonal variation in the onset of type I diabetes,[56,57,65–67] with more cases in the winter months, associated with viral infections. It is likely that such viral infections alter the process late in its course by increasing insulin requirements, thereby advancing the time of diabetes onset. In humans, the best evidence for the involvement of a specific viral agent in the initiation of autoimmunity comes from the observation that patients with congenital rubella have an increased prevalence of type I diabetes,[68,69] as well as other autoimmune diseases.[70] Coxsackievirus B infection has also been suggested as an environmental trigger,[71] although a large Swedish study found no significant difference in the levels of IgM antibodies against Coxsackievirus B types 1–5 between newly diagnosed diabetic children and population controls.[72] There is likely to be a long lag time between a triggering infection and the onset of diabetes but IgG levels were not measured in this study. It has been suggested that an infectious agent might activate autoimmunity by molecular mimicry, whereby the immune response to a viral antigen, such as the P2-C protein of Coxsackievirus B4[73] or the rubella capsid,[74] might cross-react with a beta cell antigen. Some evidence against a significant role for an infectious agent comes from Japan. Despite wide variation in the incidence rates for infectious diseases in different parts of the country, the incidence of type I diabetes is uniformly low.[75]

In animal models of type I diabetes, exposure to infectious agents may suppress rather than trigger autoimmunity. NOD mice raised in a sterile environment have an increased incidence of diabetes. Similarly, diabetes-prone BB rats housed in "viral antibody free" conditions have a higher frequency of diabetes than those housed in less stringent "specific pathogen free" conditions.[76] Specific infection with mouse hepatitis virus is associated with reduced incidence of diabetes in the NOD mouse,[77] and infection with lymphocytic choriomeningitis virus is associated with reduced incidence in both the NOD mouse and BB rat.[78,79] However, in at least one instance infection is implicated as a trigger. Kilham's rat virus, a parvovirus, has been shown to trigger beta cell autoimmunity and diabetes in the diabetes-resistant BB rat.[80] Other reports of viruses triggering diabetes in animals may involve direct viral damage of beta cells without an autoimmune mechanism.[81,82]

In humans, associations with infant feeding have been reported. Several population-based case-control studies found a protective effect associated with breast-feeding[83–85] and an increased risk associated with the early introduction of supplemental feeding.[83,84,86] A Danish study, which eliminated several possible sources of bias by using the records of postnatal health visitors, found no evidence to support an associated with the total duration of breast-feeding,[87] but did not examine the timing of introduction of supplemental feeding.

The associations with infant feeding are weak (odds ratios ~1.5),[88] but this is consistent with the effect of a common exposure acting only on genetically susceptible individuals. Several mechanisms could explain the associations with infant feeding. Breast-feeding could protect the infant from an infection. The increased caloric intake and weight gain associated with artificial feeding might cause increased insulin secretion and presentation of beta cell autoantigens.[89] Karjalainen and coworkers have suggested that intact cow's milk peptides might cross the immature gut, initiating an immune response that cross-reacts with a beta cell surface antigen.[90] Higher levels of antibodies against several components of cow's milk have been reported in children with newly diagnosed type I diabetes than in controls.[91–95] Karjalainen and coworkers reported that 100% of 142 newly diagnosed diabetic children were positive for anti–bovine serum albumin (BSA) antibodies, mostly directed against a 17 amino acid peptide called ABBOS.[90] T cell proliferation in response to the ABBOS peptide was higher in newly diagnosed patients than in controls.[96] However, these results could not be reproduced by Atkinson and coworkers,[97] who found no difference between newly diagnosed patients and controls for either anti-BSA antibodies or T cell proliferation to ABBOS. In animal studies, the addition of cow's milk to the diet of the BB rat at the time of weaning increases the incidence of diabetes,[98,99] but there are conflicting reports on the effect of cow's milk in the diet of the NOD mouse.[100,101]

A prospective cohort study of genetically susceptible individuals followed from birth is needed to confirm these associations with environmental factors. The identification of an avoidable environmental factor would clearly have major implications for prevention of the disease. A double-blind, randomized trial is planned in Finland to test the cow's milk hypothesis. This study, involving neonates with affected first-degree relatives, will test the effect of excluding cow's milk proteins from the diet in the first 9 months of life.[102]

Once Autoimmunity Is Initiated, Are Beta Cells Destroyed in a Progressive, Linear Fashion or Are There Spontaneous Remissions?

The long-term follow-up of high-titer ICA-positive relatives in the Joslin family study with serial IVGTTs suggested a model in which beta cell destruction is a progressive, linear process[103,104] (Fig. 11.2). The rate of beta cell destruction may vary widely from one individual to another. It may be so slow in some individuals that overt diabetes does not develop during the person's lifetime. Such individuals might appear to have decreased but stable beta cell function when assessed with serial IVGTTs over many years. A correlation between serial FPIR levels and the number of years to diabetes in ICA-positive relatives,[105] and the addition of IAA as a risk marker,[8] lead to the development of a "dual parameter" linear regression model.[41] In this model the time remaining before the onset of diabetes is predicted by a combination of the FPIR (reflecting the remaining beta cell mass) and the IAA level (reflecting the rate of loss of beta cells). The validity of this model and other methods of predicting diabetes risk based on combinations of markers are being evaluated in a larger data set in the collaborative ICARUS study.

Other studies, including relatives with lower titer ICA, have suggested that progression to diabetes may be less predictable.[106–108] They have suggested an alternative model, in which the rate of beta cell destruction may fluctuate, with spontaneous remission in some individuals. This model is similar to that suggested for autoimmune thyroiditis.[109] Reports of transient ICA in relatives,[106,110–113] in discordant identical twins,[114] in the general population,[115–118] and in patients initially treated for type II diabetes[108] lend support to this hypothesis. Most, but not all[106,113,115,116] of these transient ICAs have been reported in subjects with initially low titers, raising the possibility that the phenomenon may frequently be explained by variability in the ICA assay.[119] Some of these studies did not report the levels of ICA in terms of endpoint titer or JDF units.[108,110,111] However, several confirmed the change in ICA status by retesting the sera from all time points for a given subject in one assay.[106,108,111,117]

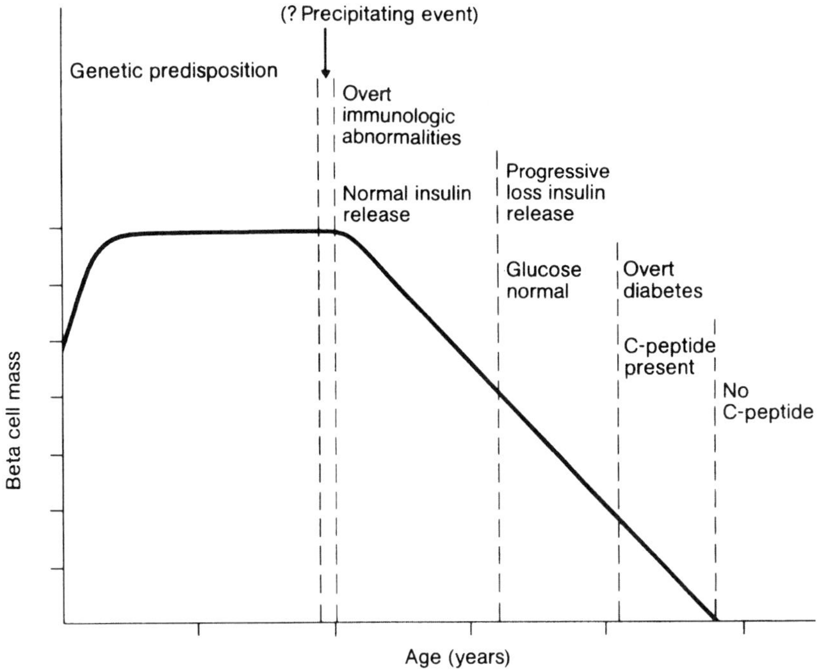

Figure 11.2. A model for the development of type I diabetes, dividing the disease into 6 stages, beginning with genetic predisposition and ending with complete beta cell destruction. Reproduced with permission from: Eisenbarth GS, *N Engl J Med*, 1986; 314:1360–1368. Copyright © **1986 by the Massachusetts Medical Society.**

Low-titer ICAs carry a reduced risk of type I diabetes, compared with high titer,[2,3] and it may be that fluctuating levels do not signify a disease process, especially if unaccompanied by other autoantibodies. Nonpersistent ICAs may represent a nonspecific immunological response associated with infection, as Helmke and coworkers reported the transient appearance of ICAs in normal schoolchildren during mumps infection.[115] The development of more reproducible assays for antibodies against biochemically defined autoantigens may improve the assessment of diabetes risk. Among those relatives followed in the Joslin family study who express more than one autoantibody, levels of IAA,[8] anti-GAD, and anti-ICA512 (unpublished data) have been remarkably stable over time.

Carel and coworkers reported that ICA-negative siblings of diabetic children have significantly lower mean FPIR than controls.[120] They suggested that autoimmune beta cell destruction may have been initiated in some of these siblings, but spontaneously remitted. However, other autoantibodies may have been present in some of the ICA-negative siblings in this study. At most, only 94% of children with newly diagnosed type I diabetes are ICA positive, using a very sensitive assay[121] but the addition of other autoantibodies may reduce the autoantibody-negative proportion. In addition, although the diet was standardized for the 3 days prior to the IVGTT, there may be differences over the longer term in the diets of children with and without a diabetic sibling that could have affected the IVGTT results.

Several lines of evidence suggest that not all individuals with autoantibodies progress to diabetes. The prevalence of ICAs among children in the general population in different countries is higher than expected from the incidence rates observed in those countries (Table 11.1). Among unselected first-degree relatives screened at the Barbara Davis Center, 26% were positive for anti-GAD antibodies,[122] compared with a 5% risk of diabetes among first-degree relatives. The frequency of anti-GAD was very high (46%) in relatives aged under 5 years. This suggests that transient evidence of autoimmunity may be present in up to half of first-degree relatives early in life, without leading to diabetes in the great majority. In this study, the anti-GAD antibodies were measured with a radioassay utilizing affinity purified porcine GAD and the upper limit of the normal range was established as the 98th percentile in 103 controls. Of note, a radioassay utilizing recombinant, in vitro translated GAD detects positive levels in only about 9% of relatives (unpublished data) and may be more specific for relatives who progress to diabetes.

Decreased insulin secretion measured with an IVGTT could be due to reduced beta cell mass or (reversible) impairment of beta cell function, or both. Inflamed islets from diabetes-prone BB rats have an enhanced insulin secretory response to glucose,[123] suggesting that reduced beta cell mass is the dominant mechanism.

Experiments with streptozotocin-treated baboons indicate that beta cell function (assessed by IVGTT) correlates with beta cell mass.[124] In humans, however, the IVGTT has several limitations. The results of beta cell function tests may vary with insulin sensitivity according to age,[120,125] physical fitness,[126] body mass index,[125,127] pubertal status,[127,128] and physical or psychological stress. Different protocols for the IVGTT give different results[129] but a standard protocol has been developed to allow meta-analyses.[130]

The interpretation of serial FPIR data is complicated by within-subject variability in the measurement. Figures 11.3A and 11.3B illustrate the course of the FPIR over time for two ICA-positive relatives. One has a clearly linear loss of secretion (Fig. 11.3A). In contrast, the other relative (Fig. 11.3B) has what appears to be a stepwise loss of secretion, with remissions and periods of recovery. However, this second pattern could equally well result from wide within-subject measurement variation, superimposed on an underlying linear loss of secretion.

Several centers have performed duplicate IVGTTs, spaced 1 or more weeks apart, on healthy volunteers. The median within-subject coefficients of variation (CV) reported for FPIR varied from 4% to 36%[125,131,132] but the CV was as high as 56% for some subjects. There are conflicting reports about whether calculating the area under the curve for insulin release improves reproducibility, compared with the sum of the 1- and 3-minute insulin levels.[125,131,132] McCulloch and coworkers studied 18 normal postpubertal subjects on two occasions separated by an average of 1 year.[106] They used an

IVGTT protocol with frequent sampling and a bolus of tolbutamide at 20 minutes, allowing the calculation of the insulin sensitivity index. The within-subject CV for the incremental area under the insulin curve (above fasting levels) from 0 to 10 minutes was 11.3%. Adjusting for the insulin sensitivity index resulted in a similar CV (10.5%). However, it is likely that adjusting for insulin sensitivity may improve reproducibility in pubertal subjects and those followed over a longer period. The subjects also underwent arginine stimulation tests (both at physiological plasma glucose concentration and with hyperglycemic clamp). The reproducibility of the response to arginine was similar to that of the response to glucose, indicating little advantage gained by the use of arginine.

Rayman and coworkers achieved highly reproducible results using retrograde venous cannulation and arterialization of the hand from which the samples are drawn,[131] but recent studies found no improvement with these techniques.[133,134] Other maneuvers that have been evaluated to improve reproducibility include placement of the intravenous line 1 hour before the test to minimize the effects of stress hormones. Allen and coworkers tested the hypothesis that catecholamine release, associated with anxiety about the test, may inhibit insulin release but found no correlation between the FPIR and plasma catecholamine levels or standardized anxiety scores.[125] However, a significant "first test effect" was observed. Among 11 normal subjects who underwent two tests, 9 had a higher FPIR on the second test.[125] One subject who fainted during the first test had a very low FPIR (2 mU/L) that became normal on a subsequent occasion.

The FPIR is a measure of beta cell function, but a measure of beta cell mass might be more useful. In the future, new ways of assessing the beta cells may be developed, including high-performance glycated hemoglobin assays and imaging with nuclear magnetic resonance (MRI) or isotopic scans. Leech and coworkers measured the HbA1c by high-performance liquid chromatography in healthy teenagers who were also tested for ICA.[135] The mean HbA1c was slightly, but significantly, higher in the ICA-positive subjects, suggesting that elevation of the HbA1c within the nornal range may be an early marker of loss of beta cell function. Signore and coworkers reported preliminary data suggesting that scans following the injection of ^{123}I-labeled interleukin-2 (IL-2) may be useful in the detection of beta cell autoimmunity.[136] A significant accumulation of tracer was detected in the pancreatic region of four newly diagnosed and two prediabetic subjects, compared with four controls. MRI has been used to detect pancreatic graft rejection.[137–139] With refinements in MRI techniques it may be possible in the future to detect insulitis or to approximate beta cell mass.

There is little information on changes in islet histology before the onset of overt diabetes in humans. However, Sutherland and coworkers studied patients with longstanding type I diabetes who received pancreatic transplants from their nondiabetic identical twins.[37] Of these, three received either delayed immunosuppression or no immunosuppression after the transplant and all three became insulin dependent again within 5 to 12 weeks. Serial biopsies of the

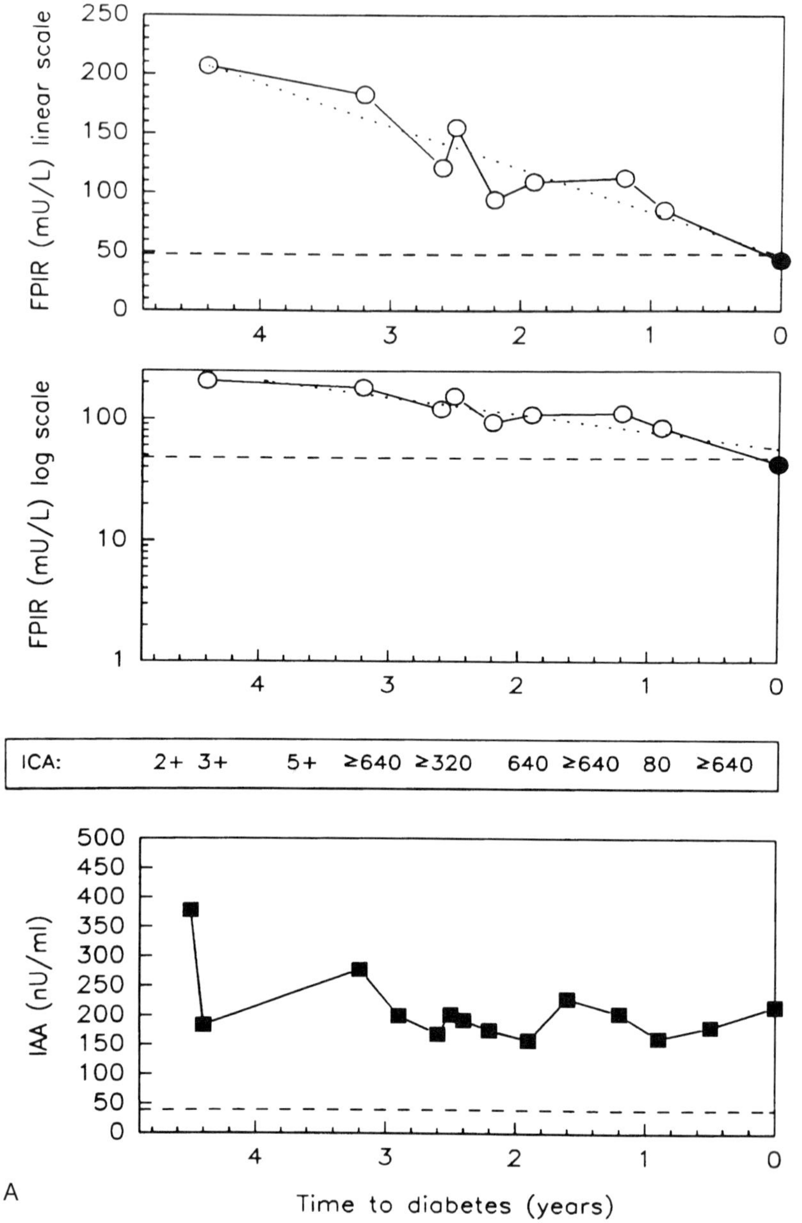

Figure 11.3. Changes in the FPIR, ICA titer and IAA level during longitudinal follow-up of two ICA-positive first-degree relatives prior to the onset of overt diabetes. The top two panels show the FPIR plotted on linear and logarithmic scales. The dashed line indicates the 1st percentile for FPIR among controls (48 mU/L) and the linear regression through the data is shown with a dotted line. *A* plots the time-course of the subject with the most linear loss of FPIR followed in the Joslin family study (onset of diabetes at age 14.4 years).

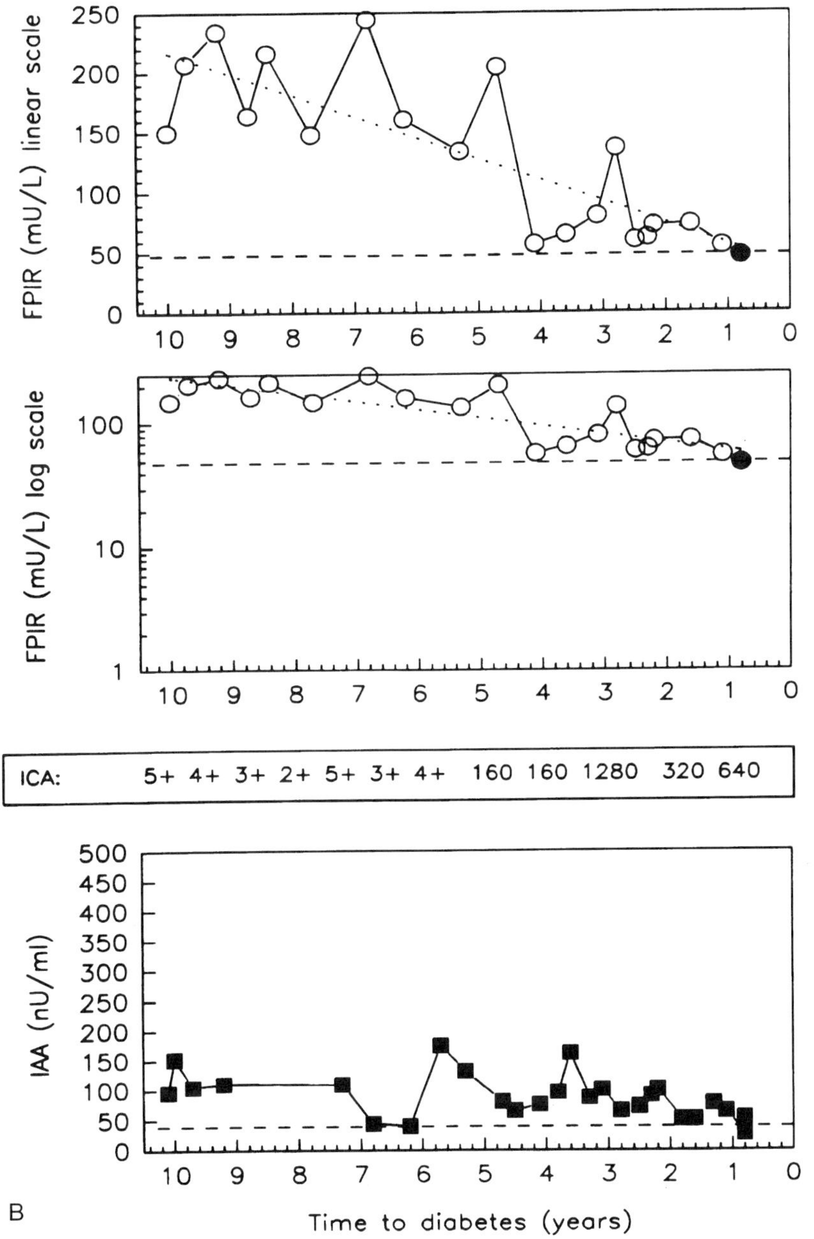

Figure 11.3 *(continued). B* plots the time course of the least linear subject (onset of diabetes at age 17.8 years). Positive ICA levels determined before the introduction of JDF units are shown on a scale of 1+ to 6+, depending on the intensity of immunofluorescence. In the lowest panel, the dashed line indicates the upper limit of normal for IAA (mean+3SD among controls).

graft revealed T cell infiltration with selective beta cell destruction, unlike graft rejection. Rather, these histological findings were consistent with reactivation of beta cell autoimmunity. Of note, the insulitis disappeared after the insulin-containing cells were destroyed.

Foulis and coworkers studied the pancreatic histology of 119 patients with type I diabetes who had died of ketoacidosis, of whom 60 had died within 1 year of diagnosis.[36] They found that insulitis is a patchy process, in which islets with or without insulitis tend to be grouped separately in different lobules. At diagnosis, the beta cells in some islets were destroyed while other islets were left untouched, but most islets were insulin deficient after a 1-year duration of diabetes. Hanafusa and coworkers performed pancreatic biopsy on seven Japanese adults, 2–4 months after the diagnosis of type I diabetes. The islets were atrophic, with reduced or absent insulin staining, but surprisingly there was hardly any lymphocytic infiltration.[140]

The diagnosis of diabetes is to some extent an arbitrary point in the natural history of the autoimmune disease. The timing of overt diabetes may be influenced by factors that increase insulin requirements, such as infections and puberty. A significant proportion of the beta cell mass may remain at diagnosis. Experiments with streptozotocin-treated baboons suggest that the FPIR may be undetectable even when about 20%–50% of beta cell mass remains,[124] although pancreatic insulin content was close to zero at this point. Autoimmune beta cell destruction continues after the diagnosis of diabetes. A temporary remission from insulin dependency may occur in up to 27% of patients, soon after diagnosis,[141] and is attributed to the beta cell rest caused by insulin treatment. Younger age at onset, male sex, high-titer ICA, severe ketoacidosis at diagnosis, and a short duration of symptoms prior to diagnosis are associated with a more rapid loss of C peptide secretion.[142] In one study a more rapid loss was seen in patients heterozygous for DR3 and DR4,[143] although another study came to the opposite conclusion,[141] and another found no significant DR associations.[142]

Conclusions

The questions discussed in this chapter cannot yet be answered with certainty. Nevertheless, significant progress has been made in recent years toward a better understanding of the events leading to type I diabetes. This information has been utilized in the planning of several large-scale intervention trials in humans that are now beginning.

We propose a model in which immunological abnormalities appear early in life in genetically susceptible individuals. This is marked by the appearance of low level, or low affinity, single autoantibodies. Autoimmunity may be activated by somatic mutation or environmental triggers. Alternatively it may be aborted by environmental factors (eg, various infections). In most individuals, these abnormalities are transient and are not associated with beta cell destruction. In some, beta cell destruction is initiated, marked by the appearance of multiple immunological abnormalities and later by measurable loss of FPIR. Genetic and environmental factors may modulate the process, affecting the rate of beta cell destruction. The loss of beta cells may be so slow in some individuals that overt diabetes does not occur during the person's lifetime. Once tolerance is broken to more than one autoantigen, the levels of autoantibodies (IAA, anti-ICA512, and anti-GAD) appear to be stable over time. The presence of more than one of these autoantibodies, combined with FPIR measurements and typing for HLA-DQ alleles, allows the identification of a subset of relatives with sufficiently high risk for type I diabetes to begin preventive trials. Studies are just beginning that will more precisely define the natural history of this process, starting from the first year of life. It is likely, but unproven, that both relatives of patients and subjects from the general population will follow a similar course.

The hypothesis that type I diabetes develops in a chronic and predictable manner forms the basis for prevention trials. It is equally important to identify those autoantibody-positive relatives who are unlikely to progress to diabetes. Knowledge about the natural history of the prediabetic period may also facilitate the diagnosis of type I diabetes. Such information becomes clinically relevant in genetic counseling, the diagnosis of diabetes in adults (type I versus type II) and in children with an unusual clinical course. It is also relevant in the evaluation of individuals with transient hyperglycemia and of potential renal donors to relatives with type I diabetes.

Evaluation of each of the above circumstances will usually include genetic, immunological, and metabolic information. The presence of the HLA haplotype DQA1*0102/DQB1*0602 is so rare among children with type I diabetes[144,145] that an alternative disorder should be considered as the cause of diabetes if this haplotype is present. Other diseases that can present as insulin-requiring diabetes in childhood include Wolfram's syndrome (DIDMOAD—diabetes insipidus, diabetes mellitus, optic atrophy, and nerve deafness),[146] the polyendocrine type I syndrome (Chapter 8), mitochondrial mutations (often associated with nerve deafness[147]), and MODY[148] (maturity onset diabetes of youth, that may be caused by mutations in the glucokinase gene).[149] The DQB1*0602 protective haplotype is likely to be present in these disorders at the normal population frequency of approximately 20%.

In adults, the presence of specific autoantibodies in a diabetic individual is probably the best available evidence of type I diabetes. At an epidemiological level, the diagnosis of type I diabetes by presence of ketoacidosis, insulin requirement, and young age of onset is useful, but for an individual may be of little value. In the past, determination of ICA was the only immunological test available. This test has high specificity but limited sensitivity. In most series high titers of ICA are present in less than 70% of new-onset patients with classic type I diabetes. The combination of three recombinant antigen based assays (IAA, anti-GAD, and anti-ICA512) appears to detect more than 98% of individuals with type I diabetes.[150] Two or more of these antibodies are present in approximately 80% of patients. As such assays become available, the detection of slow-onset type I diabetes among adults should be enhanced. Such patients will likely compose more than 10% of adults developing diabetes. Whether this will lead to the immediate institution of insulin therapy rather than oral hypoglycemic agents requires clinical trials of the potential risks and benefits of such therapy.

Of 63 children with transient hyperglycemia we have evaluated, most (89%) remain nondiabetic.[151] All of the few with ICAs or IAAs became permanently diabetic within 18 months. It is likely that the measurement of antibodies against multiple biochemically defined antigens will also improve diagnosis of this group. The IVGTT is the diagnostic test of choice in this group. Among children with resolved transient hyperglycemia, none of those with normal FPIR (greater than the 5th percentile) has progressed to diabetes. Of those with low FPIR, a subset normalizes upon repeat testing, but those remaining abnormal have all become overtly diabetic within 1 year.

An individual contemplating the donation of a kidney to a diabetic relative should have an OGTT to rule out the presence of overt diabetes, an IVGTT by ICARUS criteria, and determination of autoantibodies with assays that have high specificity and sensitivity (eg, the combination of anti-GAD, anti-insulin, and anti-ICA512). ICAs are of utility only if the laboratory performing the measurement participates in IDW proficiency workshops, with greater than 90% specificity. Most of these assays are available only in research laboratories, but this situation is likely to change rapidly with commercial laboratories performing the new autoantibody assays.

Finally, the most important reason for detecting individuals at risk for type I diabetes is the potential for preventive therapy. Large trials of preventive therapies are now under way in the United States and Europe. It is likely that with more detailed analysis and improvements in the assays available, the prediction of type I diabetes will improve further. It will be very important to begin such prediction in the general population, as the majority of new cases have no affected relative. Studies with antibodies against biochemically defined autoantigens, coupled with intravenous glucose tolerance testing, are just beginning in the general population.

References

1. Eisenbarth GS, Verge CF, Allen H, Rewers MJ. The design of trials for prevention of IDDM. *Diabetes.* 1993; 42:941–947.
2. Riley WJ, Maclaren NK, Krischer J, et al. A prospective study of the development of diabetes in relatives of patients with insulin-dependent diabetes. *N Engl J Med.* 1990; 323:1167–1172.
3. Bonifacio E, Bingley PJ, Shattock M, et al. Quantification of islet-cell antibodies and prediction of insulin-dependent diabetes. *Lancet.* 1990; 335:147–149.
4. Vardi P, Crisa L, Jackson RA, et al. Predictive value of intravenous glucose tolerance test insulin secretion less than or greater than the first percentile in islet cell antibody positive relatives of type I (insulin-dependent) diabetic patients. *Diabetologia.* 1991; 34:93–102.

5. Deschamps I, Boitard C, Hors J, et al. Life table analysis of the risk of type 1 (insulin-dependent) diabetes in siblings according to islet cell antibodies and HLA markers. An 8 year prospective study. *Diabetologia.* 1992; 35:951–957.
6. Krischer JP, Schatz DA, Riley WJ, et al. Insulin and islet cell antibodies as time dependent covariates in the development of insulin dependent diabetes: a prospective study in relatives. *J Clin Endocrinol Metab.* 1993; 77:743–749.
7. Chase HP, Garg SK, Butler-Simon N, et al. Prediction of the course of pre-type I diabetes. *J Pediatr.* 1991; 118:838–841.
8. Ziegler AG, Ziegler R, Vardi P, Jackson RA, Soeldner JS, Eisenbarth GS. Life table analysis of progression to diabetes of anti-insulin autoantibody-positive relatives of individuals with type I diabetes. *Diabetes.* 1989; 38:1320–1325.
9. Gianani R, Pugliese A, Bonner-Weir S, et al. Prognostically significant heterogeneity of cytoplasmic islet cell antibodies in relatives of patients with type I diabetes. *Diabetes.* 1992; 41:347–353.
10. Gianani R, Jackson R, Eisenbarth GS. Evidence that the autoantigen of restricted ICA is GAD. *Diabetes Res Clin Pract.* 1991; 14(suppl 1):S13. Abstract.
11. Marshall MO, Hoyer PE, Petersen JS, et al. Contribution of glutamate decarboxylase antibodies to the reactivity of islet cell cytoplasmic antibodies. *J Autoimmunity.* 1994; 7:497–508.
12. Gianani R, Rabin DU, Verge CF, et al. ICA512 autoantibody radioassay. *Diabetes.* 1995 (in press).
13. Schatz D, Krischer JP, Horne G, et al. Islet cell antibodies predict insulin-dependent diabetes in United States school age children as powerfully as in unaffected relatives. *J Clin Invest.* 1994; 93:2403–2407.
14. Bingley PJ, Bonifacio E, Shattock M, et al. Can islet cell antibodies predict IDDM in the general population? *Diabetes Care.* 1993; 16:45–49.
15. Srikanta S, Ganda OP, Soeldner JS, Eisenbarth GS. First degree relatives of patients with type I diabetes mellitus: islet cell antibodies and abnormal insulin secretion. *N Engl J Med.* 1985; 313:461–464.
16. Rewers M, LaPorte RE, King H, Tuomilehto J. Trends in the prevalence and incidence of diabetes: insulin-dependent diabetes mellitus in childhood. *World Health Stat Q.* 1988; 41:179–189.
17. Laakso M, Pyorala K. Age at onset and type of diabetes. *Diabetes Care.* 1985; 8:114–117.
18. Karjalainen J, Salmela P, Ilonen J, Surcel H-M, Knip M. A comparison of childhood and adult type I diabetes mellitus. *N Engl J Med.* 1989; 320:881–886.
19. Tuomi T, Groop LC, Zimmet PZ, Rowley MJ, Knowles WJ, Mackay IR. Antibodies to glutamic acid decarboxylase reveal latent autoimmune diabetes in adults with a non-insulin-dependent onset of diabetes. *Diabetes.* 1993; 42:359–362.
20. Ziegler AG, Vardi P, Gross DJ, et al. Production of insulin antibodies by mice rejecting insulin transfected cells. *J Autoimmunity.* 1989; 2:219–227.
21. Pilcher CC, Elliott RB. Ontogeny of islet cell and insulin autoantibodies in first degree relatives of IDDM. *Autoimmunity.* 1993; 15(suppl):78. Abstract.
22. Ziegler AG, Hillebrand B, Rabl W, et al. On the appearance of islet associated autoimmunity in offspring of diabetic mothers: a prospective study from birth. *Diabetologia.* 1993; 36:402–408.
23. Vardi P, Soloveicik L, Barzilai D, Giordanno-Galluzzo C, Seides Y, Perlman R. Insulin binding activity in cord blood of normal pregnancies. *Autoimmunity.* 1993; 15(suppl):50.

24. Vordemann J, Hillebrand B, Roll U, Ziegler AG. On the appearance of islet associated autoimmunity in offspring of diabetic mothers: a prospective study from birth. *Autoimmunity.* 1993; 15(suppl):68. Abstract.

25. Vardi P, Dib SA, Tuttleman M, et al. Competitive insulin autoantibody assay: prospective evaluation of subjects at high risk for development of type I diabetes mellitus. *Diabetes.* 1987; 36:1286–1291.

26. Vardi P, Ziegler AG, Matthews JH, et al. Concentration of insulin autoantibodies at onset of type I diabetes: inverse log-linear correlation with age. *Diabetes Care.* 1988; 11:736–739.

27. Martino GV, Tappaz ML, Braghi S, et al. Autoantibodies to glutamic acid decarboxylase (GAD) detected by an immuno-trapping enzyme activity assay: relation to insulin-dependent diabetes mellitus. *J Autoimmunity.* 1991; 4:915–923.

28. DeAizpurua HJ, Harrison LC, Cram DS. An ELISA for antibodies to recombinant glutamic acid decarboxylase in IDDM. *Diabetes.* 1992; 41:1182–1187.

29. DeAizpurua HJ, Wilson Y, Harrison LC. Glutamic acid decarboxylase (GAD) autoantibodies in preclinical insulin-dependent diabetes. *Proc Natl Acad Sci U S A.* 1992; 89:9841–9845.

30. Thivolet CH, Tappaz M, Durand A, et al. Glutamic acid decarboxylase (GAD) autoantibodies are additional predictive markers of type 1 (insulin-dependent) diabetes mellitus in high risk individuals. *Diabetologia.* 1992; 35:570–576.

31. Hagopian WA, Karlsen AE, Gottsater A, et al. Quantitative assay using recombinant human islet glutamic acid decarboxylase (GAD65) shows that 64K autoantibody positivity at onset predicts diabetes type. *J Clin Invest.* 1993; 91:368–374.

32. Dotta F, Previti M, Tiberti C, Lenti L, Pugliese G, DiMario U. Identification of the GM2-1 islet ganglioside: similarities with a major neuronal autoantigen. *Diabetes.* 1992; 41:365A. Abstract.

33. Larsson L-I, Nielsen JH, Hutton JC, Madsen OD. Pancreatic hormones are expressed on the surface of human and rat islet cells through exocytotic sites. *Eur J Cell Biology.* 1989; 48:45–51.

34. Aguilar-Diosdado M, Parkinson D, Corbett JA, et al. Potential autoantigens in IDDM: expression of carboxypeptidase-H and insulin but not glutamate decarboxylase on the β-cell surface. *Diabetes.* 1994; 43:418–425.

35. Petersen JS, Russel S, Marshall MO, et al. Differential expression of glutamate decarboxylase in rat and human islets. *Diabetes.* 1993; 42:484–495.

36. Foulis AK, LiddleCN, Farquharson MA, Richmond JA, Weir RS. The histopathology of the pancreas in type I (insulin-dependent) diabetes mellitus: a 25-year review of deaths in patients under 20 years of age in the United Kingdom. *Diabetologia.* 1986; 29:267–274.

37. Sutherland DER, Sibley R, Xu XZ, et al. Twin-to-twin pancreas transplantation: reversal and reenactment of the pathogenesis of type I diabetes. *Trans Assoc Am Physicians.* 1984; 97:80–87.

38. Arslanian SL, Becker DJ, Rabin B, et al. Correlates of insulin antibodies in newly diagnosed children with insulin-dependent diabetes before insulin therapy. *Diabetes.* 1985; 34:926–930.

39. Karjalainen J, Knip M, Mustonen a, Ilonen J, Akerblom HK. Relation between insulin antibody and complement-fixing islet cell antibody at clinical diagnosis of IDDM. *Diabetes.* 1986; 35:620–622.

40. McEvoy RC, Witt ME, Ginsberg-Fellner F, Rubenstein P. Anti-insulin antibodies in children with type 1 diabetes. *Diabetes.* 1986; 35:634–641.

41. Jackson RA, Vardi P, Herskowitz R, Soeldner JS, Eisenbarth GS. Dual parameter linear model for prediction of onset of type 1 diabetes in islet cell antibody positive relatives. *Clin Res.* 1988; 36:585A. (Abstract).
42. Castano L, Ziegler AG, Ziegler R, Shoelson S, Eisenbarth GS. Characterization of insulin autoantibodies in relatives of patients with type 1 diabetes. *Diabetes.* 1993; 42:1202–1209.
43. Zhang JZ, Davidson L, Eisenbarth GS, Weiner HL. Suppression of diabetes in nonobese diabetic mice by oral administration of porcine insulin. *Proc Natl Acad Sci (USA).* 1991; 88:10252–10256.
44. Muir A, Peck A, Clare-Salzler M, et al. Insulin immunization of non-obese diabetic mice induces a protective insulitis characterized by diminished intraislet interferon-gamma transcription. *J Clin Invest.* 1995; 95:628–634.
45. Elliott RB, Bibby NJ, Ambler G. Prevention of diabetes in the NOD mouse by insulin is unrelated to its metabolic effect. *Autoimmunity.* 1993; 15(suppl):71. (Abstract).
46. Keller RJ, Eisenbarth GS, Jackson RA. Insulin prophylaxis in individuals at high risk of type 1 diabetes. *Lancet.* 1993; 341:927–928.
47. Ujihara N, Daw K, Gianani R, et al. Identification of glutamic acid decarboxylase autoantibody heterogeneity and epitope regions in type 1 diabetes. *Diabetes.* 1994; 43:968–975.
48. Kaufman DL, Clare-Salzler M, Tian J, et al. Spontaneous loss of T-cell tolerance to glutamic acid decarboxylase in murine insulin-dependent diabetes. *Nature.* 1993; 366:69–72.
49. Tisch R, Yang X-D, Singer SM, Liblau RS, Fugger L, McDevitt HO. Immune response to glutamic acid decarboyxlase correlates with insulitis in non-obese diabetic mice. *Nature.* 1993; 366:72–75.
50. Gelber C. Paborsky L, Singer S, et al. Isolation of nonobese diabetic mouse T-cell that recognize novel autoantigens involved in the early events of diabetes. *Diabetes.* 1994; 43:33–39.
51. Olmos P, A'Hearn R, Heaton DA, Risley D, Pyke DA, Leslie RDG. The significance of concordance rate of type I (insulin dependent) diabetes mellitus in identical twins. *Diabetologia.* 1988; 31:747–750.
52. Kaprio J, Tuomilehto J, Koskenvuo M, et al. Concordance for type 1 (insulin-dependent) and type 2 (non insulin-dependent) diabetes mellitus in a population-based cohort of twins in Finland. *Diabetologia.* 1993; 35:1060–1067.
53. Savilahti E, Simell O, Koskimies S, Rilva A, Akerblom HK. Celiac disease in insulin-dependent diabetes mellitus. *J Pediatr.* 1986; 108:690–693.
54. Maclaren NK, Riley WJ. Thyroid, gastric, and adrenal autoimmunities associated with insulin-dependent diabetes mellitus. *Diabetes Care.* 1985; 8(suppl):34–38.
55. Kronenberg M, Siu G, Hood LE, Shastri N. The molecular genetics of the T-cell antigen receptor and T-cell recognition. *Annu Rev Immunol.* 1986; 4:529–591.
56. Joner G, Sovik O. Increasing incidence of diabetes mellitus in Norwegian children 0–14 years of age 1973–1982. *Diabetologia.* 1989; 32:79–83.
57. Green A, Anderson PK, Svendsen aj, Mortensen K. Increasing incidence of early onset type I (insulin-dependent) diabetes mellitus: a study of Danish male birth cohorts. *Diabetologia.* 1992; 35:178–182.
58. Soltesz G, Madacsy L, Bekefi D, Danko I, the Hungarian Childhood Diabetes Epidemiology Group. Rising incidence of type 1 diabetes in Hungarian children (1978–1987). *Diabetic Med.* 1989; 7:111–114.
59. Tuomilehto J, Rewers M, Reunanen A, et al. Increasing trend in type I (insulin-

dependent) diabetes mellitus in childhood in Finland: analysis of age, calendar time, and birth cohort effects during 1965 to 1984. *Diabetologia.* 1991; 34:282–287.
60. Drykoningen CEM, Mulder ALM, Vaandrager GJ. LaPorte RE, Bruining GJ. The incidence of male childhood type 1 (insulin-dependent)diabetes mellitus is rising rapidly in the Netherlands. *Diabetologia.* 1992; 35:139–142.
61. Nystrom L, Dahlquist G, Rewers M, Wall S. The Swedish childhood diabetes study: an analysis of the temporal variation in diabetes incidence, 1978–1987. *Int J Epidemiol.* 1990; 19:141–146.
62. Rewers M, LaPorte RE, Walczak M, Dimochowski K, Bogaczynska E. Apparent epidemic of insulin-dependent diabetes mellitus in midwestern Poland. *Diabetes.* 1987; 36:106–113.
63. Elliott RB, Pilcher C, Edgar BW. Geographic IDDM in Polynesia and Macronesia: the epidemiology of insulin dependent diabetes in Polynesian children born and reared in Polynesia, compared with Polynesian children resident in Auckland, New Zealand. Diabetes in the Young Bulletin (Proceedings of the ISGD) 1989; 20:16. (Abstract).
64. Bodansky HJ, Staines A, Stephenson C, Haigh D, Cartwright R. Evidence for an environmental effect in the aetiology of insulin dependent diabetes in a transmigratory population. *Br Med J.* 1992; 304:1020–1022.
65. Dahlquist G, Blom L, Holmgren G, et al. The epidemiology of diabetes in Swedish children 0–14 years-a six year prospective study. *Diabetologia.* 1985; 28:802–808.
66. Kostraba JN, Gay EC, Cai Y, et al. Incidence of insulin-dependent diabetes mellitus in Colorado. *Epidemiology.* 1992; 3:232–238.
67. Verge CF, Silink M, Howard NJ. The incidence of childhood IDDM in New South Wales, Australia. *Diabetes Care.* 1994; 17:693–696.
68. Menser MA, Forrest JM, Bransby RD. Rubella infection and diabetes mellitus. *Lancet.* 1978; 1:57–60.
69. Rubinstein P, Walker ME, Fedun B, Witt ME, Cooper LZ, Ginsberg-Fellner F. The HLA system in congenital rubella patients with and without diabetes. *Diabetes.* 1982; 31:1088–1091.
70. Clarke WL, Shaver KA, Bright GA, Rogal AD, Nance WE. Autoimmunity in congenital rubella syndrome. *J Pediatr.* 1984; 104:370–373.
71. Yoon JW, Austin M, Onodera T, Notkins AL. Virus-induced diabetes mellitus: isolation of a virus from the pancreas of a child with diabetic ketoacidosis. *N Engl J Med.* 1979; 300:1173–1179.
72. Tuvemo T, Dahlquist G, Frisk G, et al. The Swedish childhood diabetes study III: IgM against coxsackie B viruses in newly diagnosed type 1 (insulin-dependent) diabetic children-no evidence of increased antibody frequency. *Diabetologia.* 1989; 32:745–747.
73. Kaufman DL, Erlander MG, Clare-Salzler M, Atkinson MA, Maclaren NK, Tobin AJ. Autoimmunity to two forms of glutamate decarboxylase in insulin-dependent diabetes mellitus. *J Clin Invest.* 1992; 89:283–292.
74. Karounos DG, Simmerman L, Hickman SL, Jacob RJ. Identification of the p52-rubella related autoantigen as an insulin secretory granule protein. *Diabetes.* 1993; 42(Suppl. 1):221A. (Abstract).
75. Japan IDDM Epidemiology Study Group. Lack of regional variation in IDDM risk in Japan. *Diabetes Care.* 1993; 16:796–800.
76. Like AA, Guberski DL, Butler L. Influence of environmental viral agents on frequency and tempo of diabetes mellitus in BB/Wor rats. *Diabetes.* 1991; 40:259–262.

77. Wilbertz S, Partke HJ, Dagnaes-Hansen F, Herberg L. Persistent MHV (mouse hepatitis virus) infection reduces the incidence of diabetes mellitus in nonobese diabetic mice. *Diabetologia.* 1991; 34:2–5.
78. Oldstone MBA. Prevention of type I diabetes in nonobese diabetic mice by virus infection. *Science.* 1988; 239:500–502.
79. Dryberg T, Schwimmbeck PL, Oldstone MBA. Inhibition of diabetes in BB rats by virus infection. *J Clin Invest.* 1988; 81:928–931.
80. Guberski DL, Thomas VA, Shek WR, et al. Induction of type 1 diabetes by Kilham's rat virus in diabetes-resistant BB/Wor rats. *Science.* 1991; 254:1010–1013.
81. Yoon J-W. Role of viruses in the pathogenesis of IDDM. *Ann Med.* 1991; 23:437–445.
82. Yoon J-W, McClintock PR, Bachurski CJ, Longstreth JD, Notkins AL. Virus-induced diabetes mellitus: no evidence for immune mechanisms in the destruction of B cells by the D variant of encephalomyocarditis virus. *Diabetes.* 1985; 34:922–925.
83. Virtanen SM, Rasanen L, Aro A, et al. Infant feeding in Finnish children < 7 yr of age with newly diagnosed IDDM. *Diabetes Care.* 1991; 14:415–417.
84. Virtanen SM, Rasanen L, Aro A, et al. Feeding in infancy and the risk of type 1 diabetes mellitus in Finnish children. *Diabetic Med.* 1992; 9:815–819.
85. Mayer EJ, Hamman RF, Gay EC, Lezotte DC, Savitz DA, Klingensmith GJ. Reduced risk of IDDM among breast-fed children: The Colorado IDDM registry. *Diabetes.* 1988; 37:1625–1632.
86. Verge CF, Howard NJ, Irwig L, Simpson JM, Silink M. Environmental factors in childhood IDDM: a population-based case-control study. *Diabetes Care.* 1994 (in press).
87. Kyvik KO, Green A, Svendsen A, Mortensen K. Breast feeding and the development of type 1 diabetes mellitus. *Diabetic Med.* 1991; 9:233–235.
88. Gerstein HC. Cow's milk exposure and type I diabetes mellitus: a critical overview of the clinical literature. *Diabetes Care.* 1994; 17:13–19.
89. Johansson C, Samuelsson U, Ludvigsson J. A high weight gain early in life is associated with an increased risk of type I (insulin-dependent) diabetes mellitus. *Diabetologia.* 1994; 37:91–94.
90. Karjalainen J, Martin JM, Knip M, et al. A bovine albumin peptide as a possible trigger of insulin-dependent diabetes mellitus. *N Engl J Med.* 1992; 327:302–307.
91. Salilahti E, Akerblom HK, Tainio V-M, Koskimies S. Children with newly diagnosed insulin-dependent diabetes mellitus have increased levels of cow's milk antibodies. *Diabetes Res.* 1988; 7:137–140.
92. Yokota A, Yamaguchi Y, Ueda Y, et al. Comparison of islet cell antibodies, islet cell surface antibodies and anti-bovine serum albumin antibodies in type 1 diabetes. *Diabetes Res Clin Pract.* 1990; 9:211–217.
93. Pocecco M, Nicoloso F, Tonini G, Presani G, Marinoni S. Increases levels of cow's milk antibodies in children with newly diagnosed insulin-dependent diabetes mellitus (IDDM). *Horm Res.* 1991; 35:67. (Abstract).
94. Dahlquist G, Savilahti E, Landin-Olsson M. An increased level of antibodies to β-lactoglobulin is a risk determinant for early-onset type 1 (insulin-dependent) diabetes mellitus independent of islet cell antibodies and early introduction of cow's milk. *Diabetologia.* 1992; 35:980–984.
95. Karjalainen J, Saukkonen T, Savilahti E, Dosch HM. Disease-associated anti-bovine serum albumin antibodies in type 1 (insulin-dependent) diabetes

mellitus are detected by particle concentration fluoroimmunoassay, and not by enzyme linked immunoassay. *Diabetologia.* 1992; 35:985–990.

96. Karjalainen J, Cheung R, VanderMeulen J, Martin JM, Knip M. T-cell proliferation response against bovine albumin (BSA) follows the natural course and is restricted to the linear ABBOS sequence in insulin-dependent diabetes mellitus (IDDM). *Autoimmunity.* 1993; 15(suppl):62. (Abstract).
97. Atkinson MA, Bowman MA, Kao K-J, et al. Lack of immune responsiveness to bovine serum albumin in insulin-dependent diabetes. *N Engl J Med.* 1993; 329:1853–1858.
98. Elliott RB, Martin JM. Dietary protein: a trigger of insulin-dependent diabetes in the BB rat? *Diabetologia.* 1984; 26:297–299.
99. Daneman D, Fishman L, Clarson C, Martin JM. Dietary triggers of insulin-dependent diabetes in the BB rat. *Diabetes Res.* 1987; 5:93–97.
100. Coleman DL, Kuzava JE, Leiter EH. Effect of diet on incidence of diabetes in nonobese diabetic mice. *Diabetes.* 1990; 39:432–436.
101. Elliott RB, Reddy SN, Bibby NJ, Kida K. Dietary prevention of diabetes in the nonobese diabetic mouse. *Diabetologia.* 1988; 31:62–64.
102. Akerblom HK, Paganus A, Teramo k, et al. Primary prevention of type 1 diabetes by nutritional intervention: description of a pilot study. *Autoimmunity.* 1993; 15(suppl):58. (Abstract).
103. Srikanta S, Ganda OP, Gleason RE, Jackson RA, Soeldner JS, Eisenbarth GS. Pre-type I diabetes: linear loss of beta cell response to intravenous glucose. *Diabetes.* 1984; 33:717–720.
104. Eisenbarth GS. Type I diabetes mellitus: a chronic autoimmune disease. *N Engl J Med.* 1986; 314:1360–1368.
105. Bleich D, Jackson RA, Soeldner JS, Eisenbarth GS. Analysis of metabolic progression to type I diabetes in islet cell antibody positive relatives of patients with type I diabetes. *Diabetes Care.* 1990; 13:111–118.
106. McCulloch DK, Klaff LJ, Kahn SE, et al. Nonprogression of subclinical B-cell dysfunction among first degree relatives of IDDM patients: 5 year follow-up of the Seattle family study. *Diabetes.* 1990; 39:549–556.
107. Beer SF, Heaton DA, Alberti G, Pyke DA, Leslie RDG. Impaired glucose tolerance precedes but does not predict insulin-dependent diabetes mellitus: a study of identical twins. *Diabetologia.* 1990; 33:497–502.
108. Kobayashi T, Itoh T, Kosaka K Sato K Tsuji K. Time course of islet cell antibodies and beta cell function in non-insulin dependent stage of type I diabetes. *Diabetes.* 1987; 36:510–517.
109. Tunbridge WMG, Brewis M, French JM, et al. Natural history of autoimmune thyroiditis. *Br Med J.* 1981; 282:258–262.
110. Spencer KM, Dean BM, Tarn A, Lister J, Bottazzo GF. Fluctuating islet-cell autoimmunity in unaffected relatives of patients with insulin-dependent diabetes. *Lancet.* 1984; 1:764–766.
111. Chase HP, Voss MA, Butler-Simon N, Hoops S, O'Brien D, Doberson MJ. Diagnosis of pre-type I diabetes. *J Pediatr.* 1987; 111:807–812.
112. Thivolet C, Beaufrere B, Betuel H, et al. Islet cell and insulin antibodies in subjects at high risk for development of type I (insulin-dependent) diabetes in first degree relatives of diabetic patients. *Diabetologia.* 1991; 34:186–191.
113. Thivolet C, Beaufrere B, Geburher L, Chatelain P, Orgiazzi J, Francois R. Autoantibodies and genetic factors associated with the development of type 1

(insulin-dependent) diabetes in first degree relatives of diabetic patients. *Diabetologia.* 1991; 34:186–191.
114. Millward BA, Alviggi L, Hoskins PJ, et al. Immune changes associated with insulin-dependent diabetes may remit without causing the disease: a study in identical twins. *Br Med J.* 1986; 292:793–796.
115. Helmke K, Otten A, Willems WR, et al. Islet cell antibodies and the development of diabetes mellitus in relation to mumps infection and mumps vaccination. *Diabetologia.* 1986; 29:30–33.
116. Landin-Olsson M, Karlsson A, Dahlquist G, et al. Islet cell and other organ-specific autoantibodies in all children developing type 1 (insulin-dependent) diabetes mellitus in Sweden during one year and in matched control children. *Diabetologia.* 1989; 32:387–395.
117. Karjalainen JK. Islet cell antibodies as predictive markers for IDDM in children with high background incidence of disease. *Diabetes.* 1990; 39:1144–1150.
118. Levy-Marchal C, Tichet J, Farjardy I, Gu XF, Dubois F, Czernichow P. Islet cell antibodies in normal French schoolchildren. *Diabetologia.* 1992; 35:577–582.
119. Landin-Olsson M. Precision of the islet-cell antibody assay depends on the pancreas. *J Clin Lab Anal.* 1990; 4:289–294.
120. Carel JC, Boitard C, Bougneres PF. Decreased insulin response to glucose in islet cell antibody-negative siblings of type 1 diabetic children. *J Clin Invest.* 1993; 92:509–513.
121. Pilcher CC, Elliott RB. A senstive and reproducible method for the assay of human islet cell antibodies. *J Immunol Methods.* 1990; 129:111–117.
122. Yu L, Gianani R. High prevalence of GAD autoantibody (GAA) in first degree relatives less than age 10 (Abstract, 1994 ADA meeting). *Diabetes.* (in press).
123. Santiago JV. Insulin therapy in the last decade. *Diabetes Care.* 1993; 16(suppl 3):143–154.
124. McCulloch DK, Koerker DJ, Kahn SE, Bonner-Weir S, Palmer JP. Correlations of in vivo beta-cell function tests with beta-cell mass and pancreatic insulin content in streptozocin-treated baboons. *Diabetes.* 1991; 40:673–679.
125. Allen HF, Jeffers BW, Klingensmith GJ, Chase HP. First-phase insulin release in normal children. *J Pediatr.* 1993; 123:733–738.
126. Arslanian S, Austin A. Determinants of first and second phase insulin secretion in healthy adolescents. *Pediatr Res.* 1993; 3(suppl):S74. Abstract.
127. Cutfield WS, Bergman RN, Menon RK, Sperling MA. The modified minimal model: application to measurement of insulin sensitivity in children. *J Clin Endocrinol Metab.* 1990; 70:1644–1650.
128. Smith CP, Williams AJK, Thomas JM, et al. The pattern of basal and stimulated insulin responses to intravenous glucose in first degree relatives of type I (insulin-dependent) diabetic children and unrelated adults aged 5 to 50 years. *Diabetologia.* 1988; 31:430–434.
129. Colman PG, Stewart V, Kean J, et al. Comparison of two commonly used standard IVGTTs. *Diabetes Care.* 1992; 15:1053–1055.
130. Bingley PJ, Colman P, Eisenbarth GS, et al. Standardization of IVGTT to predict IDDM. *Diabetes Care.* 1992; 15:1313–1316.
131. Rayman G, Clark P, Schneider AE, Hales CN. The first-phase insulin response to intravenous glucose is highly reproducible. *Diabetologia.* 1990; 33:631–634.
132. Smith PJ, Tarn AC, Thomas JM, et al. Between and within subject variation of the first phase insulin response to intravenous glucose. *Diabetologia.* 1988; 31:123–125.

133. McNair PD, Colman PG, Alford FP, Harrison LC. Reproducibility of the first phase insulin response (FPIR) in the intravenous glucose tolerance test (IVGTT) is not improved by retrograde cannulation and arterialisation or by the use of a lower glucose dose. *Autoimmunity.* 1993; 15(suppl):62. Abstract.

134. Rowe RE, Leech NJ, McCulloch DK. Does drawing blood from a retrogradely cannulated hand vein improve reproducibility in the intravenous glucose tolerance test (IVGTT)? *Autoimmunity.* 1993; 15(suppl):79. Abstract.

135. Leech NJ, Rowe RE, Bucksa J, McCulloch DK. HbA1c may be an early indicator of islet cell dysfunction. *Autoimmunity.* 1993; 15(suppl):75. Abstract.

136. Signore A, Chianelli M, Ferretti E, Multari G, Andreani D, Pozzilli P. New tools for imaging insulitis in pre diabetes. *Autoimmunity.* 1993; 15(suppl):64. Abstract.

137. Yuh WTC, Wiese JA, Abu-Yousef MM, et al. Pancreatic transplant imaging. *Radiology.* 1988; 167:679–683.

138. Kelcz F, Sollinger HW, Pirsch JF. MRI of the pancreas transplant: lack of correlation between imaging and clinical status. *Mag Res Med.* 1991; 21:30–38.

139. del Pilar Fernandez M, Bernardino ME, Neylan JF, Olson RA. Diagnosis of pancreatic transplant dysfunction: value of gadopentetate dimeglumine-enhanced MR imaging. *AJR.* 1991; 156:1171–1176.

140. Hanafusa T, Miyazaki A, Miyagawa J, et al. Examination of islets in the pancreas biopsy specimens from newly diagnosed type I (insulin-dependent) diabetic patients. *Diabetologia.* 1990; 33:105–111.

141. Martin S, Pawlowski B, Greulich B, Ziegler AG, Mandrup-Poulsen T, Mahon J. Natural course of remission in IDDM during 1st yr after diagnosis. *Diabetes Care.* 1992; 15:66–73.

142. Schiffrin A, Suissa S, Weitzner G, Poussier P, Lalla D. Factors predicting course of β-cell function in IDDM. *Diabetes Care.* 1992; 15:997–1001.

143. Knip M, Ilonen J, Mustonen A, Akerblom HK. Evidence for an accelerated B-cell destruction in HLA-Dw3/Dw4 heterozygous children with type I (insulin-dependent) diabetes. *Diabetologia.* 1986; 29:347–351.

144. Baisch JM, Weeks T, Giles R, Hoover M, Stastny P, Capra JD. Analysis of HLA-DQ genotypes and susceptibility in insulin-dependent diabetes mellitus. *N Engl J Med.* 1990; 322:1836–1841.

145. Erlich HA, Griffith RL, Bugawan TL, Ziegler R, Alper C, Eisenbarth GS. Implication of specific DQB1 alleles in genetic susceptibility and resistance by identification of IDDM siblings with novel HLA-DQB1 allele and unusual DR2 and DR1 haplotypes. *Diabetes.* 1991; 40:478–481.

146. Karasik A, O'Hara C, Srikanta S, et al. Genetically programmed selective islet beta-cell loss in diabetic subjects with Wolfram syndrome. *Diabetes Care.* 1989; 12:135–138.

147. Kadowaki T, Kadowaki H, Mori Y, et al. A subtype of diabetes mellitus associated with a mutation of mitochondrial DNA. *N Engl J Med.* 1994; 330:962–968.

148. Bowden DW, Gravius TC, Akots G, Fajans SS. Identification of genetic markers flanking the locus for maturity-onset diabetes of the young on human chromosome 20. *Diabetes.* 1992; 41:88–92.

149. Froguel P, Zouali H, Vionnet N, et al. Familial hyperglycemia due to mutations in glucokinase: definition of a subtype of diabetes mellitus. *N Engl J Med.* 1993; 328:697–702.

150. Verge CF, Gianani R, Yu L, et al. Prediction of type I diabetes in first degree relatives using a combination of antibodies against defined autoantigens (insulin, GAD65 and ICA512). *Pediatr Res.* 1995; 37:110A. Abstract.

151. Herskowitz-Dumont R, Wolfsdorf JI, Jackson RA, Eisenbarth GS. Distinction between transient hyperglycemia and early insulin-dependent diabetes mellitus in childhood: a prospective study of incidence and prognostic factors. *J Pediatr.* 1993; 123:347–354.
152. Notsu K, Oka N, Note S, Nabeya N, Kuno S, Sakurami T. Islet cell antibodies in the Japanese population and in subjects with type I (insulin-dependent) diabetes. *Diabetologia.* 1985; 28:660–662.
153. Boehm BO, Manfras B, Seissler J, et al. Epidemiology and immunogenetic background of islet cell antibody positive nondiabetic schoolchildren: Ulm-Frankfurt population study. *Diabetes.* 1991; 40:1435–1439.
154. Diabetes Epidemiology Research International Group. Geographic patterns of childhood insulin-dependent diabetes mellitus. *Diabetes.* 1988; 37:1113–1119.
155. Levy-Marchal C, Papoz L, DeBeaufort C, et al. Incidence of juvenile type 1 (insulin-dependent) diabetes mellitus in France. *Diabetologia.* 1990; 33:465–469.
156. Bruning GJ, Grobbee DE, Scheffer GJ, et al. Ten year follow-up study of islet cell antibodies and childhood diabetes mellitus. *Lancet.* 1989; 1:1100–1103.
157. Green A, Gale EAM, Patterson CC, for the Eurodiab ACE Study Group. Incidence of childhood-onset insulin-dependent diabetes mellitus: the Eurodiab ACE study. *Lancet.* 1992; 339:905–909.
158. Bergua M, Sole J, Marion G, et al. Prevalence of islet cell antibodies, insulin antibodies and hyperglycemia in 2291 school children. *Diabetologia.* 1987; 30:724–726.
159. Serrano Rios M, Moy CS, Martin Serrano R, et al. Incidence of type 1 (insulin-dependent) diabetes mellitus in subjects 0–14 years of age in the Comunidad of Madrid, Spain. *Diabetologia.* 1990; 33:422–424.
160. Elliott RB, Pilcher CC, McGregor MA. Protection from diabetes in normal school children using nicotinamide. *Autoimmunity.* 1993; 15(suppl):57. Abstract.
161. Scott RS, Brown LJ, Darlow BA, Forbes LV, Moore MP. Temporal variation in incidence of IDDM in Canterbury, New Zealand. *Diabetes Care.* 1992; 15:895–899.
162. Rowe RE, Leech NJ, Nepom GT, McCulloch DK. High genetic risk for IDDM in the Pacific Northwest: first report from the Washington State diabetes prediction study. *Diabetes.* 1994; 43:87–94.
163. Dokheel TM, The Pittsburgh Diabetes Epidemiology Research Group. An epidemic of childhood diabetes in the United States? *Diabetes Care.* 1993; 16:1606–1611.
164. Colman PG, McNair PD, Caudwell JP, Howard NJ, Colaguri S, Harrison LC. Screening of an apparent 'hot spot' of IDDM for markers of preclinical IDDM. *Autoimmunity.* 1993; 15(suppl):31. Abstract.
165. Bingley PJ, Gale EAM. Incidence of insulin dependent diabetes in England: a study in the Oxford region, 1985–6. *Br Med J.* 1989; 298:558–560.
166. Landin-Olsson M, Palmer JP, Lernmark A, et al. Predictive value of islet cell and insulin autoantibodies for type I (insulin-dependent) diabetes mellitus in a population-based study of newly-diagnosed diabetic and matched control children. *Diabetologia.* 1992; 35:1068–1073.
167. Tuomilehto J, Lounamaa R, Tuomilehto-Wolf E, et al. Epidemiology of childhood diabetes mellitus in Finland—background of a nationwide study of type 1 (insulin-dependent) diabetes mellitus. *Diabetologia.* 1992; 35:70–76.
168. Verge CF, Gianani R, Yu L, et al. Late progression to diabetes and evidence for

chronic beta cell autoimmunity in identical twins of patients with type I diabetes. *Diabetes.* 1995 (in press).

169. Pugliese A, Moromisato R, Awdeh Z, et al. HLA-DQB1*0602 is associated with dominant protection from diabetes even among islet cell antibody positive first degree relatives of patients with insulin-dependent diabetes. *Diabetes.* 1995; 44:608–613.

12

Clinical Trials for the Prevention of Type I Diabetes

H. Peter Chase
Anthony R. Hayward

The real issues for strategies to prevent type I diabetes are the anticipated duration of the prophylaxis, the effectiveness of prophylaxis, the toxicity of treatment, and the complexity of the treatment regimen. If, as seems likely in man, the propensity to develop insulin-dependent diabetes mellitus (IDDM) is lifelong, then young people at risk for the disease will have to be treated for many decades. If disease susceptibility, on the other hand, depends on specific environmental factors, then prophylaxis might be tailored to match these circumstances. Longstanding evidence that the complications of diabetes are delayed by good control has recently been confirmed by the Diabetes Control and Complications Trial. This means that the benefits, inconveniences, and toxicity of diabetes prophylaxis have to be weighed against the potential for good control. These are likely to be related issues, because adherence to a prophylactic regimen may well require the same degree of commitment (or compliance) as does maintaining a good glycosylated hemoglobin level using existing treatments for a person with diabetes. If this is the case, then the majority of patients may fail to benefit from a prophylaxis approach, just as they fail to achieve good control with available treatments. Faced with this dilemma, a rational approach would be to determine how effectively diabetes can be prevented. There are no secure data in humans yet, while there is a superfluity of data from animal models. The problem with these results, which are reviewed in the next section, is the ease with which it is possible to prevent diabetes in non-obese diabetic (NOD) mice and BioBreeding (BB) rats. The likelihood that interventions that work in rodents may not work in man must be borne in mind.

Animal Models for IDDM Prevention

In both BB rats and NOD mice, pancreatic beta cells are destroyed by immunological mechanisms. The strengths of these models for human IDDM are discussed in Chapter 3 and extend to the characterization of several genetic predisposing factors and to the identification of pathogenic T cell clones. The weaknesses of the animal models stem mainly from our ignorance of the mechanisms by which autoimmunity is triggered or sustained in the experimental animals or, for that matter, in man. Both animal strains have been bred to maximize their incidence of diabetes and, in addition, most laboratories house their animals under conditions that yield the highest number of diabetics. Nevertheless, some 20% of female NOD mice escape even under "optimal" diabetogenic conditions. Whether the environmental factors that operate to protect these mice have parallels in humans is unknown. This ignorance limits the conclusions that can be drawn from the diverse interventions that prevent IDDM in experimental models. With this caveat, the general approaches that have proved effective in animals are summarized in Table 12.1.

Clinical Trials for the Prevention of Type I Diabetes

The recognition of insulin-dependent (type I) diabetes mellitus as an immunological disease led to the first controlled trials of intervention using nonspecific immunosuppressive treatments in subjects already diagnosed with diabetes. Cyclosporin A (CyA) and prednisone-azathioprine were tried initially because they had been effective in animals. These early trials were important because they showed that insulin dependency could be delayed for a period while immunosuppression was maintained. They also showed that the natural history of IDDM progression was reinstituted following withdrawal of immunosuppression.

Trials of prophylaxis in individuals with recent-onset diabetes are based on the view that beta cell destruction is a gradual process and that an intercurrent stress precipitates symptoms (and loss of glucose homeostasis) before all insulin-making potential is lost. Unfortunately, 90 percent of islets have already been destroyed by the time diabetes is diagnosed.[1] Thus, the best possible outcome of trials in people who already have diabetes is prolonging the time when small amounts of insulin continue to be made, rather than prevention of diabetes. Benefit to the subject under these circumstances might come not from discontinuing insulin shots but from simplifying daily blood glucose control, lowering glycosylated hemoglobin levels, and reducing the risk for diabetes complications. Benefit of this type is conjectural and is unlikely to appeal to recent-onset diabetics unless the preventive regimen is simple and safe.

A different approach for prophylaxis trials is to concentrate on individuals identified as prediabetic by the criteria described below. The best possible

Table 12.1. Interventions Preventing IDDM in Animal Models

Strategy	*Specificity*	*Animal*	*Conclusion*
Immune suppression	None	NOD & BB	Nonspecific suppression of cell-mediated immunity (eg, with cyclosporin or rapamycin) prevents IDDM in these animals, but the degree of immunosuppression required would be unacceptable for long-term human treatments.[47–50]
	CD4 cells	NOD	CD4 depletion prevents IDDM at least transiently. Nondepleting CD4 antibody may have a longer action, as has been found in transplantation.[51]
Transplantation	None	NOD & BB	Mice that receive grafts of marrow, dendritic cells, fetal liver,[52] and thymus[53,54] are spared.
Immune stimulation	None	NOD	Interventions that activate T cells, ranging from injection of monoclonal antibodies[55] or even attenuated myco bacterial organisms,[5,56] may have this effect.
Oral tolerance	Insulin	NOD	Mice fed insulin have been shown to have delayed or reduced onset of diabetes.[46]
Other diets and nutritional therapies	None	NOD	These diets can be divided into those with a hypothesized mechanism, such as radical scavenging, and those that are nutritionally special.[57–65]
Cytokines		NOD	These agents alter levels or activities of interleukins.[66–68]
Hormones	Unknown	NOD	Hormones may have numerous effects.[69,70]

NOD = nonobese diabetic mouse
BB = BioBreeding rat

outcome in prediabetic individuals (whose glucose homeostasis is not so impaired so as to make them symptomatic) would be the maintenance of insulin production and a life free of insulin replacement. Ascertainment of individuals with a high likelihood of developing diabetes is currently by screening first-degree relatives of affected individuals. The yield, about 4.3% of those screened, is very small in relation to the number of individuals developing type I diabetes per year. Prevention trials in recent-onset cases are therefore likely to continue to be important until better screening methods, applicable to entire populations, are developed.

Trials in Newly Diagnosed Subjects

Cyclosporin A

Two methods of prolonging insulin production have been successful to date. The first was the administration of CyA.[2,3] The effects of this agent were greatest when started within 6 weeks of initiation of insulin therapy, and the treatment had to be continued for at least 6 months and, preferably, for 1 year to show benefit. Unfortunately, the effects of CyA on T cells are lost when the CyA is discontinued. As CyA is nephrotoxic, it has been concluded[3] "that additional studies with CyA alone, in subjects with newly diagnosed IDDM, are no longer warranted." Despite this rather negative conclusion, the impact of the trials with CyA should not be underestimated. The initial promise of immunosuppression as a means to prevent diabetes stimulated interest in the early diagnosis of diabetes and led, ultimately, to screening approaches by which prediabetes could be recognized. The fact that some participants in the trials could maintain glycosylated hemoglobin (HbA1) levels in the normal range for months while on CyA showed for the first time that the destruction of beta cells could be slowed even if not halted. A major limitation of CyA therapy in new-onset diabetic patients is the relapse to hyperglycemia within 3 years even if CyA was continued. Relapses occurred despite the maintenance of C peptide secretion. This suggested the relapses resulted from insufficient beta cell mass at the initiation of therapy rather than ineffective immunosuppression. The trials also stimulated awareness of the cost/benefit ratio of interventions to prevent diabetes. The costs in the context of CyA were high, as the drug is expensive, and even with careful and expensive monitoring of blood levels, renal damage still occurred. Thus the costs were felt to outweigh the benefits.

Biostater

The second method to prolong endogenous insulin production is to infuse exogenous insulin to control blood glucose levels tightly with the Biostator machine.[4] Although Biostator machines are no longer commercially available, the stress of keeping the patient constantly in bed for 14 days with large needles in place would probably have prevented widespread acceptance of this treatment.

Immunostimulation. A third approach to prolonging insulin production in the newly diagnosed diabetic is through immunostimulation. This strategy is based on the lower incidence of diabetes in NOD mice stimulated immunologically with agents as diverse as allogeneic cells or bacillus Calmette-Guérin (BCG).[5] The mechanism for the protection is not clear, though stimulation and expansion of populations of T cells making IL4 or IL10 has been suggested.[5] In the absence of evidence linking BCG antigens with those expressed on the islet cell surface, the mechanism of action may well be immunologically nonspecific. We are currently exploring the possibility that immune stimulation after the onset of diabetes might reduce insulin requirements or increase C peptide synthesis when measured 1 year after vaccination with the attenuated mycobaterium, BCG. Vaccination with BCG is already known to be safe and immunogenic, and a preliminary human study gave some evidence for benefit.[6] On the basis of this result, we are pursing a double-blind study employing two medical teams, one to manage the diabetes and one to give and read the BCG and placebo vaccines. Entry is restricted to subjects within 8 weeks of clinical onset, or within 16 weeks if the islet cell antibody (ICA) test is positive, who are between ages 5 and 18 years and who have negative human immunodeficiency virus (HIV) and purified protein derivative (tuberculin) (PPD) tests. The result of this randomized placebo-controlled trial will be known late in 1996.

Treatments to halt islet cell destruction and prevent diabetes would ideally be started before the beta cell mass is significantly compromised. Nevertheless, detecting partial benefit in recent-onset diabetics would be useful if it pointed to an intervention that could be used with greater efficiency in subjects with pre–type I diabetes. Ultimately the focus of the prevention of diabetes must be in patients with pre–type I diabetes (hereafter referred to as prediabetes), and the remainder of this chapter reviews progress that is being made towards this goal.

Identification of Subjects with Pre-Type I Diabetes

Prediabetes describes the period when islet cell destruction is in progress but glucose homeostasis has not been lost. The best definition of prediabetes is an individual actually followed to the development of diabetes. Subjects are currently identified as being at high risk by the sequence of events summarized below:

1. They are ascertained by their relationship to a diabetic individual (usually a first-degree relative).
2. Their serum has tested positive for immunological markers of islet-specific immunity (the presence of antibodies associated with islet beta cells).
3. Their first-phase insulin production (see Metabolic Testing, below) is low enough to give at least a 50% risk for diabetes within the next 5 years.

These selection criteria in effect reproduce two of the factors thought to be important in the etiology of type I diabetes: genetic predisposition and the development of autoimmunity. The outcome of trials currently being started in high-risk individuals (to be referred to as prediabetics) are likely to influence treatment strategies for a decade, so it is worth considering the strengths and weaknesses of the selection criteria in detail.

Genetics

MHC Genes. When one pair of identical twins develops type I diabetes, the second twin has a 30–50% risk of also developing diabetes (see Chapter 7). The finding that fewer than 100% of second twins become diabetic suggests that additional factors, probably environmental, contribute to the pathogenesis of type I diabetes. Similarly, a higher risk for diabetes was shown for siblings (approximately a 5% risk) or for offspring when the father had diabetes (approximately 12% risk) or when the mother had diabetes (approximately a 6% risk).[7] The strongest genetic associations are with the human leukocyte antigen (HLA) system. Approximately 95% of people with type I diabetes have either DR3 or DR4 (compared to 50% of the general population), and 53% have the DR3, 4 combination (compared to 6% of the general population).[8] An 8-year prospective study[9] found a 70% risk for developing diabetes in ICA-positive siblings with DR3, 4, compared with a 37% risk in ICA-positive siblings who were negative for DR3, 4.

Much of the contribution from HLA DR4 stems from linkage with an HLA DQ antigen, 0302. This allele lacks aspartic acid at position 57 of the DQB chain (Asp-negativity) and increases the risk for type I diabetes.[10,11] In Finland, Asp-negativity was found in 74.5% of patients with type I diabetes compared to 18% of controls.[12] Other HLA antigens are also associated with a very low incidence of diabetes (see Chapter 7). Thus, genetic screening is likely to play an important part in identifying subjects who could be enrolled in prevention trials. The present generation of trials will enroll high-risk individuals identified among first-degree relatives of index cases. Because 70–90% of patients have no first-degree relative with diabetes,[13] this creates a potential for significant ascertainment bias. For example, first-degree relatives of diabetics presenting in infancy are likely to be underrepresented merely because family sizes are small and parents may be discouraged from having more children where the first has a time-consuming and emotionally demanding condition. First-degree relatives of parents who developed diabetes after 40 years of age may be overrepresented merely because family size will not have been limited in response to parental disease. How important these sources of bias are will depend on the diversity of genes contributing to disease susceptibility.

Non-MHC Genes. Animal studies indicate that at least two and perhaps as many as five different genes contribute to susceptibility to diabetes. An advantage to identifying prediabetics by screening first-degree relatives is that selection for non-HLA genes is likely to occur in parallel. The development of multiple markers for polymorphisms on each human chromosome is making the identification of non-MHC genes predisposing to diabetes possible, so that screening of the general population will be possible in the long term. Until this is possible it is likely that identifying prediabetics by kinship is the only feasible approach.

As more genetic markers associated with susceptibility and protection are identified it will be important to apply them retrospectively to the prevention protocols where high-risk people are initially identified with immunological tests. For example, if immunological and metabolic tests indicate a high risk for diabetes and the subject is entered into a prevention protocol, it will be important to make sure that relevant genes are similarly divided in numbers of subjects with HLA/DR3, 4 and DQB Asp-negativity. Cells might also be saved for other markers that may be shown to be good predictors in future years, as this area of research is advancing rapidly.

Immunological

Because the incidence of diabetes in identical twins of type I diabetics is less than 50%, additional selection criteria are needed to identify subjects for prevention studies. Some reports have suggested that the degree of ICA positivity is the best predictor for advancement to insulin dependence.[14–16]

Others consider ICA positivity only to be an indicator that damage has occurred to the islet, and insist that a metabolic test (see below) be done to determine the amount of damage. We previously noted that nine of 10 first-degree relatives advancing to diabetes had ICA titers greater than or equal to 80 JDF units, making this a high-risk finding.[17] However, six other first-degree relatives of diabetics had similar titers of ICA but had not advanced to diabetes over a 6-year period. Thus, the high titer result might have high specificity, but poor predictive value (10 of 16 subjects). Also, subjects with lower titers of ICA obviously also develop diabetes, although the percentages are not as high. Bruining and coworkers[18] noted that only four of eight children found to have positive ICAs in a general population (not first-degree relatives) developed diabetes in a 10-year period. Another 3 of 4806 children initially negative for ICA also developed diabetes. Thus, whether screening first-degree relatives or the general population, it would seem that a second test, more specific for quantity of damage, would be important.

ICA assays are difficult to quantitate and this leads to interlaboratory differences. Factors that are likely to limit the reproducibility of the assay between laboratories include (1) the quality of the human pancreas chosen for the assay and (2) interobserver differences for a subjective endpoint. Nevertheless, the Third International Workshop on ICA concluded, "The indirect immunofluorescent (IFL) test for ICA is still the most useful screen for identifying people at risk for Type I diabetes, and, until such time as the relevant antigens are identified and purified in large quantities, it remains the method of choice for its detection".[19]

More recently, other antibodies have been identified in the blood of newly diagnosed subjects (and pre–type I subjects). These include autoantibodies to insulin (IAA),[20–22] glutamic acid decarboxylase (GAD),[23–25] and ICA69.[26] Although some increase in risk has been shown for people who have two positive antibody tests rather than just one,[22] none of these additional tests has significantly increased the accuracy of detecting prediabetes in first-degree relatives of index cases compared with the use of the ICA test alone. Testing for multiple autoantibodies may be more important for screening populations not confined to first-degree relatives; only large-scale (and ideally prospective) studies are likely to decide this issue. The methodology for most of these tests is currently being refined so they will be suited for transfer to routine laboratories. Most researchers in this area hope that the widely used ICA test can be replaced in the 1990s by more quantitative endpoints.

Metabolic Testing

The interval between finding an autoantibody in a first-degree relative of a diabetic and the development of diabetes can exceed 10 years. Prospective studies where the success of an intervention will not be known for more than 10 years are clearly not practical, so a further selection for subjects with extensive beta cell destruction is usual. Direct measurement of the functional mass of islet cells is not possible and the best approximation comes from the intravenous glucose tolerance test (IVGTT). Srikanta and coworkers[27] were the first to show that the sum of the 1- and 3-minute insulin levels had some predictive value. Our own experience confirmed the predictive value of a very low first-phase insulin response (FPIR) on IVGTT (<25 μU/ml) in children.[28] A later report[17] noted predictability for different levels of FPIR in first-degree relatives under age 18 years who had two or more positive ICA tests (Table 12.2). Vardi and coworkers[29] found 15 of 17 (88%) ICA-positive first-degree relatives to develop insulin dependence if their FPIR fell to <48 μU/ml (the first percentile at the Joslin Diabetes Center). In contrast, only 3 of 18 (17%) with values above this level developed insulin dependence.

Little is known about the replicate errors, either within subject or between subjects, of the IVGTT. The test needs to be performed with the utmost accuracy in timing and consistency.[30,31] It should be performed after an overnight fast of uniform duration. Some people vary in their response and the downward progression of the FPIR is not always linear.[28] Finally, the results are age-dependent, particularly in prepubertal versus pubertal children.[32] Despite the problems listed above, the FPIR test is of value in predicting time to insulin dependence in first-degree relatives of diabetics who are ICA positive. It will therefore be important to relate the outcomes of diabetes prevention trials with the FPIR level required for the study entry. Comparison between trials with different FPIR entry criteria may prove to be impossible, particularly if the efficacy of different prevention strategies is affected by the amount of damage already sustained by beta cells.

Trials Using Subjects with Pre–Type I Diabetes

A recent NIH consensus report on prevention of type I diabetes concluded: "The general consensus from the meeting was that indeed there is method-

Table 12.2. FPIR* and Time to Diabetes[17]

FPIR* (μU/ml)	Time to diabetes (months)	
	Mean time	95th percentile
< 67	19	57
< 46	14	21
< 30	4.6	18

*FPIR = First phase insulin response (sum of 1-minute + 3-minute insulin levels) on intravenous glucose tolerance testing.

ology that can identify, with near certainty among first-degree relatives of type I diabetic patients, those who will develop diabetes and that immune intervention therapy before the onset of symptoms might prevent the disease from occurring".[33]

It is now generally accepted that prediabetes can be accurately diagnosed in a select high-risk group of subjects. The justification for identifying this high-risk group comes from their potential recruitment into protocols to test strategies to prevent diabetes. These high-risk subjects are, however, so rare that no center is likely to identify more than 20 subjects suitable to enter a prevention trial in any one year. Our own power estimates indicated that high-risk prediabetics (with two ICA tests positive at 40 JDF units and two FPIRS <60 μU/ml) would have to be randomized into control and test groups of 60 subjects each in order to have an 80% chance for detecting a statically significant difference after 3 years. Such sample sizes are a major complication in planning interventions for subjects who are likely to develop diabetes within 3 to 5 years. Identifying prediabetics is very expensive (we estimate $1,200 per subject, allowing for lab tests and two IVGTT tests), so a cost-effective approach requires extensive and international collaboration. The use of the relatively small number of subjects available is also most efficient if trials throughout the world are coordinated to determine if initial pilot trial data can be confirmed. The two pilot trials published to date that show some promise in preventing diabetes in prediabetics used nicotinamide[34] or a combination of intravenous (IV) and subcutaneous insulin.[35] Larger-scale studies of each are now planned.

Nicotinamide

The mechanism of nicotinamide protection is currently unknown. Nicotinamide was initially shown to prevent diabetes in NOD mice.[36] Nicotinamide inhibits poly (ADP-ribose) synthetase[37] and, at high concentrations, can act as a free radical scavenger.[38] Pretreatment with nicotinamide prevents the decrease in proinsulin synthesis in islets from rats treated with alloxan or streptozotocin.[37] It also inhibits the activated macrophage killing of beta cells in vitro,[39] and the expression of class 2 major histocompatibility complex (MHC) on beta cells caused by the cytokines, tumor necrosis factor (TNF), and interferon gamma.[40] These are all processes thought to be a part of the immune-mediated destruction of beta cells found in the human disease. A recent workshop report summarizes the biological actions and therapeutic potential of nicotinamide.[41]

A pilot study of nicotinamide was undertaken jointly between Auckland, NZ, and Denver, USA.[34] Among 14 treated subjects, only one developed diabetes after a mean of 17 months of treatment, whereas eight untreated subjects were all insulin-dependent after a mean of 17 months. All subjects were less than 16 years old when diabetes was detected by ICA screening and all had ICA titers equal to or greater than 80 JDF units. All subjects had a FPIR of less than 67 μU/ml (the 5th percentile of normal). On further (unpublished) follow-up of approximately 5 years, 3 of 4 subjects in Denver (all of who had a FPIR <30 μU/ml) and 5 of 10 Auckland subjects (most with the higher FPIR levels) had become insulin dependent. This pilot trial was weakened by the fact that all the control subjects were followed in Denver. The result, with 8 of the initial 14 patients being insulin dependent after 5 years, may indicate that nicotinamide merely delays the onset of diabetes rather than achieving a sustainable prevention. Nevertheless, nicotinamide is likely to be harmless, can be taken in pill form, is inexpensive, and can easily be compared to placebo tablets.

Nicotinamide will next be evaluated in a German trial headed by Dr. Hubert Kolb,[42] and in the European Nicotinamide Diabetes Intervention Trial (ENDIT) study under the direction of Dr. Edwin Gale.[43] The German trial is named "DENIS" for Deutsche Nicotinamide Intervention Study. It is a 3-year trial that is similar to the ENDIT study except it involves 74 youths, ages 3 to 12 years at entry, half of whom will receive the nicotinamide and half the placebo. The ENDIT trial will be double blind, randomized, and placebo controlled. Enrollment will be open to the first-degree relatives of patients with type I diabetes (sibling, child, parent) who have at least two ICA-positive tests, one of which is equal to or greater than 20 JDF units, drawn 3–12 months apart. An IVGTT will be performed by the ICARUS protocol[31] and used for the subsequent meta-analysis but not for randomization. An oral glucose tolerance test (OGTT) will be performed as a two-point test (0 min and 2 h capillary blood glucose) to rule out diabetes mellitus by World Health Organization (WHO) criteria.[44] Demographic information will be collected following the example of the ICARUS questionaire. Follow-up procedures will be by yearly FPIR with ICA and IAA tests. C peptide levels or other markers of beta cell function may be tested yearly. The dose of nicotinamide will be 1.2 g/M^2.

There will be joint monitoring of adverse effects. All subjects will have blood work at admission (complete blood count, gamma GT, AST, ALT, serum bilirubin, creatinine, BUN, uric acid) and then repeated at 5 weeks to 3 months after baseline and every 6 months from baseline thereafter. The primary outcome measure will be the incidence of diabetes mellitus by WHO criteria. The OGTT will be done at least once per year.

Insulin

The mechanism by which insulin might delay or prevent diabetes is unknown. It was initially hypothesized that the beta cells were being allowed to "rest" and might therefore be less prone to immunological attack. Whether this view is correct or whether additional mechanisms, such as induction of specific tolerance, contribute remains to be determined. The initial study of insulin in subjects with prediabetes was reported from the Joslin Clinic.[35] Five subjects, ages 7 to 14 years, were treated with 5 days of IV insulin aimed at keeping blood glucose levels between 3.3 and 4.2 mmol/L (60–76 mg/dl). Outpatient daily insulin was divided into two subcutaneous injections consisting of human regular and ultralente insulin in the morning and lente insulin at bedtime. The total dose was approximately 0.2 units/kg body weight per day. The children's lifestyles were not restricted during the outpatient treatment and severe hypoglycemia was not a problem. After a mean of 3.04 years, only one of the five treated subjects was insulin dependent, compared to all seven subjects who had refused the treatment.

The very small number of subjects treated is a weakness of this pilot trail, as was the inclusion of two subjects with FPIR levels of 76 and 83 μU/ml in the treatment arm. The use of subjects who refused treatment as a control group is not ideal and none of the controls had an FPIR above 49 μU/ml. Additional points of concern relate to the difficulty of treatment and the reluctance of ICA-positive parents to enter into the study. Measurement of blood glucose on subjects every 15 to 20 minutes for 5 days while IV insulin is given is a level of intensiveness outside routine care. Nevertheless, a group of investigators in the United States opted to evaluate IV and subcutaneous insulin in a multicenter trial under the auspices of the National Institutes of Health (NIH). The criteria for randomization into this trial are summarized in Table 12.3.

Table 12.3. U.S. Diabetes Prevention Trial (DPT 1) Eligibility Criteria for High-Risk Protocol

First-degree relatives: 4 to 45 years (inclusive)
Second-degree relatives: 4 to 20 years (inclusive)
ICA ≥10 JDF units (2 of 3 times in series)
Not DQA1 0102, DQB1 0602
IVGTT criteria:
A. Siblings and offspring 4 to 45 years (or 2nd-degree relatives 4–20 years):
Age 4–7: <60 μU/ml (sum 1+3 min [2 of 3])
Age ≥8: <100 μU/ml (2 of 3)
B. Parents (≤45 y): <60 μU/ml (2 of 3)
OGTT not diabetic (NDDG adult criteria)

ICA= Islet cell antibodies
IVGTT= Intravenous glucose tolerance test
OGTT= Oral glucose tolerance test
NDDG= National Diabetes Data Group

The insulin prophylaxis study will require approximately 400 subjects (by sample size calculations done three different ways). Half of the subjects will receive IV insulin for 4 days once yearly for 3 to 5 years and 0.125 U/kg body weight of ultralente insulin subcutaneously twice daily. The other half will receive no treatment. There will be 10 centers throughout the United States, and the structure will be similar to that used for the Diabetes Control and Complications Trial. The ICA, insulin, HLA, and IAA tests will be done in single-reference laboratories. The outcome criterion for this trial is a diabetic oral glucose tolerance test by the adult National Diabetes Data Group criteria[45] after discontinuing insulin (in the treated group) for days.

A second study will give insulin by mouth to subjects at lower risk for diabetes. As of this writing, oral insulin has been shown to have an effect in NOD mice,[46] but it has not yet been tested in humans.

Conclusions

The fact that diabetes can be successfully managed, and the development of complications delayed, by good control of blood glucose has placed significant constraints on treatments intended to prevent diabetes. Global immunosuppression protocols, of the type used for transplant recipients, clearly carry an unacceptable morbidity. Immunologists caring for patients with autoimmune diseases have a need to establish organ-specific immunological tolerance that is just as pressing as that facing transplant surgeons. The two approaches that are currently being explored seem very speculative when viewed in relation to the complexity of immunoregulation or the development of autoimmunity. The animal models of type I diabetes should be a fruitful ground for treatments designed to prevent diabetes in humans. In reality it has been difficult to realize this expectation. One obstacle has been the ease with which diabetes is prevented in NOD mice. For example, interventions that have succeeded in mice include special diets, injection with male sex hormones, and even the failure to exclude common mouse viruses from colonies. It is very difficult to judge the cost-effectiveness of preventive strategies in mouse colonies.

With the limitations of animal models in mind, it seems likely that much of the development of prevention approaches will have to be done in humans. Constraints on research funding on both sides of the Atlantic have increased the pressure for collaboration beyond local and national boundaries. In the event that an effective intervention is found, one can only hope that it can be adopted without chauvinistic bias. All in all, the initiation of two large multicenter trials to determine whether type I diabetes can be prevented promises to make this decade an exciting one.

References

1. Gepts W, de May J. Islet cell survival determined by morphology: an immunocytochemical study of the islets of Langerhans in juvenile diabetes mellitus. *Diabetes.* 1978; 27:251–261.
2. Stiller CR, Dupre J, Gent M, Jenner MR, Keown PA, Laupacis A, Martell R, Rodger NW, Graffenried B, Wolfe MJ. Effects of cyclosporine immunosuppression in insulin-dependent diabetes mellitus of recent onset. *Science.* 1984; 223:1362–1367.
3. Chase HP, Butler-Simon N, Garg SK, Hayward A, Klingensmith GJ, Hamman RF, O'Brien D. Cyclosporine A for the treatment of new-onset insulin-dependent diabetes mellitus. *Pediatrics.* 1990; 85:241–245.
4. Shah SC, Malone JI, Simpson NE. A randomized trial of intensive insulin therapy in newly diagnosed insulin-dependent diabetes mellitus. *N Engl J Med.* 1989; 320:550–554.
5. Harada M, Kishimoto Y, Makino S. Prevention of overt diabetes and insulitis in NOD mice by a single BCG vaccination. *Diabetes.* 1990; 8:85–90.
6. Shehadeh N, Calcinaro F, Bradley BJ, Bruchlim I, Vardi P, Lafferty KJ. Effect of adjuvant therapy on development of diabetes in mouse and man. *Lancet.* 1994; 343:706–707.
7. Warram HH, Krolewski AS, Gottlieb MS, Kahn CR. Differences in risk of insulin-dependent diabetes in offspring of diabetic mothers and diabetic fathers. *N Engl J Med.* 1984; 311:149–152.
8. Ludvigsson J, Lindblom B. Human lymphocyte antigen DR types in relation to early clinical manifestations in diabetic children. *Pediatr Res.* 1984; 18:1239–1241.
9. Deschamps I, Boitard C, Hors J, Busson M, Marcelli-Barge A, Mogenet A, Robert JJ. Life table analysis of the risk of type 1 (insulin-dependent) diabetes mellitus in siblings according to islet cell antibodies and HLA markers: an 8 year prospective study. *Diabetalogia.* 1992; 35:951–957.
10. Morel PA, Dorman JS, Todd JA, McDevitt HO, Trucco M. Aspartic acid at position 57 of the HLA-DQ beta chain protects against type I diabetes: a family study. *Proc Natl Acad Sci USA.* 1988; 854:8111–8115.
11. Baisch JM, Weeks T, Giles R, Hoover M, Stastny P, Capra JD. Analysis of HLA-DQ genotypes and susceptibility in insulin-dependent diabetes mellitus. *N Engl J Med.* 1990; 322:1836–1841.
12. Reijonen H, Ilonen J, Knip M, Akerblom H. HLA-DQB1 alleles and absence of Asp 57 as susceptibility factors of IDDM in Finland. *Diabetes.* 1991; 40:1640–1644.
13. Bingley PJ, Bonifacio E, Gale EAM. Perspectives in diabetes: can we really predict IDDM? *Diabetes.* 1993; 42:213–220.
14. Bonifacio E, Bingley PJ, Shattock M, et al. Quantitative islet cell antibody measurement assists in the prediction of insulin-dependent diabetes. *Lancet.* 1990; 35:147–149.
15. Riley WJ, Maclaren NK, Krisher J, et al. A prospective study of the development of diabetes in relatives of patients with insulin-dependent diabetes. *N Engl J Med.* 1990; 323:1167–1172.
16. Karjalainen JK. Islet cell antibodies as predictive markers for IDDM in children with high background incidence of disease. *Diabetes.* 1990; 39:1144–1150.
17. Chase HP, Garg SK, Butler-Simon N, Klingensmith G, Norris L, Ruskey CT,

O'Brien D. Prediction of the course of pre-type I diabetes. *J Pediatr.* 1991; 118:838–841.

18. Bruining GJ, Grobbee DE, Scheffer GJ, DeBruyn AM, Molenaar JL, Bruining HA, Valkenburg HA. Ten year follow-up study of islet-cell antibodies and childhood diabetes mellitus. *Lancet.* 1989; 1:1100–1102.
19. Bonifacio E, Boitard C, Gleichman H, Shattock MA, Molenaar JL, Bottazzo G-F. Assessment of precision, concordance, specificity, and sensitivity of islet cell antibody measurements in 41 assays. *Diabetologia.* 1990; 33:731–736.
20. Palmer JP, Asplin CM, Clemons P, Lyen K, Taipati O, Raghu P, Paquette TL. Insulin antibodies in insulin-dependent diabetics before insulin treatment. *Science.* 1983; 222:1337–1339.
21. McEvoy RC, Witt ME, Ginsberg-Fellner F, Rubenstein P. Anti-insulin antibodies in children with type I diabetes. *Diabetes.* 1986; 35:634–641.
22. Ziegler AG, Ziegler R, Vardi P, Jackson RA, Soeldner JS, Eisenbarth GS. Life table analysis of progression to diabetes of anti-insulin autoantibody-positive relatives of individuals with type I diabetes. *Diabetes.* 1989; 38:1320–1325.
23. Baekkeskov S, Aanstoot H, Christgau S, Reetz A, Solimena M, Cascaiho M, Folli F, Richter-Olesen H, Decamilli P. Identification of the 64K autoantigen in insulin-dependent diabetes as the GABA-synthesizing enzyme glutamic acid decarboxylase. *Nature.* 1990; 347:151–156.
24. Atkinson MA, Maclaren NK, Scharp DW, Lacy PE, Riley WJ. 64000 Mr autoantibodies as predictors of insulin-dependent diabetes. *Lancet.* 1990; 335:1357–1360.
25. Barmeier H, McCulloch DK, Neifing JL, Warnock G, Rajotte RV, Palmer JP, Lernmark A. Risk for developing type I (insulin-dependent) diabetes mellitus and presence of islet 64K antibodies. *Diabetologia.* 1991; 34:727–733.
26. Pietropaolo M, Castano L, Babu S, Buelow R, Kuo YS, Martin S, Martin A, Powers AC, Prochazka M, Naggert J, Leiter EH, Eisenbarth GS. Islet cell autoantigen 69 KD (ICA69). *J Clin Invest.* 1992; 92:359–369.
27. Srikanta S, Ganda OP, Gleason RE, Jackson RA, Soeldner JS, Eisenbarth GS. Pre-type I diabetes: linear loss of beta cell response to intravenous glucose. *Diabetes.* 1984; 33:717–720.
28. Chase HP, Voss MA, Butler-Simon N, Hoops S, O'Brien D, Doberson MJ. Diagnosis of pre-type I diabetes. *J Pediatr.* 1987; 111:807–812.
29. Vardi P, Crisa L, Jackson RA. Predictive value of intravenous glucose tolerance test insulin secretion less than or greater than the first percentile in islet cell antibody positive relatives of type I (insulin-dependent) diabetic patients. *Diabetologia.* 1991; 34:93–102.
30. Ad Hoc Expert Committee. Prevention of type 1 diabetes mellitus. *Diabetes Care.* 1990; 13:1026–1027.
31. Bingley PJ, Colman P, Eisenbarth GS, Jackson RA, McCulloch DK, Riley WJ, Gale EAM. Standardization of IVGTT to predict IDDM. *Diabetes Care.* 1992; 15:1313–1316.
32. Allen HF, Jeffers BW, Klingensmith GJ, Chase HP. First phase insulin release in normal children. *J Pediatr.* 1993; 123:733–738.
33. Ad Hoc Expert Committee. Position statement: prevention of type I diabetes mellitus. *Diabetes.* 1990; 39:1151–1152.
34. Elliott RB, Chase HP. Prevention or delay of type I (insulin-dependent) diabetes mellitus in children using nicotinamide. *Diabetologia.* 1991; 34:362–365.

35. Keller RJ, Eisenbarth GS, Jackson RA. Insulin prophylaxis in individuals at high risk of type I diabetes. *Lancet.* 1993; 341:927–928.
36. Yamada K, Nonaka K, Hanafusa T, Miyazaki A, Toyoshima H, Tarui S. Preventive and therapeutic aspects of large dose nicotinamide injections on diabetes associated with insulitis: an observation in nonobese diabetic (NOD) mice. *Diabetes.* 1982; 31:749–753.
37. Uchigata Y, Yamamoto H, Nagai H, Okamoto H. Effect of poly(ADP-ribose) synthetase inhibitor administration to rats before and after injection of alloxan and streptozotocin on islet proinsulin synthesis. *Diabetes.* 1983; 32:316–318.
38. LeDoux SP, Hall CR, Forbes PM, Patton NJ, Wilson GL. Mechanisms of nicotinamide and thymidine protection from alloxan and streptozotocin toxicity. *Diabetes.* 1988; 37:1015–1019.
39. Kolb H, Burkart, Appels B, Hannenberg H, Kantwerk-Funke G, Kiesel U, Schraermeyer U. Essential contribution of macrophages to islet cell destruction in vivo and in vitro. *J Autoimmun.* 1990; 3:1–4.
40. Yamada K, Miyajima E, Nonaka K. Inhibition of cyotokine-induced MHC class II but not class I molecule expression on mouse islet cells by niacinamide and 3-aminobenzamide. *Diabetes.* 1990; 39:1125–1130.
41. Pociot F, Reimers JI, Anderson HU. Nicotinamide-biological actions and therapeutic potential in diabetes prevention. *Diabetologia.* 1993; 36:574–576.
42. Diabetes-Forchunginstitut an der Universität Düsseldorf, Auf'm Hennekamp 65, D-40225 Dusseldorf, Germany.
43. Department of Diabetes and Metabolism, St Batholomew's Hospital, London, EC1A 7BE.
44. World Health Organization Technical Report Series. Report of a WHO Study Group. *Diabetes Mellitus.* 1985; 727:1–99.
45. National Diabetes Data Group. Classification and diagnosis of diabetes mellitus and other categories of glucose intolerance. *Diabetes.* 1979; 28:1039–1057.
46. Zhang JZ. Davidson L, Eisenbarth GS, Weiner HL. Suppression of diabetes in nonobese diabetic mice by oral administration of porcine insulin. *Proc Natl Acad Sci USA.* 1991; 88:10252–10256.
47. Baeder WL, Sredy J, Sehgal SN, Chang JY, Adams LM. Rapamycin prevents the onset of insulin-dependent diabetes mellitus)IDDM) in NOD mice. *Clin Exp Immunol.* 1992; 89:174–178.
48. Pacheco-Silva A, Bastos MG, Muggia RA, Pankewyez O, Nichols J, Murphy JR, Strom TB, Rubin-Kelly VE. Interleukin 2 receptor targeted fusion toxin (DAB486-IL-2) treatment blocks diabetogenic autoimmunity in nonobese diabetic mice. *Eur J Immunol.* 1992; 22:697–702.
49. Maki T, Ichikawa T, Blanco R, Porter J. Long-term abrogation of autoimmune diabetes in nonobese diabetic mice by immunotherapy with anti-lymphocyte serum. *Proc Natl Acad Sci USA.* 1992; 89:3434–3438.
50. Hayward AR, Shriber M. Reduced incidence of insulitis in NOD mice following anti-CD3 injection: requirement for neonatal injection. *Autoimmunity.* 1992; 5:59–67.
51. Hutchings P, O'Reilly L, Parish NM, Waldmann H, Cooke A. The use of a non-dependent anti-CD4 monoclonal antibody to re-establish tolerance to beta cells in NOD mice. *Eur J Immunol.* 1992; 22:1913–1918.
52. Sanhadji K, Touraine JL, Aitouche A, Vicari A, Chargui J, Goillot E. Fetal liver cell transplantation in various murine models. *Bone Marrow Transplant.* 1992; 9:77–82.

53. Clare-Salzler MJ, Brooks J, Chai A, Van Hette K, Anderson C. Prevention of diabetes in non-obese diabetic mice by dendritic cell transfer. *J Clin Invest.* 1991; 90:741–748.
54. Georgin HM, Mandel TE. Reduced incidence of diabetes in nonobese diabetic mice transplanted with thymus from diabetes-resistant donors. *Transplant Proc.* 1992; 24:203–204.
55. Yagi H, Matsumoto M, Kishimoto Y, Makino S, Harada M. Possible mechanism of the preventive effect of BCG against diabetes mellitus on NOD mouse: suppression of pathogenesis by macrophage transfer from BCG-vaccinated mice. *Cell Immunol.* 1991; 138:142–149.
56. Qin HY, Sadelian MW, Hitchon C, Lauzon J, Singh B. Complete Freund's adjuvant–induced T cells prevent the development and adoptive transfer of diabetes in nonobese diametic mice. *J Immunol.* 1993; 150:2072–2080.
57. Hoorfar J, Buschard K, Dagnaes-Hansen F. Prophylactic nutritional modification of the incidence of diabetes in autoimmune non-obese diabetic (NOD) mice. *Br J Nutr.* 1993; 69:597–607.
58. Williams AJK, Beales PE, Krug J, Procaccini E, Signore A, Xu S, Gale EAM, Pozzilli P. Tolbutamide reduces the incidence of diabetes mellitus, but not insulitis, in the non-obese-diabetic mouse. *Diabetologia.* 1993; 36:487–492.
59. Mandel TE, Koulmanda M, Mackay IR. Prevention of spontaneous and cyclophosphamide-induced diabetes in non-obese diabetic (NOD) mice with oral 2-acetyl-4- tetrahydroxybutylimidazole (THI), a componenet of caramel colouring III. *Clin Exp Immunol.* 1992; 88:414–419.
60. Mathieu C, Laureys J, Sobis H, Vandeputte M, Waer M. Bouillon R 1,25-dihydroxyvitamin D3 prevents insulitis in NOD mice. *Diabetes.* 1992; 41:1491–1495.
61. Hayward AR, Shriber M, Sokol R. Vitamin E supplemenatation reduces the incidence of diabetes but not insulitis in NOD mice. *J Lab Clin Med.* 1992; 119:503–507.
62. Rabinovitch A, Suarez WL, Power RF. Lazaroid antioxidant reduces incidence of diabetes and insulitis in nonobese diabetic mice. *J Lab Clin Med.* 1993; 121:603–607.
63. Rabinovitch A, Suarez WL, Power RF. Combination therapy with an antioxidant and a corticosteroid prevents autoimmune diabetes in NOD mice. *Life Sci.* 1992; 51:1937–1943.
64. Reddy S, Bibby NJ, Elliott RB. Early noicotinamide treatment in the NOD mouse: effects on diabetes and insulitis suppression and autoantibody levels. *Diabetes Res.* 1990; 15:95–102.
65. Uehara Y, Shimizu H, Sato N, Shimomura Y, Mori M, Kobayashi I. Probucol partially prevents development of diabetes in NOD mice. *Diabetes Res.* 1991; 17:131–134.
66. Seino H, Takahashi K, Satoh J, Zhu XP, Sagara M, Masuda T, Nobunaga T, Funahashi I, Kajikawa T, Toyota T. Prevention of autoimmune diabetes with lymphotoxin in NOD mice. *Diabetes.* 1993; 42:398–404.
67. Rapoport MJ, Jaramillo A. Zipris D, Lazarus AH, Serreze DV, Leiter EH, Cyopick P, Danska JS, Delovitch TL. Interleukin 4 reverses T cell proliferative unresponsiveness and prevents the onset of diabetes in nonobese diabetic mice. *J Exp Med.* 1993; 178:87–99.
68. Formby B, Jacobs C, Dubuc P, Shao T. Exogenous administration of IL-1 alpha

inhibits active and adoptive transfer autoimmune diabetes in NOD mice. *Autoimmunity.* 1992; 12:21–27.

69. Fox HS. Androgen treatment prevents diabetes in nonobese diabetic mice. *J Exp Med.* 1992; 175:409–412.
70. Hawkins T, Gala RR, Dunbar JC. The effect of neonatal sex hormones manipulation on the incidence of diabetes in nonobese diabetic mice. *Proc Soc Exp Biol Med.* 1993; 202:201–205.

13
Theoretical Essays

Kevin J. Lafferty and George S. Eisenbarth, Editors

A. The Development of Autoimmune Diabetes: Theoretical Aspects

Kevin J. Lafferty

The nonobese diabetic (NOD) mouse develops type I diabetes spontaneously and the disease is associated with lymphocytic infiltration of the pancreatic islet and eventual destruction of islet β-cells. This destructive process is quite specific, with α-cells and other cellular components of the pancreatic islets initially being spared. The disease process represents a form of tissue-specific autoimmunity. It is associated with the development of antibodies specific for islet components such as insulin glutamic acid decarboxylase (GAD) and other islet-cell antigens (see Chapter 2). Although such antibodies become elevated with the development of disease, there is no evidence that antibodies of themselves are pathogenic.[1] The disease process appears to represent a form of cell-mediated immunity dependent on CD4 T cell activity, and it has been demonstrated that disease develops in mice whose capacity to produce humoral immunity has been blocked.[1]

Initiation of Disease

The specificity of the disease process resulting in damage to only the β-cells of the islet suggests that the pathogenic process may involve a cytotoxic T cell attack directed at some β-cell–specific antigen. The development of disease is dependent on the activity of both CD4 and CD8 T cells[2,3] and it is reasonable to suggest that the CD4 cell is behaving as a helper cell required for the activation of the cytotoxic CD8 T cell that in turn initiates islet damage. However, studies carried out at the Barbara Davis Center demonstrated that although both CD4 and CD8 T cells are required for the initiation of disease, the immunological specific effector cell is the CD4 T cell (see Chapter 5).[3,4] Pancreatic islet–reactive T cell clones have been isolated from the NOD mouse and in all cases these cells have proved to express the CD4 phenotype (see Chapter 4). Such cloned CD4 T cells have the capacity to initiate disease in the absence of CD8 T cell function.[5,6] Thus, while there is no question that the CD8 T cell plays an essential role in the development of disease, this cell does not appear to be the immunologically specific effector cell. Ann Cooke has shown this cell to be required early in the process of disease development, indicating that the CD8 T cell has an accessory or helper function in the activation of the CD4 effector of the autoimmune response.[7] There are examples where CD8 T cells can modify the activation of CD4 T cells and this process is mediated via active involvement of the antigen-presenting cell (APC).[8] There is also evidence[9] that the early activated CD8 T cell produces high levels of interferon gamma (IFN-γ) and in this way forces the CD4 T cell response toward the production of IFN-γ and interleukin-2 (IL-2) (Th1 phenotype). The balance between Th1 and Th2 CD4 T cell activation plays a critical role in determining whether or not the autoimmune response generated will be destructive (see below).

There has been considerable speculation concerning factors responsible for the initiation of the disease process. Susceptibility to diabetes both in humans and in the animal models is determined by the major histocompatibility complex (MHC) genotype; the disease-prone character is determined by genes in the class II region of the MHC complex (see Chapter 3). However, although susceptibility to the development of diabetes is under genetic control, the clinical disease itself is not solely determined by genotype. Thus, in the case of identical twins there is only a 30–40% concordance for disease. In the NOD mouse model, where all individuals are genetically identical as the result of inbreeding, disease develops in only 20–40% of male NOD animals and approximately 80% of females. The observation that the incidence of disease increases when animals are maintained under specific pathogen-free conditions indicated an environmental contribution to the development of disease.[10] The negative correlation with infection was an unexpected finding; one notion relating to the development of this disease was that the process resulted from a cross-reactive immune response to some environmental pathogen.[11] If this were the case, one would expect the disease incidence to fall when animals were spared the immunological challenge of environmental pathogens.

Another interesting characteristic of the disease process is that although clinical disease is seen only in a proportion of animals in the NOD colony, all animals of the NOD genotype have pathology in their pancreas. That is, all animals express autoimmunity and show the development of lymphocytic infiltrates around islet tissue within the pancreas.[12] There is, however, a difference between animals that develop clinical disease and those that have insulitis but do not go on to develop overt diabetes. In the latter case, the lymphocytes accumulate around the outside of the islet and rarely penetrate within the islet itself. In the former situation there is extensive invasion of islets by mononuclear cells and associated destruction of islet β-cells.[12] It is worth noting that following destruction of islet β-cells the lymphocytic infiltrate disappears from the pancreas and one is left with small pseudo-islets made up predominantly of α-cells with little or no lymphocytic accumulation around the tissue. We must conclude therefore that the disease process is dependent on the recognition of some β-cell–associated antigen that is not expressed by other cells within the islet.

Studies carried out in transgenic animals where particular viral antigens are expressed in islet β-cells demonstrate that neither the expression of foreign antigens nor the possession of T cells specific for such antigens is a sufficient requirement for the precipitation of the disease.[13] The initiation of disease requires the "appropriate" presentation of antigen to an immune system that has potentially reactive T cells. We do not fully understand what is involved in "appropriate" antigen presentation. What we know is that infection of animals with a particular virus can lead to islet destruction when some viral antigens are expressed on islet β-cells. However, the development of a destructive process is not always seen in such situations. Variability appears to depend on the genetic background of the animal and the nature of the virus used in such studies.[13]

What is now becoming clear is that two distinct forms of autoimmune response can be observed. There is the response that leads to islet damage and the development of diabetes, which we can define as destructive autoimmunity. There is also a form of response that leads to pathology and associated lymphocyte accumulation around pancreatic islets but that is a nondestructive process and does not lead to clinical disease. The coexistence of the potential for either destructive or nondestructive autoimmunity in animals of a defined genotype suggests the development of diabetes is a stochastic process. That is, although we can precisely define the kinetics of the disease process and the proportion of animals in any group that will express overt diabetes at any given time (provided we are dealing with a colony maintained under controlled conditions), we are unable to specify beforehand exactly which animals will become diabetic. That is, we are unable to predict which animals will undergo the destructive process and which will develop nondestructive autoimmunity before the process is well under way. Clearly, environmental conditions have a large influence on the proportion of animals that fall into either of these groups. This is why animals of the same genotype held under conventional laboratory conditions have a much lower incidence of disease than those maintained under specific pathogen-free conditions.

We do not precisely know what is responsible for the development of the disease process leading to clinical diabetes. We know that the genotype—specifically the class II MHC antigen type—in both animals and humans is a major factor controlling the disease-prone character. However, possession of the disease-prone genotype is not in itself a sufficient requirement for the development of disease. Moreover, T cells with the capacity to recognize and respond to islet autoantigens can exist in animals that do not develop clinical diabetes. All we can say with any confidence is that disease develops in disease-prone animals and individuals following "appropriate" stimulation of the immune system. The problem is to define what is meant by the term "appropriate stimulation."

Pathogenesis of the Disease Process

When it comes to understanding the basis of the pathogenic process involved in islet β-cell destruction and the development of IDDM we are on somewhat firmer ground. As was mentioned above, the disease process is a T cell–dependent phenomenon in which both CD4 and CD8 T cells are required for the initiation of disease but where the CD4 T cell is the immunologically specific effector cell. CD4 T cells of the disease-prone individual are probably not interacting directly with antigen expressed on islet β-cells. Such antigens would be presented in association with class II MHC antigens; that is, in a form which does not favor CD4 T cell recognition. The CD4 T cells are most likely to be interacting with antigen derived from β-cells and processed by class II MHC-bearing antigen-presenting cells. This process would lead to the development and expression of cell-mediated immunity in which cytokine production by the inflammatory cells is a major pathogenic event leading to islet destruction.

There is evidence that free radical production is involved in this process. Both superoxide production by activation macrophages and nitric oxide production by islets in response to IL-1 appear to be involved in the pathogenic process (see Chapter 5). The Okamoto hypothesis provides the most useful model for understanding the involvement of free radical damage in the disease process (see Chapter 5). According to this hypothesis free radicals initiate DNA damage, which in turn activates the DNA repair enzyme (poly ADP-ribose synthetase) that is involved in DNA repair. This enzyme uses cellular NAD in the process and as a result depletes the β-cells' radical scavenging capacity. The cycling of this process results in β-cell death. One prediction of this model is that iron-chelating agents such as desferrioxamine, which block the conversion of superoxide to the more damaging hydroxyl radical, and specific inhibitors of the DNA repair enzyme such as nicotinamide, may be used to regulate this destructive process. Experimental evidence is consistent with such predictions.[14]

It has been suggested that nicotinamide is an agent that may be used to prevent the development of diabetes in a clinical situation. Certainly this agent is effective in animal models. However, the Okamoto hypothesis indicates that the effect of nicotinamide is to block the DNA repair enzyme. This process may lead to the development of oncogenic change because of interference with the DNA repair process. Earlier studies that examined the effect of nicotinamide on streptozotocin-induced diabetes indicated that nicotinamide could prevent the induction of diabetes by this agent.[15] However, animals protected in this way were tumor prone and a significant proportion developed β-cell adenomas later in life. Any use of nicotinamide for the control of autoimmune diabetes in a clinical situation should be approached with considerable caution.

Exposure to environmental pathogens can have a marked effect on the development of diabetes in disease-prone animals. Environmental stimulation of the immune system leads to a decrease in the proportion of animals that go on to develop clinical disease. Immunostimulation of disease-prone animals with agents such as complete Freund's adjuvant or the vaccine BCG has been shown to block the development of diabetes in disease-prone NOD animals.[16,17] Immunostimulation with either of these agents blocks the development of disease both when administered early, that is, soon after weaning, or quite late in the pathogenic process. Animals vaccinated at 85 days of age (clinical disease is first expressed from 90 days on) do not go on to develop clinical disease.[17] Such immunostimulation does not inhibit the development of autoimmunity. It does, however, force the autoimmune response along the nondestructive pathway.[17] Although such animals are protected from the development of overt diabetes they remain disease prone, and administration of cyclophosphamide can acutely result in the development of diabetes in these animals.[17]

These observations emphasize the need to view the immune system as an integrated network regulated by both positive and negative influences. Although "appropriate" stimulation of the immune system can lead to the development of diabetes in disease-prone animals, it is now also clear that other forms of immunostimulation can negatively regulate this process. This positive and negative regulation of immune function is correlated with the nature of cytokine production in either destructive or nondestructive lesions.[12] In the former case, leukocytes within destructive lesions are producing IFN-γ in high proportion and they contain relatively low numbers of IL-4–producing T cells (high proportion of Th1 cells). The nondestructive lesion, on the other hand, has a much smaller proportion of IFN-γ producing cells and a higher ratio of IL-4–producing cells (high proportion of Th2 cells). More direct evidence for cytokine involvement in this process comes from studies in which antibodies to IL-10 and IL-4 were used in an attempt to reverse the protective effect of immunostimulation. In these studies antibody treatment was shown to reverse the protective adjuvant effect (Calcinaro et al, unpublished data).

Although the mechanism of the adjuvant effect is not fully understood, the fact that quite marked effects have been obtained in animal models using both complete Freund's adjuvant and the more benign BCG vaccine has prompted clinical testing of BCG vaccination in newly diagnosed diabetic individuals. A preliminary clinical study of this kind has provided evidence that BCG vaccination may alter the natural history of the disease process in humans.[17] These studies were carried out in an unblinded fashion and used historical controls and must, therefore, be considered as preliminary observations. Further studies carried out in a blinded fashion are required to establish whether or not BCG vaccination can alter the pathogenesis of diabetes in humans. If such studies are positive it may be possible to prevent the development of clinical disease in humans by immunostimulation as is the case in the experimental model.

The development of spontaneous diabetes as seen both in animals and humans is an autoimmune process dependent on the development of islet specific cell–mediated immunity. β-cell destruction is the result of inflammatory tissue damage and the specificity of this process appears to reflect the sensitivity of β-cells to radical damage. The class II MHC antigen genotype of both animals and humans regulates their disease-prone status. However, whether or not clinical disease develops in such individuals is the result of a balance between positive and negative regulation within the immune system. Such regulation is associated with differential cytokine production. Thus, appropriate stimulation of the immune system can lead either to the development of diabetes or to the development of nondestructive autoimmunity. This latter observation may provide the means for safe regulation of diabetes in disease-prone individuals.

References

1. Bendelac A, Boitard C, Bedossa P, Bazin H, Bach JF, Carnaud C. Adoptive T cell transfer of autoimmune nonobese diabetic mouse diabetes does not require recruitment of host B lymphocytes. *J Immunol.* 1988; 141:2625–2628.
2. Miller BJ, Appel MC, O'Neil JJ, Wicker LS. Both the lyt-2^+ and L3T4^+ T cell subsets are required for the transfer of diabetes in nonobese diabetic mice. *J Immunol.* 1988; 140:52–58.
3. Wang Y, Pontesilli O, Gill RG, La Rosa FG, Lafferty KJ. The role of CD4+ and CD8+ T cells in the destruction of islet grafts by spontaneously diabetic mice. *Proc Natl Acad Sci USA.* 1991; 88:527–531.
4. Christianson SW, Shultz LD, Leiter EH. Adoptive transfer of diabetes into immunodeficient NOD-scid/scid mice: relative contributions of CD4+ and CD8+ T lymphocytes from diabetic versus prediabetic NOD.NON-thy-1a donors. *Diabetes.* 1993; 42:44–55.
5. Bradley BJ, Haskins K, La Rosa FG, Lafferty KJ. CD8 T cells are not required for islet destruction induced by a CD4+ islet-specific T-cell clone. *Diabetes.* 1992; 41:1603–1608.
6. Wegmann DR, Shehadeh N, Lafferty KJ, Norbury-Glaser M, Gill RG, Daniel D. Establishment of islet-specific T-cell lines and clones from islet isografts placed in spontaneously diabetic NOD mice. *J Autoimmun.* 1993; 6:517–527.
7. Hutchings PR, Simpson E, O'Reilly LA, Lund T, Waldmann H, Cooke A. The

involvement of Ly2+ T cells in beta cell destruction. *J Autoimmun.* 1990; 3:101–109.
8. Gill RG, Lafferty KJ. A novel form of T-T collaboration requiring the active participation of the antigen presenting cell. *Ann NY Acad Sci.* 1989; 532:421–425.
9. Kemeny DM, Noble A, Holmes BJ, Diaz-Sanchez D. Immune regulation: a new role for the CD8+ T cell. *Immunol Today.* 1994; 15:107–110.
10. Wilberz S, Partke HJ, Dagnaes-Hansen F, Herberg L. Persistent MHV (mouse hepatitis virus) infection reduces the incidence of diabetes mellitus in non-obese diabetic mice. *Diabetologia.* 1991; 34:2–5.
11. Jahnke U, Fischer EH, Alvord Jr EC. Sequence homology between certain viral proteins and proteins related to encephalomyelitis and neuritis. *Science.* 1985; 229:282–284.
12. Shehadeh NN, LaRosa F, Lafferty KJ. Altered cytokine activity in adjuvant inhibition of autoimmune diabetes. *J Autoimmun.* 1993; 6:291–300.
13. Scott B, Lo D. Peripheral tolerance and the CD4 cell. In: Bluthmann H, Ohashi P, eds. *Analysis of the Immune System Utilising Transgenesis and Targeted Mutagenesis.* Orlando: Academic Press; 1993.
14. Nomikos IN, Prowse SJ, Carotenuto P, Lafferty KJ. Combined treatment with nicotinamide and desferrioxamine prevents islet allograft destruction in NOD mice. *Diabetes.* 1986; 35:1302–1304.
15. Rakieten N, Gordon BS, Beaty A, Cooney DA, Davis RD, Schein PS. Pancreatic islet cell tumors produced by the combined action of streptozotocin and nicotinamide. *Proc Soc Exp Biol Med.* 1970; 137:280–283.
16. Sadelain MWJ, Qin H-Y, Lauzon J, Singh B. Prevention of type 1 diabetes in NOD mice by adjuvant immunotherapy. *Diabetes.* 1990; 39:583–589.
17. Shehadeh NN, Calcinaro F, Bradley BJ, Bruchlim I, Vardi P, Lafferty KJ. Effect of adjuvant therapy on development of diabetes in mouse and man. *Lancet.* 1994; 343:706–707.

B. Pathogenesis of Type I Diabetes

George S. Eisenbarth

As contained within the chapters of this text, there is a wealth of new information concerning the pathogenesis of type I diabetes. With this new information comes not only a better understanding of the disease and increased ability to predict the disorder in man, but also additional and refined questions. Answers to several crucial questions are lacking and thus, similar to most autoimmune disorders, any schema to integrate current knowledge will be incomplete and require considerable speculation. As a framework for asking additional questions and directing a search for what I believe to be crucial pathogenic events, I offer the following hypotheses.

Any complete pathogenic schema must account for the phenomena illustrated in the figure (13.1). Beginning at the end of the process that leads to type I diabetes, it is now clear that patients with type I diabetes and animals such as the nonobese diabetic (NOD) mouse produce autoantibodies and T cells reactive with a relatively large series of autoantigens[1] including insulin, glutamic acid decarboxylase (GAD), ICA512, etc. What is even more striking is that T cell clones derived from the NOD mice recognize more than one protein, and that different CD4 clones recognizing different proteins are sufficient to transfer diabetes into NOD/*scid* mice. This statement can be derived by combining the studies of Haskins and coworkers on diabetogenic clones reacting with as yet none of the characterized autoantigens[2,3] and the studies of Wegmann and coworkers on clones derived from islet infiltrates that recognize a B chain insulin peptide. Thus, in the NOD mouse, and importantly within islets, pathogenic T cell clones are present that are sufficient to cause disease in mice lacking both B and T cells. The simplest hypothesis is that at least a subset of such clones are not secondary to islet destruction and are themselves the rate-limiting factor for development of type I diabetes. It is likely that such clones will follow classic rules of T cell recognition (eg, trimolecular complex of major histocompatibility complex [MHC], peptide, and T cell receptor) but this assumption has not yet been formally proven. Thus, understanding the etiology of type I diabetes involves elucidating the factors that initiate and regulate the generation of such clones.

Type I diabetes develops only in the setting of genetic susceptibility. This

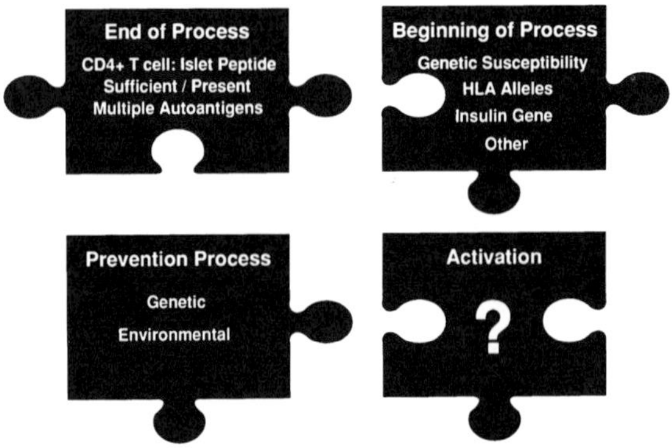

Figure 13.1

is well demonstrated for man,[4] the NOD mouse,[5] and the BioBreeding (BB) rat.[6] Genes within the major histocompatibility complex are essential for disease in all three.[7,8] In both the BB rat and the NOD mouse, genes outside of the MHC are also essential. In the BB rat, an autosomal recessive immunodeficiency allele on chromosome 4 increases the risk of diabetes by approximately 1000-fold.[7,9] In this strain, however, disease can readily be induced in nonlymphopenic BB rats (the DR [diabetes resistant] BB rat) following the injection of poly-IC and antibodies to the T cell surface antigen RT6, or by infection with Kilham rat virus.[10–12] Thus, given appropriate environmental factors, part of the genetic susceptibility for diabetes can be bypassed. In the BB rat model, activation of autoimmunity can be suppressed by normal immune function. This is also true for the NOD mouse and man. In the NOD mouse, which has a deletion of the I-E alpha gene (homologous to DR of man),[8,13] transgenic replacement of this deletion prevents diabetes. In man, the DQ molecule DQA1*0102/DQB1*0602 protects from diabetes in all populations studied to date.[14,15] This protection is dominant over susceptibility such that approximately 20% of individuals in the United States carry this allele, while less than 1.5% of insulin-dependent diabetics are DQB1*0602 positive. The only patient with insulin-dependent diabetes we have observed with this allele has an immunodeficiency syndrome, polyendrocrine type I (see Chapter 8), and thus may not be able to generate a protective immune response associated with DQB1*0602. In addition, approximately 12% of ICA-positive first-degree relatives of patients with type I diabetes carry DQB1*0602, but in our studies none has progressed to diabetes. This allele does not prevent all autoimmunity and is, for example, a high-risk allele for multiple sclerosis. Thus, within the MHC are alleles protecting from and associated with type I diabetes. One can speculate that these alleles, by the islet peptides that they bind and the type of immune response they engender (eg, Th1 versus Th2), can either increase or decrease the risk of type I diabetes.

In humans, in addition to MHC alleles, it is clear that polymorphisms of regulatory sequences of the insulin gene influence disease risk.[16] The area of most interest appears to be a region of variable nucleotide tandem repeats 3′ of the insulin gene.[17,18] "Protection" from diabetes, depending on the specific insulin gene allele, shows imprinting in several populations. To date, insulin is the only beta cell–specific autoantigen. For example, in human islets, glucagon-producing cells that are not destroyed express GAD.[19] Thus, the simplest hypothesis is that insulin gene polymorphisms influence autoimmunity directed at insulin and this molecule is central to beta cell destruction. The ability of NOD T cells reactive to an insulin peptide to destroy normal beta cells within a *scid* mouse enhances the importance of this specific antigen. One speculative manner by which insulin gene polymorphisms may regulate development of anti-insulin autoimmunity is by influencing either the timing or, for example, thymic expression of insulin during ontogeny, thereby inducing tolerance to insulin.

In humans, similar to both animal models, it is very likely that there are genes outside of the MHC and insulin gene that are essential for disease pathogenesis. A subset of such "autoimmune" or "anti-autoimmune" genes (which are potentially inactivated to induce disease) are probably responsible for the polyendocrine autoimmune syndromes. Type I diabetes is associated with other autoimmune diseases such as Addison's disease, myasthenia gravis, and Graves' disease. I believe we will not understand the pathogenesis of type I diabetes until such genes are mapped and defined. Such genes may simply be enzymes influencing T cell function and tolerance, surface receptors, lymphokines, or any of a large number of potential molecules influencing immune function. It is noteworthy that the BB rat develops thyroiditis and the NOD mouse sialitis, indicating that in these animal models defects in immune regulation not restricted to islets are present. It is my contention that until such genes are identified, our pathogenic hypotheses will be far from complete.

If genetic susceptibility is so important, why are all identical twins of patients with type I diabetes not concordant for the disease? This question has been addressed by the hypothesis essays of Lafferty and Talmage. A large number of relatively nonspecific environmental factors appear capable of diverting or abrogating autoimmunity. Environmental factors influencing type I diabetes appear to act in the first few years of life and may act not to trigger the disease but to suppress disease. This would be consistent with the findings in both the BB rat and the NOD mouse that gnotobiotic environment increases dramatically the development of diabetes. It is remarkable that a single injection of Freund's adjuvant prevents diabetes for the life of a NOD mouse.[20] We have recent evidence that more than 45% of first-degree relatives of patients with type I diabetes less than age 10, but none of 20 normal children, transiently express anti-GAD autoantibodies. This leads to the hypothesis that for the great majority of relatives, anti-islet autoimmunity begins but is abrogated. Despite such "nonproductive" autoimmunity, the disease early in life becomes predictable by the pattern and types of autoantibodies expressed. In particular, with the expression of a series of autoantibodies, for most individuals progression to diabetes is very likely. To date, the only identified exception to this rule is the expression of GAD ICA and anti-insulin autoantibodies in DQB1*0602 positive relatives.[21]

The above observations lead to the hypothesis that activation of anti-islet autoimmunity is a function of the developing immune system in the presence of a non-MHC genetic defect, limited extra islet insulin production (eg, not in thymus), MHC alleles targeting anti-islet immunity, and requires no environmental activation. T cells reacting at the site of highest insulin concentration (the islets) are sufficient to activate disease. Once beta cell destruction is initiated it can progress or be suppressed. If it progresses, many islet-related molecules become the target of autoimmunity and a cascade of destruction is initiated. This implies that the process is antigen driven and critically dependent upon events within islets, which is consistent with exogenous insulin therapy preventing insulitis in the BB rat,[22] NOD mouse,[23,24] and potentially man.[25]

The above hypothesis contains within it (1) a search for relatively common autoimmune genes related to type I diabetes and polyendrocrine autoimmunity; (2) speculation that the process is antigen driven and that the key autoantigen is insulin; (3) speculation that no exogenous or endogenous non-islet factor is required for activation and thus the search for environmental triggers will continue to be futile; (4) environmental factors that deviate or suppress autoimmunity will be difficult to identify (many of them) but will be important; and (5) the common assumption that T cell recognition of peptides with specific MHC alleles (the trimolecular complex) is central to disease pathogenesis.

Problems with the above global hypothesis include the following. (1) The lack of identification of the loci and genes associated with polyendocrine autoimmunity and the observation that only 10% of patients with type I diabetes have an overt additional autoimmune disease[26] (nevertheless, many patients with type I diabetes express, for example, antigastric and antithyroid autoantibodies without overt disease). There appears to be a hierarchy of autoimmunity, such that with rare diseases (eg, myasthenia gravis and Addison's disease) there are almost always additional autoimmune diseases. The difference between polyendocrine autoimmunity and type I diabetes may result from allelic differences, homozygosity for disease alleles, or more likely more than one predisposing "autoimmune" gene. (2) Studies of glutamic acid decarboxylase indicate that in the NOD mouse it is the first antigen recognized by T cells; there is a suggestion that induction of "tolerance" to GAD prevents diabetes.[27,28] Within the islets of the NOD mouse, responses to GAD do not precede insulin-reactive T cell clones (unpublished observations, Wegmann et al) and to date, only a few of the T cell clones that transfer disease to NOD/*scid* mice respond to GAD. A large number of immunizations and environmental manipulations prevent diabetes of the NOD mouse, and it is thus likely that apparently protective responses can be generated by intravenous and intrathymic injection of many peptides. (3) Insulin expression within the thymus with potential imprinting of thymic expression has not yet been demonstrated. (4) Transgenic NOD mice with a random Vbeta element develop diabetes and insulitis at a rate equal to that of nontransgenic mice.[29] If recognition of peptides in the trimolecular complex is essential for disease, even with the expected escape of a subset of clones in this transgenic model, why is the time course of disease not altered? Breeding of the RAG mutation onto this transgenic background should most directly test the alternative hypothesis that, though T cells with intact T cell receptors are essential for disease, targeting is not Vbeta sequence dependent. If NOD mice with the Vbeta and Valpha transgenes develop diabetes in the absence of endogenous T cell receptor rearrangement, the above global hypothesis is simply wrong and alternative destructive and targeting mechanisms must be considered (eg, macrophages) or other T cell elements may determine reactivity with islet molecules (eg, common Valpha sequences).

The progress during the past decade and the current intensity of study of type I diabetes makes one optimistic that the questions posed above will be answered and we will both understand and be able to manipulate the autoimmunity that leads to type I diabetes.

References

1. Atkinson MA, Maclaren NK. Islet cell autoantigens in insulin-dependent diabetes. *J Clin Invest.* 1993; 92:1608–1616.
2. Haskins K, McDuffie M. Acceleration of diabetes in young NOD mice with a CD4+ islet-specific T cell clone. *Science.* 1990; 249:1433–1436.
3. Bradley BJ, Haskins K, La Rosa FG, Lafferty KJ. CD8 T cells are not required for islet destruction induced by a CD4+ islet-specific T-cell clone. *Diabetes.* 1992; 39:96–103.
4. Erlich HA, Bugawan TL, Scharf S, Nepom GT, Tait B, Griffith RL. HLA-DQB sequence polymorphism and genetic susceptibility to IDDM. *Diabetes.* 1990; 39:96–103.
5. Ghosh S, Palmer SM, Rodrigues NR, et al. Polygenic control of autoimmune diabetes in nonobese diabetic mice. *Nature Genetics.* 1993; 4:404–409.
6. Jacob HJ, Pettersson A, Wilson D, Mao Y, Lernmark A, Lander ES. Genetic dissection of autoimmune type I diabetes in the BB rat. *Nature Genetics.* 1992; 2:56–60.
7. Jackson RA, Buse JB, Rifai R, et al. Two genes required for diabetes in BB rats. *J Exp Med.* 1984; 159:1629–1631.
8. Hattori M, Buse JB, Jackson RA, et al. The NOD mouse: recessive diabetogenic gene within the major histocompatibility complex. *Science.* 1986; 231:733–735.
9. Janeway CA Jr. The T cell receptor as a multicomponent signalling machine: CD4/CD8 coreceptors and CD45 in T cell activation. *Annu Rev Immunol.* 1992; 10:645–674.
10. Guberski DL, Thomas VA, Shek WR, et al. Induction of type 1 diabetes by Kilham's rat virus in diabetes-resistant BB/Wor rats. *Science. 1991*254; 1010:1013.
11. Gottlieb PA, Berrios JP, Mariani G, et al. Autoimmune destruction of islets transplanted into RT6-depleted diabetes-resistant BB/Wor rats. *Diabetes.* 1990; 39:643–646.

12. Rossini AA, Greiner DL, Friedman HP, Mordes JP. Immunopathogenesis of diabetes mellitus. *Diabetes Rev.* 1993; 1:43–75.
13. Nishimoto H, Kikutani H, Yamamura K, Kishimoto T. Prevention of autoimmune insulitis by expression of I-E molecules in NOD mice. *Nature.* 1987; 328:432–434.
14. Baisch JM, Weeks T, Giles R, Hoover M, Stastny P, Capra JD. Analysis of HLA-DQ genotypes and susceptibility in insulin-dependent diabetes mellitus. *N Engl J Med.* 1990; 322:1836–1841.
15. Erlich HA, Griffith RL, Bugawan TL, Ziegler R, Alper C, Eisenbarth GS. Implication of specific DQB1 alleles in genetic susceptibility and resistance by identification of IDDM siblings with novel HLA-DQB1 allele and unusual DR2 and DR1 haplotypes. *Diabetes.* 1991; 40:478–481.
16. Julier C, Hyer RN, Davies J, et al. Insulin-IGF2 region encodes a gene implicated in HLA-DR4-dependent diabetes susceptibility. *Nature.* 1991; 354:155–159.
17. Lucassen AM, Julier C, Beressi J-P, et al. Susceptibility to insulin dependent diabetes mellitus maps to a 4.1 kb segment of DNA spanning the insulin gene and associated VNTR. *Nature Genetics.* 1993; 4:305.
18. Pugliese A, Bain SC, Todd JA, Awdeh ZL, Alper CA, Eisenbarth GS. INS polymorphisms on chromosome 11 in type I diabetes. *Autoimmunity.* 1993; 15(suppl):32. Abstract.
19. Petersen JS, Russel S, Marshall MO, et al. Differential expression of glutamic acid decarboxylase in rat and human islets. *Diabetes.* 1993; 42:484–495.
20. Sadelain MWJ, Qin H-Y, Lauzon J, Singh B. Prevention of type I diabetes in NOD mice by adjuvant immunotherapy. *Diabetes.* 1990; 39:583–589.
21. Yu L, Gianani R. GAD autoantibody levels in ICA positive relatives with restricted ICA. *Diabetes.* 1985; 28:933–935.
22. Gottsfredsen CF, Buschard K< Frandsen EK. Reduction of diabetes incidence of BB Wistar rats by early prophylactic insulin treatment of diabetes-prone animals. *Diabetologia.* 1985; 28:933–935.
23. Atkinson M, Maclaren N, Luchetta R, Burr I. Insulitis and diabetes in NOD mice reduced by prophylactic insulin therapy. *Diabetes.* 1990; 39:933–937.
24. Zhang JZ, Davidson L, Eisenbarth GS, Weiner HL. Suppression of diabetes in nonobese diabetic mice by oral administration of porcine insulin. *Proc Natl Acad Sci U S A.* 1001; 88:10252–10256.
25. Keller RJ, Eisenbarth GS, Jackson RA. Insulin prophylaxis in individuals at high risk of type I diabetes. *Lancet.* 1993; 341:927–928.
26. Landin-Olsson M, Karlsson FA, Lernmark A, Sundkvist G, and the Diabetes Incidence Study in Sweden Group. Islet cell and thyrogastric antibodies in 633 consecutive 15- to 34-yr-old patients in the diabetes incidence study in Sweden. *Diabetes.* 1992; 41:1022–1027.
27. todd JA, Bell JI, McDevitt HO. HLA-DQ beta gene contribution to susceptibility and resistance to insulin dependent diabetes mellitus. *Nature.* 1987; 329:599–604.
28. Kaufman DL, Clare-Salzler M, Tian J, et al. Spontaneous loss of T-cell tolerance to glutamic acid decarboxylase in murine insulin-dependent diabetes. *Nature.* 1993; 366:69–72.
29. Lipes MA, Rosenzweig A, Tan K, et al. Progression to diabetes in NOD mice with transgenic T cell receptors. *Science.* 1993; 259:1165–1169.

C. The New Math of Diabetes: When Th1 – Th2 = Th0

Donald Bellgrau and Daniel P. Gold

Thymus-derived T lymphocytes are required for diabetes mellitus to occur; elimination of antibody production does not protect against disease, indicating that T, not B, lymphocytes are the major players in the immune-mediated destruction of insulin-producing beta cells. How T cells contribute to diseases is not known, but experimental evidence indicates that there may be a "regulatory" T cell defect. A consequence of such a defect is that an "unregulated" immune response is free to destroy insulin-producing islet beta cells.

Two important questions to be answered are (1) what is the nature of the regulatory defect and (2) what are the characteristics of the cells normally under regulation, ie, the autoreactive cells? One view is that the regulators and regulated populations are encompassed in two subsets of peripheral T cells termed Th1 and Th2. Although it is an oversimplification to ascribe homogeneous characteristics to Th1 and Th2 populations, a generic view is that Th1 T cells are involved in "cell-mediated immune responses" associated with IL-2 and interferon gamma production while Th2 cells drive the humoral response associated with IL-4 production. A popular view is that a Th1/Th2 imbalance alters the immune homeostasis of protective versus inductive lymphokines. More specifically, in autoimmune diabetes it may be that a Th2 deficit can shift the immune response heavily toward the Th1 subset.[1] The inference is that it is the Th2 regulators that control the Th1 mediators of autoreactivity. Therefore at least one diabetogenic gene should influence Th2 function. Indeed, in our studies of the diabetes prone BB rat (BB-DP) we have obtained experimental evidence indicating that the BB-DP regulatory defect occurs as a consequence of diminished numbers of the Th2 T cells and that this characteristic is linked to the inheritance of a known diabetogenic gene.[2]

Is a shift in the Th1/Th2 ratio enough to cause disease? Because diabetic susceptibility is polygenic the answer is almost certainly no. In fact, genetic studies in the rat, where the gene responsible for diminished Th2 T cells is fixed on other genetic backgrounds, indicate that this diabetes susceptibility gene is necessary but not sufficient for disease.[3] A second candidate for a genetic influence is the effector population. As mentioned above, the logical extension of the Th1/Th2 "imbalance leading to autoimmunity" paradigm is to propose that the Th1 subset contains the effectors of beta cell destruction. However, experimental evidence does not fit easily with ascribing beta cell destruction to Th1 T cells. First, injection of interleukin-2 (IL-2), a dominant cytokine of this subset, does not exacerbate diabetic disease. In fact, injecting diabetes-prone animals with IL-2 actually prevents diabetes. Second, in both human and murine models of diabetes there a deficit in IL-2 production associated with disease-prone individuals.[4–6] Therefore, while we agree that impairing the Th2 arm of the immune response is a predisposing factor in diabetes we do not believe that the effector cells that benefit from the release from regulation are Th1 cells.

If not Th1, then what? The autoreactivity in the BB-DP is associated with a broad cytokine profile high in both IL-4 and interferon gamma, ruling against Th2, and low levels of IL-2, ruling against Th1. Cell surface phenotype analyses of the autoreactive subset indicate that the effectors are more juvenile/immature than peripheral Th1 and Th2 T cells.[7] This population proliferates to self antigen in vitro and expresses a limited T cell receptor Vbeta chain family usage.[8] Experiments in the mouse have ascribed these properties to a medullary thymocyte subset termed Thy0 for thymic Th0.[9] Th0 are though to be the peripheral precursors of the Th1 and Th2 subsets.[10]

Although no information exists on the way in which mouse Thy0 retain their autoreactivity, our data on what we believe is the Thy0 equivalent in the rat provide some clues. In the BB-DP, the effector subset appears to be unusually resistant to apoptosis,[11] defined by crosslinking CD4 followed by direct stimulation of the T cell receptor. Normally this CD4 crosslinking protocol induces apoptosis/programmed cell death in greater than 95% of CD4+ peripheral T cells from normal rats. The BB-DP effector population is also resistant to anergy induction following presentation with an exogenous source of superantigen.[12] Anergy in this setting is defined as an inability to proliferate in vitro to an antigen to which the T cells were previously exposed in vivo. In total we interpret the resistance to apoptosis and anergy as characteristics of T cells that escape the selection process that normally deletes autoreactive T cells. Whether other diabetes susceptibility genes impart these resistance characteristics or they are characteristics of Thy0 in general is yet to be determined. However we favor the hypothesis that the enhanced resistance to tolerizing signals is driven by a diabetogenic gene.

In summary we believe that there is a defect in the Th2 T cell subset that is created by a diabetogenic gene. This regulatory defect uncovers an autoreactive T cell subset that is not a Th1 but is rather a Th0, most probably a thymic Th0. This autoreactive population, released from regulation by the deficit in Th2 function, is the diabetogenic effector population. Whether it is intrinsically autoreactive or is influenced by other diabetogenic genes is not known. Besides overt autoreactivity, this population may be characterized as expressing limited TCR Vbeta chain usage, possibly associated with the nature of the thymic selecting antigens, and resistance to tolerizing signs that likely permit escape from the normal negative selection process involved in the deletion of overtly autoreactive thymocytes. The resistance to tolerizing signals manifested in the resistance to apoptotic death and resistance to anergy may be imparted by a diabetogenic gene distinct from the one that controls the regulatory T cell deficit.

References

1. Fowell D, Mason D. Evidence that the T cell repertoire of normal rats contains cells with the potential to cause diabetes: characterization of the $CD4^+$ T cell subset that inhibits this autoimmune potential. *J Exp Med.* 1993; 177:627–636.
2. Gold DP, Shaikewitz T, Mueller D, Redd J, Sellin KS, Pettersson A, Lernmark A, Bellgau D. T cells from BB-DP rats show a unique cytokine MRNA profile associated with the Iddm susceptibility gene, CYP. Submitted.
3. Jacob HJ, Pettersson A, Wilson D, Mao Y, Lernmark A, Lander E. Genetic dissection of autoimmune type 1 diabetes in the BB rat. *Nature Genetics.* 1992; 2:56–60.
4. Serreze DV, Leiter EH. Defective activation of T suppressor cell function in nonobese diabetic mice. *J Immunol.* 1988; 140:3801.
5. Keller R, Eisenbarth GS, Jackson RA. Insulin prophylaxis in individuals at high risk of type 1 diabetes. *Lancet.* 1993; 341:927–928.
6. Zielaskek J, Burkart V, Naylor P, Goldstein A, Kiesel U, Kolb U. Interleukin-2 dependent control of disease development in spontaneously diabetic BB rats. *Immunology.* 1990; 69:209–214.
7. Groen H, Van Der Berk J, Nieuwenhuis P, Kampinga J. Peripheral T cells in diabetes prone (DP) BB rats are CD45R-negative. *Thymus.* 1989; 14:145.
8. Gold D, Bellgrau D. Identification of a limited T-cell receptor B chain variable region repertoire associated with diabetes in the BB rat. *Proc Natl Acad Sci U S A.* 1991; 88:9888.
9. Hayakawa K, Lin BT, Hardy RR. Murine thymic $CD4^+$ T cell subsets: a subset (Thy0) that secretes diverse cytokines and overexpresses the VB8 T cell receptor gene family. *J Exp Med.* 1992; 176:269–274.
10. Firestein GS, Roeder WD, Laxer JA, Townsend KS, Weaver CT, Hom JT, Linton J, Torbett BE, Glasebrook AL. A new murine $CD4^+$ T cell subset with an unrestricted cytokine profile. *J Immunol.* 1989; 143:518–525.
11. Bellgrau D, Redd J, Sellins ks. Peculiar T cell signalling does not preclude positive selection in the diabetes prone BB rat. *Diabetes.* 1994; 43:47–52.
12. Sellins KS, Gold DP, Bellgrau D. Resistance to tolerance induction in the diabetes prone BioBreeding rat as one manifestation of abnormal responses to superantigens. (Submitted.)

D. Why Doesn't Everyone Develop Autoimmune Diabetes?

David W. Talmage and Richard J Sanderson

The islet cells of the pancreas are particularly vulnerable to autoimmune attack because they are more easily destroyed by nonspecific oxidants and inflammation than other tissues.[1] For this reason the autoimmune process in the pancreas does not require T cells or antibody specific for surface membrane antigens. A cellular inflammation (insulitis) in response to any tissue antigen (eg, cytoplasmic protein) will apparently do the job. What prevents the immune system from responding to these self proteins?

We know that a key organ in the development of tolerance to self is the thymus, where both positive and negative selection of T cells occur.[2] The most important negative selection is the deletion of T cells with the ability to respond to self major histocompatibility complex (MHC) antigens. The MHC antigens responsible for the deletion are on the surface of antigen-presenting cells (APCs), probably macrophages and dendritic cells.

Positive selection in the thymus greatly increases the frequency of T cells with low affinity for MHC antigens. However, this low affinity would have to be below the threshold required to activate T cells in order to escape the process of negative selection described above. Positive selection explains why T cell responses are more easily generated to peptides complexed to self MHC antigens than to not-self MHC antigens. The quilt of low-level affinity to self MHC antigens requires only a few tufts of high affinity to specific peptides to exceed the threshold required for activation.[3] thus, T cells with affinity for islet cell peptides not found in the thymus should be particularly available for activation, because they would receive positive but not negative selection in the thymus. So what prevents an immune response to these islet-specific proteins?

The answer to the last question is that there must be an extra-thymic process or processes to suppress the response to selfpeptides not present in the thymus. And we have evidence that such an extra-thymic suppression does take place. Cultured islet or thyroid grafts, which survive for long periods in allogeneic hosts, induce a resistance to rejection in their hosts, called tolerance.[4] This is an active process that takes weeks to months to develop, and although difficult to transfer, the tolerance has been successfully transferred through parabiosis.[5] This tolerance suppresses the rejection of new grafts as well as old and also prevents the rejection of grafts after the transfer of activated immune cells specific for the graft.

If tolerance can be acquired to foreign antigens, then it must also be possible to acquire tolerance to self antigens. We do not believe that this acquired tolerance to self antigens is due to blocking antibody. Although antibody to foreign MHC antigens has been detected in graft recipients, antibody to minor antigens, which are usually tissue-specific peptides, has not been detected. And the acquired tolerance to cultured grafts develops to minor antigens as well as major.[4]

Our proposal is based on the fact that in addition to their specificity, T cells can be divided into several classes based on the lymphokines they produce.[6,7] One class of T cells, called Th1 cells, produces both interleukin-2 (IL-2) and interferon gamma, two lymphokines that are necessary for the cellular infiltration and rejection processes of delayed-type hypersensitivity (DTH). Other T cells make other lymphokines and are collectively called Th2 cells, although they probably do not constitute a homogeneous group. Unfortunately, there are currently no surface markers capable of identifying the lymphokine-producing class of T cells and investigators have had to rely on the production of a specific lymphokine to identify T cell class in this way.

Our proposal is that Th1 and Th2 cells represent mutually suppressing classes of T cells.[8] Thus, if either class becomes dominant in the T cell response to a particular peptide, it suppresses the response of the other class. According to this proposal, tolerance is not due so much to the absence of a T cell response but to the dominance of Th2 cells in that response. A number of different findings seem to point in this direction. It has long been known that antibody production and delayed hypersensitivity appear to be mutually exclusive. Recently, Sanderson has shown that IL-4, a product of Th2 cells that is required for most antibody responses, inhibits the clustering of lymphocytes that occurs in response to PMA and calcium ionophore.[9] LaRosa and coworkers have shown that the infiltration that occurs in NOD mice made resistant to the development of diabetes by the injection of complete Freund's adjuvant (CFA) has a significantly higher content of IL-4–producing cells than the infiltrate of uninjected mice.[10] All of these findings suggest that IL-4 suppresses the production of interferon and IL-2 by Th1 cells.

Our proposal that IL-4 inhibits the production of interferon should be easily testable. If this hypothesis should be confirmed, then the following model of tolerance to tissue-specific selfpeptides would seem likely.

The Proposed Model

Th1 and Th2 cells are mutually suppressing. Thus, one or the other cell population tends to become dominant in the T cell response to a particular peptide. The outcome depends on the dose of antigen and the manner in which it is presented. In a normal individual not susceptible to diabetes, the response to self peptides is dominated by Th2 cells. This is probably also true with viral and bacterial antigens. The production of IL-4 by Th2 cells enables the animal to make a quick antibody response that is essential to resistance to the microbial antigens. At the same time damaging autoimmune DTH to self peptides is avoided; there is also relatively little autoantibody production to self peptides, because most of these are too small to induce such a response. Antibody responses to the larger protein MHC antigens are avoided because T cells specific for these antigens are deleted by the negative selection in the thymus.

In an individual susceptible to diabetes, the specific clones of Th2 cells that are needed to induce tolerance to certain self peptides (eg, islet cell peptides) are deleted in the thymus or blocked from leaving because of a cross-reaction with a particular MHC class II antigen. In the absence of these specific Th2 cells, the specific clone of Th1 cells is free to expand and produce interferon, which activates the inflammatory macrophages that kill the islet cells by some nonspecific process.

A number of predictions of the model are easily testable. Already mentioned is inhibition of IL-2 and interferon by IL-4. IL-4 injected along with islet transplants in diabetic NOD mice should inhibit the recurrence of diabetes. Anti–Il-4 given to NOD mice made diabetes resistant by the injection of CFA should develop diabetes anyway. The lymphocytic infiltration around cultured grafts in tolerant animals should be relatively rich in Th2 cells.

The model also has the advantage of explaining a puzzling phenomenon that has been known for some time. This is the apparent mutual exclusion of antibody production and delayed hypersensitivity. If IL-4 is suppressive for Th1 cells, then this means that the helper factor required for antibody production is paradoxically suppressing the development of delayed hypersensitivity. The only explanation for such a strange behavior is that this action has some benefit to the organism, such as preventing the development of autoimmunity. The recent demonstration that anti–IL-4 can block the development of tolerance supports this proposal.[11]

References

1. LaRosa FG. Abrogation of mouse pancreatic islet allograft rejection by a four-day culture. *Transplantation.* 1988; 46:330–333.
2. Marrack P, Lo D, Brinster R, Palmiter R, Burkly L, Flavell R, Kappler J. The effect of thymic environment on T cell development and tolerance. *Cell.* 1988; 53:627–634.
3. LaRosa FG, Talmage DW. Cellular and molecular biology of tissue transplantation. *Cell Biol Rev.* 1988; Springer International, University of Basque Country.
4. LaRosa FG, Talmage DW. Tolerance to cultured allografts protects third party

grafts containing new MHC and common minor antigens. *Transplantation.* 1987; 43:314–316.

5. LaRosa FG, Smilek D, Talmage DW, Lafferty KJ, Bauling P, Ammons TJ. Evidence that tolerance to cultured thyroid allografts is an active immunological process. *Transplantation.* 1992; 53:903–913.
6. Hsieh CS, Macatonia SE, Tripp CS, Wolf SF, O'Garra A, Murphy KM. Development of T_H1 $CD4^+$ T cells through IL-12 produced by Listeria induced macrophages. *Science.* 1993; 260:547–549.
7. Scott P. IL-12: Initiation cytokine for cell-mediated immunity. *Science.* 1993; 260:496–497.
8. Heinzel FP, Sadick MD, Holaday BJ, Coffman RL, Locksley RM. Reciprocal expression of interferon gamma or interleukin 4 during the resolution or progression of murine Leishmaniasis: evidence for the expansion of distinct helper T cell subsets. *J Exp Med.* 1991; 169:59.
9. Sanderson RJ. Unpublished observations.
10. Shehadeh NN, LaRosa FG, Lafferty KJ. Altered cytokine activity in adjuvant inhibition of autoimmune diabetes. *J Autoimmunity.* 1993; 6:291–300.
11. Schurmans S, Heusser CH, Qin HY, Merino J, Brighouse G, Lambert PH. In vivo effects of anti IL-4 monoclonal antibody on neonatal induction of tolerance and on an associated autoimmune syndrome. *J Immunol.* 1990; 145:2465–2473.

Appendix

Selected Type I Diabetes Research Resources

S. Babu
D. Stenger

A. Monoclonal Anti-Islet Antibodies

1. Anti-human c peptide MON 5021: Anti-insulin MON 5023:
   Caltag Laboratories
   436 Rozzi Place
   South San Francisco, CA 94080

2. A2B5: ATCC CRL 1520* (American Type Tissue Collection)
   Islet and neuronal ganglioside (all vertebrates)[1]

3. 3G5: ATCC CRL 1814*
   Pancreatic islet and neuronal ganglioside[2]

4. 4F2C13: ATCC CRL 1520*
   Human islet cell surface/proliferating cells 80:40 surface heterodimer[3]

   *American Type Culture Collection
   c/o Sales and Marketing Department
   12301 Parklawn Dr.
   Rockville, MD 20852

5. HISL1 Human islets[4]
   George S. Eisenbarth, MD, PhD
   Barbara Davis Center
   4200 E. 9th Ave., Box B140
   Denver, CO 80262

B. Hybridomas producing monoclonal antibodies

Anti GAD-1[5]: Anti GAD-6[6]:	Developmental Studies Hybridoma Bank Dept. of Biology University of Iowa Iowa City, IA 57767
Anti GAD-1[5]:	ATCC HB 184 American Type Culture Collection c/o Sales and Marketing Department 12301 Parklawn Dr. Rockville, MD 20852

C. Autoantigen Plasmids

1. Human islet GAD65 cDNA for in vitro transcription and translation[7]:	Thomas Dyrberg, MD Novo-Nordisk A/S Novo Alle DK-2880 Bagsværd Denmark
2. Human islet GAD65 cDNA clone[8,9]:	Åke Lernmark, PhD Robert H. Williams Laboratory Department of Medicine RG-20 University of Washington Seattle, WA 98195
3. GAD65 cDNA clone[10]: GAD67 cDNA clone[10]:	Allan J. Tobin, PhD Department of Biology UCLA 405 Hilgard Avenue Los Angeles, CA 90024
4. ICA69 clone[11]:	George S. Eisenbarth, MD, PhD Barbara Davis Center 4200 E. 9th Ave., Box B140 Denver, CO 80262
5. ICA512bdc clone	George S. Eisenbarth, MD, PhD Barbara Davis Center 4200 E. 9th Ave., Box B140 Denver, CO 80262

D. Autoantigen Determination

1. ICA[12] and IAA[13] proficiency:	Noel K. Maclaren, MD Univ. of Fla. College of Medicine Dept. of Pathology & Laboratory Medicine P.O. Box 100275 Gainesville, FL 32610-0275

2. IDS Autoantibody Workshop (1995)

   Charles Verge
   Barbara Davis Center for Childhood Diabetes
   Box B140, 4200 E. 9th Ave.
   Denver, CO 80262

3. ICARUS (Islet Cell Antibody Register User's Study)[14]:

   E. A. M. Gale, MA, FRCP
   St. Bartholomew's Hospital Centre for Clinical Research
   Dept. of Diabetes and Metabolism
   59 Bartholomew Close, West Smithfield
   London EC1A 7BE
   England

E. Genetic Resources

1. EBV cell lines/DNA from multiplex families with type I diabetes:

   Human Biological Data Interchange
   2401 Walnut Street, Suite 406
   Philadelphia, PA 19013

   British Diabetic Association
   Warren Repository
   10 Queen Anne Street
   London, W1M 0BD

2. Microsatellite markers:
   Mouse and Human:

   Research Genetics
   2130 Memorial Parkway SW
   Huntsville, AL 35801

3. HLA typing:
   Amplitype DQα Typing Kit (#N808-0056)

   Applied Biosystems
   761 Main Ave.
   Norwalk, CT 06859

F. Animal Models

1. NOD mice[15]:

   Taconic Farms, Inc.
   273 Hover Ave.
   Germantown, NY 12526

2. NOD *scid* mice[16]:

   Edward H. Leiter, PhD
   Jackson Laboratory
   Bar Harbor, ME 04609

3. BB rats[17]: Arthur A. Like, MD
Univ. of Massachusetts Med. Ctr.
55 Lake Ave. N.
Worcester, MA 01655

G. Human Tissue Pancreata

National Disease Research Interchange
2401 Walnut Street
Suite 408
Philadelphia, PA 19104

References

1. Eisenbarth GS, Shimizu K, Bowring MA, Wells S. Expression of receptors for tetanus toxin and monoclonal antibody A2B5 by pancreatic islet cells. *Proc Natl Acad Sci U S A.* 1982; 79:5066–5070.
2. Powers AC, Rabizadeh A, Akeson R, Eisenbarth GS. Characterization of monoclonal 3G5 and utilization of this antibody to immobilize pancreatic islet cell gangliosides in a solid phase radioassay. *Endocrinology.* 1984; 114:1–6.
3. Srikanta S, Telen M, Posillico JT, Dolinar R, Krisch K, Haynes BF, Eisenbarth GS. Monoclonal antibodies to a human islet cell surface glycoprotein: 4F2 and LC7-2. *Endocrinology.* 1987; 120:2240–2244.
4. Srikanta S, Krisch K, Eisenbarth GS. Islet cell protein defined by monoclonal islet cell antibody HISL-19. *Diabetes.* 1986; 35:300–305.
5. Gottlieb DL, Chang Y-C, Schwob JE. Monoclonal antibodies to glutamic acid decarboxylase. *Proc Natl Acad Sci USA.* 1986; 83:8808–8812.
6. Chang Y-C, Gottlieb DL. Characterization of the proteins purified with monoclonal antibodies to glutamic acid decarboxylase. *J Neurosci.* 1988; 8:2123–2130.
7. Petersen JS, Hejnaes KR, Moody A, Karlsen AE, Marshall MO, Hoier-Madsen M, Boel E, Michelsen BK, Dyrberg T. Detection of GAD_{65} antibodies in diabetes and other autoimmune diseases using a simple radioligand assay. *Diabetes.* 1994; 43:459–467.
8. Karlsen AE, Hagopian WA, Grubin CE, Dube S, Disteche CM, Adler DA, Bärmeier H, Mathewes S, Crant FJ, Foster DC, Lernmark Å. Cloning and primary structure of a human islet isoform of glutamic acid decarboxylase from chromosome 10. *Proc Natl Acad Sci USA.* 1991; 88:8337–8341. GenBank accession #M74826.
9. Grubin CE, Daniels T, Toivola B, Landin-Olsson M, Hagopian WA, Li L, Karlsen AE, Boel E, Michelsen B, Lernmark Å. A novel radioligand binding assay to determine diagnostic accuracy of isoform-specific glutamic acid decarboxylase antibodies in childhood IDDM. *Diabetologia.* 1994; 37:344–350.
10. Bu D-F, Erlander MG, Hitz BC, Tillakaratne NJ, Daufman DL, Wagner-McPherson CB, Evans GA, Tobin AJ. Two human glutamate decarboxylases, 65kDa GAD and 67kDa GAD, are each encoded by a single gene. *Proc Natl Acad Sci USA.* 1992; 89:2115–2119. GenBank accession #M81882 (GAD65) and #M81883 (GAD67).

11. Pietropaolo M, Castano L, Babu S, Buelow R, Kuo YL, Martin S, Martin A, Powers AC, Prochazka M, Naggert J, Leiter EH, Eisenbarth GS. Islet cell autoantigen 69kDa (ICA69): molecular cloning and characterization of a novel diabetes-associated autoantigen. *J Clin Invest.* 1993; 92:359–371. GenBank accession #L01100.
12. Lernmark Å, Molenaar JL, van Beers WA, Yamaguchi Y, Nagataki S, Ludvigsson J, Maclaren NK. The Fourth International Serum Exchange Workshop to standardize cytoplasmic islet cell antibodies: The Immunology and Diabetes Workshops and participating laboratories. *Diabetologia.* 1991; 34:534–535.
13. Greenbaum CJ, Wilkin TJ, Palmer JP. Fifth International Serum Exchange Workshop for Insulin Autoantibody (IAA) Standardization: The Immunology and Diabetes Workshops and participating laboratories. *Diabetologia.* 1992; 35:798–800.
14. Bingley PJ, Colman P, Eisenbarth GS, Jackson RA, McCulloch DK, Riley WJ, Gale EA. Standardization of IVGTT to predict IDDM. *Diabetes Care.* 1992; 15:1313–1316.
15. Makino S, Kunimoto K, Muraoka Y, Mizushima Y, Katagiri K, Tochino Y. Breeding of a non-obese diabetic strain of mice. *Exp. Anim.* 1980; 29:1–13.
16. Prochazka M, Gaskin HR, Shultz LD, Leiter EH. The nonobese diabetic scid mouse: model for spontaneous thymomagenesis associated with immunodeficiency. *Proc Natl Acad Sci USA.* 1992; 89:3290–3294.
17. Nakhooda AF, Like AA, Chappel CI, Murray FT, Marliss EB. The spontaneously diabetic Wistar rat: metabolic and morphologic studies. *Diabetes.* 1977; 26:100–112.

Index